AF766078

Glaxo

Presented to your unit
with the compliments of
your local representative from
Glaxo Laboratories Limited.

With best wishes for 1992.

FOR SUBSCRIBERS OUTSIDE USA AND CANADA

ANNUAL OF GASTROINTESTINAL ENDOSCOPY

☐ 1991 and all future annuals at 25% discount. Please send me the 1991 annual and all future annuals at 25% discount from the normal price: £45 (SAVE £15)

☐ 1990 annual only with 25% discount. Price: £33.75 (SAVE £11.25)

☐ 1991 annual only at full price: £60

RELATED PUBLICATIONS

GASTROINTESTINAL ENDOSCOPY DATABASE 1991

☐ £120 (includes postage and packing)

UK residents add 17.5% VAT

Diskette size ☐ 5 1/4" ☐ 3 1/2"

SLIDE ATLAS OF GASTROINTESTINAL ENDOSCOPY 1991

☐ £120 (includes postage and packing)

120 top quality slides in black and white and full colour, with slide notes displayed in an attractive binder

Guarantee: Your money will be refunded, if we receive your cancellation and undamaged goods back within 30 days of receipt of order

Name ....

Address ....

....

Postcode .... Country ....

Cheque enclosed payable to Current Science Ltd

☐ Visa ☐ MasterCard ☐ Am Ex ☐ Please send an institutional invoice

Card No | | | | | | | | | | | | | | | | | Exp Date | | | | |

Amount payable .... Date ....

Signature ....

Personal subscriptions must be paid by personal cheque or credit card. Please allow 4 to 6 weeks for delivery. All subscriptions run on a calendar-year basis.

Please send me further information on: .... (see below)

FOR SUBSCRIBERS WITHIN USA AND CANADA ONLY

ANNUAL OF GASTROINTESTINAL ENDOSCOPY

☐ 1991 and all future annuals at 25% discount. Please send me the 1991 annual and all future annuals at 25% discount from the normal price: US$71.25 (SAVE US$23.75)

☐ 1990 annual only with 25% discount. Price :US$60 (SAVE US$20)

☐ 1991 annual only at full price: US$95

RELATED PUBLICATIONS

GASTROINTESTINAL ENDOSCOPY DATABASE 1991

☐ US$200 (includes postage and packing)

Diskette size ☐ 5 1/4" ☐ 3 1/2"

SLIDE ATLAS OF GASTROINTESTINAL ENDOSCOPY 1991

☐ US$200 (includes postage and packing)

120 top quality slides in black and white and full colour, with slide notes displayed in an attractive binder

Guarantee: Your money will be refunded, if we receive your cancellation and undamaged goods back within 30 days of receipt of order

Name ....

Address ....

....

Zip .... Country ....

Check enclosed payable to Current Science

☐ Visa ☐ MasterCard ☐ Am Ex ☐ Please send an institutional invoice

Card No | | | | | | | | | | | | | | | | | Exp Date | | | | |

Amount payable .... Date ....

Signature ....

Personal subscriptions must be paid by personal check or credit card. Please allow 4 to 6 weeks for delivery. All subscriptions run on a calendar-year basis.

Please send me further information on: ....(see below)

IS CURRENT OPINION IN YOUR LIBRARY'S COLLECTION?

Current Science/Current Biology, 34-42 Cleveland Street, London W1P 5FB

Please send a sample of the journal shown below:

Clinical review journals in:

☐ Anaesthesiology
☐ Cardiology
☐ Dentistry
☐ Gastroenterology
☐ Infectious Diseases
☐ Lipidology
☐ Neurology & Neurosurgery
☐ Obstetrics & Gynecology
☐ Oncology
☐ Ophthalmology
☐ Orthopaedics
☐ Pediatrics
☐ Psychiatry
☐ Radiology
☐ Rheumatology
☐ Urology

Biology review journals in:

☐ Biotechnology
☐ Cell Biology
☐ Genetics & Development
☐ Immunology
☐ Neurobiology
☐ Structural Biology

☐ Current Biology

Peer- review journals:

☐ AIDS
☐ Coronary Artery Disease
☐ Journal of Hypertension
☐ European Journal of Gastroenterology & Hepatology

☐ 1991 Catalogue

To the librarian at my institution:

Librarian's Name ....

Library ....

Address ....

....

Zip/Postcode .... Country ....

with my recommendation to subscribe:

Your name ....

Your title ....

Address ....

....

Zip/Postcode .... Country ....

AIRMAIL

Affix
Stamp

CURRENT SCIENCE
SUBSCRIPTIONS
34-42 CLEVELAND STREET
LONDON W1P 5FB
UNITED KINGDOM

NO POSTAGE
NECESSARY
IF MAILED
IN THE
UNITED STATES

BUSINESS REPLY MAIL
FIRST CLASS PERMIT NO. 33925 PHILADELPHIA, PA

Postage Will Be Paid By Addressee

CURRENT SCIENCE
20 NORTH 3rd STREET
PHILADELPHIA
PA 19106-2113
USA

AIRMAIL

Affix
Stamp

CURRENT SCIENCE
SUBSCRIPTIONS
34-42 CLEVELAND STREET
LONDON W1P 5FB
UNITED KINGDOM

Annual of Gastrointestinal Endoscopy

illustrated in color

Annual of Gastrointestinal Endoscopy

illustrated in color

Editors

PB Cotton
Duke University Medical Center,
Durham, North Carolina, USA

GNJ Tytgat
Academic Medical Centre,
Amsterdam, The Netherlands

CB Williams
St Mark's and St Bartholomew's Hospitals,
London, UK

1991

CS
CURRENT
SCIENCE

Published by Current Science Ltd,
34–42 Cleveland Street, London W1P 5FB, UK

Copyright ©1991 by Current Science Ltd. All rights reserved. No part of this publication may be reproduced, stored in a retrieval system or transmitted by any form or by any means without the prior permission of the copyright holders.

British Library Cataloguing-in-Publication Data:

Annual of gastrointestinal endoscopy. – 1991 –
1. Man. Gastrointestinal tract. Endoscopy
616.3'307545

ISSN 0952-6293
ISBN 1-870485-32-7

Contents

Literature scanner

M Jacyna

Current Science

John Dalton (Managing Editor); Maurizia Merati (Illustrations); Mauricio Moreno (Database); Informat Computer Communications Ltd (Typesetting).

Preface

We hope that you will find the 1991 *Annual of Gastrointestinal Endoscopy* interesting and helpful. The principle behind the *Annual* is simple enough – choose experts and let them select and write a critique of the previous year's literature in their field. There are a few snags in realizing the formula, however, which the keen-eyed reader may notice.

First, we are committed to publication as early as possible in the year. Our chosen experts work over the Christmas holiday period to make a deadline very early in the New Year – so that a few articles published late may inevitably be overlooked. Second, we favour a new 'three-tier' ranking scheme for articles by which each reviewer makes a personal judgement as to those articles that are considered 'outstanding' (••), are 'of interest' (•) or deserve only a brief, but honourable, mention; these criteria, and the decision whether those articles of lesser interest should be listed with or without a summary comment, have been rather variably applied. Finally, there is mild discord as to whether the *Annual* should include every conception relating to gastrointestinal endoscopy during the year (including all single-case reports, some 'Letters to the Editor' and those grandiose-sounding series – which prove on reading to be worthy only of annihilation); alternatively, should the reviews, and their reference annotations, concentrate mainly on key papers, with expanded coverage of them?

Individual reviewers this year have handled their strategies slightly differently, which we have accepted so as to avoid any delay in publication. We think that the result is acceptably comprehensive and readable. Gastrointestinal endoscopy is a fast-evolving practical discipline and the hope of the Editors is that the *Annual* should evolve to combine the best attributes of a useful 'restaurant guide' to the related literature, reflecting current authoritative opinion whilst not becoming an undigested, and indigestible, catalogue.

PB Cotton,
Durham,
USA,

GNJ Tytgat,
Amsterdam,
The Netherlands,

CB Williams,
London,
UK

© Current Science Ltd ISBN 1-870485-32-7 ISSN 0952-6293

Endoscopy unit design and organization: commentary

P.B. Cotton* and M. Schaffner†

*Director of Endoscopy and †Head Nurse, Gastroenterology Unit,
Duke University Medical Center, Durham, North Carolina, USA

Twenty years ago, gastrointestinal endoscopy was for most gastroenterologists a peripheral activity involving only a few procedures each week, one or two endoscopes, casual facilities and a single part-time assistant or nurse. Subsequent dramatic developments in diagnostic and therapeutic applications have turned endoscopy into a major industry. Many gastroenterologists (certainly trainees) think of endoscopy in terms of individual procedures and patients, and are primarily concerned with indications, techniques and results. However, 'toys have turned into tools, and the excitements of conception have fathered a service obligation' [1]. Increasing numbers of us have to wrestle with the broader problems involved in developing and managing endoscopy departments. Many hospitals and clinics are now striving to develop state of the art facilities in which to provide optimal patient services. Some centers have as many as 10 procedure rooms, dozens of endoscopists, and a small army of nurses and supporting staff, including radiological, electronic and audiovisual technicians, secretaries, data analysts, aids, porters (messengers), cleaners, and so on. Planning, building (or refurbishing) and managing such units are complex tasks for which only recently have some sources of guidance become available [1–9].

We are increasingly asked to advise on the crucial issues of design and staff structure, and here give some overall comments. The principles involved are equally applicable to small and multidisciplinary units.

Factors influencing design

There are many factors that should be considered in the planning phase in order to arrive at an appropriate floor plan and balance of activities.

- The current numbers of endoscopy procedures and breakdown by type, complexity, need for fluoroscopy and X-ray film taking (endoscopic retrograde cholangiopancreatography)-ERCP.
- Whether any procedure rooms may be shared now or in the future with other disciplines (e.g. for bronchoscopy and transesophageal echocardiography).
- The ratio of outpatients to inpatients (usually about 3:1) and the source of the inpatients. The site must be convenient for outpatients, but preferably also for examination and treatment of ill inpatients. At some institutions, geography dictates a need for two units: a large outpatient unit, and a smaller inpatient focus near the main ward floors and intensive care unit.
- The need for non-endoscopy procedure space, e.g. for manometry, function studies, ultrasonography, lithotripsy.
- Prediction of the procedure volumes about 3 years after opening.
- Whether the unit is to be self-contained with its own reception/recovery facilities, or part of a larger ambulatory unit in which these peripheral functions are shared.
- Whether trainees will be using the unit, and whether the faculty will be full or part-time. Both factors influence the time taken for procedures, and turn-around efficiency.
- The philosophy behind developing a new unit (and the perceived inadequacies of the old one). This will influence priority given to different functions, e.g. patient privacy and comfort, teaching space, disinfection, etc.
- The way patients are handled outside of the procedure rooms. There are many opinions and systems, which provide different degrees of privacy. Some luxurious units have individual rooms for each patient in which they are assessed, undress, recover, dress and are interviewed before discharge; relatives can wait in this room. However, such facilities need a high nursing ratio to supervise patients recovering from sedation. At the other end of the spectrum are units in which there are only recovery bays where patients undress, recover, and dress. Low-level interviews and discussions take place in the bays, but there should be one or two interview rooms available for private consultation. A few separate dressing areas in addition will increase flexibility. If possible, patients waiting for procedures should be separated from those recovering, and the recovery area should not be a corridor for other traffic.
- Sedation practice. Endoscopists giving heavy sedation need more recovery space and staff.
- Whether or not to install radiography equipment. Some radiologists resist the idea of having major equipment outside the main radiography department, and there are downsides: quite apart from the cost, there are issues of maintenance,

©Current Science Ltd ISBN 1-870485-32-7 ISSN 0952-6293

technical help and processing – and what happens when the machine goes down. However, many endoscopy units now do sufficient ERCP procedures and fluoroscopy to justify having their own equipment. Digital radiographic images are improving to the level at which they may be acceptable for ERCP. Digital equipment (especially the C-arm variety) is simple to install and manage. A film processing area must be provided if regular radiography machines are used.

Some general principles

There are several features that we commonly emphasize when reviewing floor plans. There must be a central focus of the unit – like the bridge of a ship or cockpit of an airplane. The captain or pilot is the charge nurse of the day, assisted by a secretary/receptionist. Essentially, this focus is a nursing station where all the management decisions of the day are made, and where doctors and all other staff know they can get answers to their questions. The procedure schedule for the day will be displayed in this area. Furthermore, it is useful to have a dry marker board on which to indicate who is in charge for the day, which nurses and doctors are working in which rooms, announcements about meetings and visitors, which may affect the schedule – as well as social news (birthdays, babies, etc.). If at all possible, the nurse station should be contiguous (or back on to) the recovery area to facilitate communication and give some potential for overlapping responsibilities.

Cleaning and disinfection need more space than most planners imagine. These functions should be centralized rather than performed in the procedure rooms, particularly because of the toxic aspects of glutaraldehyde (which mandate high-volume venting). Approximately 400 square feet will be required in a five procedure room unit. This area should be set up so that the nurse can walk into one end with dirty instruments, and out of the other with clean equipment.

It is essential to explain to those installing radiography equipment exactly how it will be used. Radiography engineers like to place their machines in the center of the room like a piece of sculpture to be admired – this wastes space – and they rarely appreciate that you will be using the table the wrong way round – i.e. with the endoscopist and radiologist on the same side. Beware, siting mistakes are uncomfortable and expensive to change.

Procedure rooms are like kitchens. They do not need to be vast. Indeed, small may be beautiful and convenient if ergonomically planned [2, 3]. The problem is that we cannot predict what new equipment will suddenly need to be added. It is somewhat easier to be flexible if rooms are oblong rather than square, and if there is adequate storage space elsewhere. In a big unit it is convenient to have a mixture of small 'standard' rooms (10 feet × 15 feet can be sufficient) and larger 'flexible' rooms, as well as any radiography rooms.

Except for radiography procedures (and laparoscopy), there is no need to have fixed examination tables; modern recovery stretchers are satisfactory, and facilitate patient transfer.

Equipment such as TV monitors and intravenous supports should be ceiling-hung wherever possible. Obviously the monitor site(s) must be chosen for the convenience of doctors and nurses. Most planners underestimate the need for storage areas, for accessory equipment, endoscope cases, carts, stretchers, intravenous poles, and so on. The anesthesiology department should be consulted to make sure that general anesthetics can be given easily and safely in the area.

Staffing

Assisting with gastrointestinal endoscopy is a task for trained professional nurses. Unfortunately, this fact has been recognized only slowly in many countries. Nursing staff carry a major responsibility for patient safety; in difficult procedures they can make all the difference between triumph and disaster. There must be one properly trained nurse assistant in each procedure room, with two for any complex endoscopies such as ERCP and therapy [9]. There must be one nurse in charge of the unit for the day, and at least one other handling the recovery area – depending on the volume. Someone will be working in the 'back hall', cleaning, disinfecting, and packaging for sterilization. Not all of the staff need to be of registered nurse grade.

Shortage of nurses has encouraged many managers to explore the most efficient 'mixes' of staff, and to become innovative in recruiting [10, 11]. Lower-level staff can be trained to perform cleaning and disinfection effectively, and to assist with recovery duties. However, the procedure-related nurses should maintain their skills in handling those functions, and may rotate through these areas.

As emergency procedures performed out of hours are often the most difficult and dangerous (as well as most worthwhile) it is essential to have gastrointestinal nursing staff on 24-hour call. This will also ensure a more consistent approach to cleaning and disinfection of endoscopic equipment for patient safety [8].

The extent to which the nurse manager is involved in actual procedures will depend on the size of the unit. In a department with four or five procedure rooms, the nurse manager should allocate at least half of his or her time for office and managerial activities. The amount of secretarial assistance will depend upon the methods employed for scheduling and reporting. An appropriate technologist must be available if radiography equipment is in use, not only to assist with the procedures, but also to help in maintaining and monitoring radiation safety standards.

Organization

The endoscopy unit will be run jointly by a medical director and nurse manager, supported by a secretary/manager. They are responsible for forward planning, efficiency and safety of the day-to-day activities, discipline and staff morale. In particular, the nurse manager will be largely responsible for setting the tone for the unit and the spirit of the team. He or she will determine whether it is a source of pride and fun – or embarrassment and drudgery. Staff morale will be maximized by having frequent discussion meetings, formal written procedure manuals, continuing education opportunities, and prospective quality assurance studies of medical and nursing aspects of unit activity. Systems must be devised for maintaining detailed statistics of unit activity, budgetary issues and trends. Use of a 'relative value scale' provides a more accurate reflection of workload than a simple tally of endoscopy numbers [4, 6].

Conclusion

Endoscopy units have become more and more like operating theater suites: specially designed facilities in which highly trained medical and nursing staff perform often complex (and potentially dangerous) procedures with high-tech equipment. Failure to provide this total environment is a disservice to our discipline, and to our patients. It is no longer adequate to do only what local circumstances permit, but essential to press for the resources to make practicable that which is necessary [1].

References

1 Cotton PB, Williams CB: *Practical Gastrointestinal Endoscopy. Third Edition.* Blackwell Scientific Publications, 1990.
2 Overholt BF, Chobanian SJ. *Office Endoscopy.* Williams and Wilkins, 1990.
3 Waye JD, Rich ME: *Planning and Endoscopy Unit for Suite and Office.* Igaku-Shoin, 1990.
4 **Endoscopy suite design.** *Endosc Rev* 1990, May, 11-88.
5 *Guidelines for Establishment of Gastrointestinal Endoscopy Areas.* ASGE Publication No. 1003, revised 3/86.
6 Sivak MA. **The endoscopy unit.** In: *Gastroenterologic Endoscopy.* WB Saunders, 1988.
7 **Provision of Gastrointestinal Endoscopy and Related Services for a District General Hospital.** British Society of Gastroenterology, 1990.
8 Schaffner M. **Infection Control Issues in the Gastrointestinal endoscopy unit.** *Gastroenterology Nursing,* Spring 12(4), 1990.
9 **Monitoring and Safety Recommendations.** *SGNA News,* March 1990.
10 Lassiter S. **Staff Nurse Retention: Strategies for Success.** *J Neurosci Nursing,* 21(2), April 1989.
11 Belmer FT, McKnight P. **Management Strategies to Minimize Nursing Turnover.** *Health Care Management Review,* 14(1), Winter 1989.

The use of monitoring during endoscopy: commentary

D. Fleischer

Division of Gastroenterology, Georgetown University Hospital, Washington, DC, USA

Introduction

Continuous electrocardiographic monitoring. Continual blood pressure monitoring. Pulse oximetry. End-tidal carbon dioxide. What will we be monitoring next? Electroencephalography? Pulmonary wedge pressure? Tumescence? Where will it all end? With the incidence of immediate complications for endoscopic procedures still at an exceptionally low rate, there is a tendency to ask rhetorically: 'are monitors really needed at all?' And if so, perhaps we need not go the full nine yards. In order to best address the issue, it is useful to examine two concepts. First, what is meant by the term'monitoring'? Second, how do the physicians make decisions about how they practice medicine?

Monitoring

Ironically, the word monitoring may be as much part of the problem as the actual activity is part of the solution. Monitoring means different things to different individuals. A generic dictionary definition of monitoring is simply 'to watch, observe, or check on a person or thing.' The more literal definition in the specific medical sense would relate to taking measurements: for example, measuring and recording blood pressure, pulse, respiratory rate, cardiac rhythm, oxygen saturation, or carbon dioxide content. However, monitoring could also be construed in the more general medical sense as making observations: assessing the patient's clinical status by noting the degree of sedation, skin color, or ease of respiration. A very different definition of monitoring is often taken by regulatory or accrediting agencies to mean 'noting the process, for example, assessing the quality of care that an individual patient receives and/or the quality of care that was delivered to the patient'. This last broader definition relates to the assessment of structure, function and outcome, matters that are essential components of quality assurance.

The physician must therefore be clear on what he or she means when the question of monitoring during endoscopy is raised. To better examine that question, a review of how physicians make decisions will be useful.

Physician decision making

Figure 1 lists the different parameters that come into play when doctors are asked to decide. These same factors would be relevant to the clinical determination whether or not a sessile colonic polyp should be removed or when a physician is determining what monitoring is required for an endoscopic procedure.

- Instinct
- Personal experience
- Experience of others:
  - Colleagues
  - Publications:
    - Anecdotal
    - Randomized trials
  - Courses
- Socioeconomic
- Legal
- National recommendations

Fig. 1. Factors used by physicians in making decisions.

Instinct and personal experience

Some things just 'seem right'. It seems inherently obvious that, if a patient is being sedated and an endoscope is being delivered through one of the gateways to the digestive tract, some form of monitoring should occur. One's instinct cannot be separated from one's personal experience, so that if on a previous occasion a patient had an unexplained cardiac arrest during a colonoscopy, that physician would be more likely to consider monitoring the next patient than the physician who had performed 100 consecutive colonoscopies without any recognized difficulty.

Experience of others

Just as no man is an island (Langerhans not excluded), in most cases our medical decisions are influenced by what other physicians do. Because the local experience is important, we often discuss our activities with our colleagues and there grows up a conventional wisdom that 'that's the way we do things around here.' In addition, we subscribe to numerous publications (and on some occasions, we even read them rather than simply pile them on our desks). It is not uncommon for information in those publications to influence what we do. Although we may even change our practice based on an anecdotal report in a respected medical journal, it is more common that we pattern our clinical practices on the basis of the results of published randomized, double-blinded, controlled studies. The thoughtful physician reads the methodology segment and tries to determine how much like his own patient the study population is. We tend to be influenced by scientific evaluations that relate to the needs of our patients. Finally, we learn about the experience of others from courses and videotapes. If a credible speaker with a breadth of experience believes that we should monitor our patients, then that is likely to influence the physician who has not yet made up his mind about what degree of monitoring is appropriate.

As we do care about what our colleagues do, we should be aware of what they do with regard to monitoring. In order to make this information more concrete, the focus will now move to electronic monitoring (electrocardiography [EKG], pulse oximetry, etc.).

In 1989, a survey was sponsored by the American Society for Gastrointestinal Endoscopy. Keeffe and O'Connor [1] surveyed members of the Society. At that time, 54% of those surveyed used EKG monitoring on a routine basis. Additionally, 65% used pulse oximetry regularly. In a less formal survey conducted by the author at a national course in February 1991, more than 95% of the physicians used pulse oximetry routinely. Clearly, there is a trend towards using more, not less, electronic monitoring.

Socioeconomic and legal considerations

It is not surprising that business concerns are influencing decisions about monitoring, as it is hard for any physician today not to be influenced by financial factors. In some areas of the USA, physician insurers reduce malpractice coverage rates for physicians who use pulse oximetry during endoscopic procedures. Though there is no evidence to establish the fact that monitoring of this nature affects patient outcomes, the insurance companies find reason to give a positive incentive to physicians who choose to use pulse oximeters.

What are the expenses involved in electronic monitoring? Although numbers will vary from country to country, in the USA it is possible to buy a high-quality pulse oximeter for approximately $2000; to purchase a continual blood pressure monitoring machine for $1000 to $3000; and to purchase a cardiac monitor for approximately $4000. As equipment is used more frequently, some of the prices are being reduced. Practically speaking it would be possible to have a pulse oximeter, an automatic sphygnomanometer, and a cardiac monitoring system for between $5 and $10 000. Different physicians will determine that none, some, or all of these devices are required.

Perhaps the most persuasive argument that electronic monitoring should be used is the legal concern. For better or for worse, defensive medical practices and the need to appear prepared are practice considerations. Rightly or wrongly, the physician who had used monitoring during an endoscopic procedure in which a patient complication occurred would be less vulnerable to a malpractice challenge if he or she had been monitoring the patient during the procedure. Although there are a few things that raise the hackles on a physician's back more, it is a fact of life in the 1990s that medicolegal factors do influence the way that we practice medicine. And I have made the comment in several settings 'that the way we do medicine is far more likely to be influenced by legal precedents than it is by randomized, controlled studies in the *New England Journal of Medicine.*' This is one of the reasons why I believe that universal rather than selective monitoring is appropriate.

National recommendations

Although they are not developed as legal documents, the recommendations of national societies do carry great weight. They are, in fact, the most important determinant in guiding physicians. The recommendations of the American Society of Gastrointestinal Endoscopy have addressed many areas. A guideline regarding monitoring of patients receiving conscious sedation for gastrointestinal endoscopy was developed by the Standards of Practice Committee in 1989. It can be summarized as follows:

(1) A well-trained gastrointestinal assistant, working closely with the physician, who observes the patient's status during endoscopic procedures, is the most important part of the monitoring process.
(2) The use of extracorporeal equipment to monitor patients may be a useful adjunct to patient surveillance, but is never a substitute for clinical assessment.
(3) The amount of monitoring should be proportional to the perceived risk to the individual patient undergoing each specific procedure.
(4) The minimal clinical monitoring for all sedated patients should include heart rate, blood pressure, and respiratory rate.
(5) The proper role of pulse oximetry and continuous EKG monitoring is controversial. Given the cost of the equipment and the manpower to use it, the best decision as to whether it should be used would be based on data exhibiting that such monitoring affects patient outcomes. Such data do not exist.
(6) However, in those situations in which the individualized need of the patient indicates that more frequent assessment of cardiac rhythm or oxygen saturation will complement the clinical assessment, use of EKG monitoring or pulse oximetry may be beneficial.

In devising these guidelines, the Committee took a very pragmatic approach to the role of electronic monitoring. As the fifth summary point above relates, they underscored the fact that the role of monitoring was controversial and, as clear patient outcome data did not exist, they attempted to provide guidance without mandating a specific practice.

Conclusions

This review is all well and good, but what should physicians do in real life? The answer will, of course, vary from situation to situation but is a matter that I have sorted out in my own mind.

I believe that one well-trained gastrointestinal assistant can handle straightforward endoscopic procedures, but that when the endoscopic task is complex, the assistant will be required to provide hands-on assistance during the endoscopic procedure and a second assistant should be available to monitor the patient. I also believe that some form of electronic monitoring should be used for all patients. In the endoscopy suite in which I work, all patients have cardiac monitoring, continual automatic blood pressure monitoring, and pulse oximetry. I believe that a high degree of patient safety would be likely if fewer than all three of these devices were to be used. It will be noted that I stated that I believe that monitoring should be the same for all patients: that is, the same equipment should be used for the 92-year-old man with heart disease and the 46-year-old woman without heart disease who are undergoing colonoscopy. Although statistically the 92-year-old man is more at risk for a cardiorespiratory misadventure, there is some risk, albeit small, in the younger patient, and as I am persuaded by the argument that no clinician is good enough to tell in each case who will have a problem, they both should be monitored. Also, one's legal vulnerability is reduced if the cardiorespiratory event occurred in the patient who was monitored rather in one who was not.

Closing section

Coming to grips with monitoring for gastrointestinal endoscopy has been a difficult task. Physicians tend to resist change when they feel that it is being mandated by normedical forces over which they have little control. But, in the end, what physicians really want is that which is best for their patients. Monitoring is indeed a form of quality control and my instincts tell me that that is a good thing.

References

1 Keeffe E., O'Connor K. 1989 ASGE Survey of Sedation and Monitoring Practices during Endoscopy. *Gastrointest Endosc* (in press).

Endoscopy of the oesophagus

G.N.J. Tytgat

Department of Gastroenterology, Academic Medical Centre, Amsterdam, The Netherlands

No true highlights were published during the past year in endoscopic oesophagology. Nevertheless, useful information was published in several areas but this was to a large extent confirmatory in nature, consolidating previous knowledge.

Introduction

In this review the most pertinent studies published during 1990 will be commented upon. For convenience, they are subdivided into diagnostic oesophageal endoscopy; therapy of non-malignant oesophageal obstruction; oesophageal endoscopy of neoplastic lesions and therapeutic endoscopy for malignant oesophageal obstruction. Literature pertaining to oesophageal varices and sclerotherapy was not covered as this is reviewed in the chapter on Hemorrhage. Similarly, publications on oesophageal endosonography were not covered so as to prevent duplication with the chapter on Endosonography.

Diagnostic oesophageal endoscopy for inflammatory and non-inflammatory conditions

Gastrooesophageal reflux disease remains the leading cause of oesophageal inflammation. The severity of the mucosal abnormalities largely determines the response to therapy [1•]. Staging the degree of endoscopic abnormality will become increasingly important because the choice of acid-suppressive therapy should be guided by the degree of endoscopic abnormality. Certainly for circumferential damage, the healing capabilities of H_2-receptor antagonists are often insufficient and therapy with proton-pump inhibitors should be advised.

Prolonged, rather severe reflux is generally considered the main mechanism leading to the development of a columnar-lined oesophagus. Not only acid and pepsin is involved, but presumably also bile and/or pancreatic juice, as a columnar-lined oesophagus may develop after total gastrectomy. Rarely, other mechanisms appear to be involved. I have seen a patient with periarteritis nodosa whose mid-oesophagus infarcted. The lesion ultimately healed with a patch of columnar mucosa. Repeated mucosal injury by prolonged polychemotherapy with mucositis-inducing drugs can also lead to columnar metaplasia in the absence of reflux. Moreover, a patient was recently described who received polychemotherapy for breast cancer and later developed a bleeding oesophageal ulcer within a columnar-lined segment which was not present before the start of the chemotherapy [2•]. As the proliferative rate of the columnar mucosa is faster than that of the squamous mucosa, one wonders whether that is not the mechanism leading to proximal extension of columnar gastric-type mucosa after damage of the proliferative zone of the squamous mucosa. Attempts continue to search for methods to revert columnar metaplasia in the oesophagus. Recently retinoids were tried because they are considered essential for normal cellular growth and differentiation. However, administration of 13-*cis*-retinoic acid led to oesophageal ulceration in two out of 10 patients, in addition to inflammatory changes in the others [3•].

Acquired immunodeficiency syndrome (AIDS) continues to dominate the literature on oesophageal infection. The leading cause of infection and oesophagitis is *Candida*. Although oral thrush has been reported to be a marker of oesophageal candidiasis, examination of specimens obtained by directed oesophageal brushing and endoscopy is reported to be the best method for diagnosing oesophageal candidiasis [4]. However, routine endoscopy of patients with AIDS and oesophageal symptoms may burden the endoscopic services. The value of blind brushing was therefore further evaluated. A sheeted brush was introduced into a 16 French (F) nasogastric tube, inserted orally to a distance of 35 cm. The brush was then extended outside the sheet and the nasogastric tube moved up and down and rotated for about 20 s. After repositioning the brush into the sheet, the whole assembly was pulled out. The sensitivity of the blind brushing method was excellent (96%), with a specificity of 87%. The procedure was considered to be simple, required less than 3 min and was tolerated well by the patients. It eliminates the need for expensive equipment and specialized manpower by retaining a high diagnostic yield compared with endoscopy [5•].

Another patient presented with the initial infection of the human immunodeficiency virus [6•] (Fig. 1). The oesophageal lesions mimicked a herpetic infection. Seroconversion occurred several days later. Reports continue of large or giant oesophageal ulcers in AIDS patients for which no cause can be found. Empiric therapy has included sucralfate, acyclovir, H_2-recptor antagonists and corticosteroids (Fig. 2). Corticosteroid therapy may not be without risk. Such large idiopathic ulcers may cause massive haemorrhage [7•]. Severe oesophageal mycobacterial infection in AIDS was described as causing the formation of sinus tracts and fistulas, lead-

© Current Science Ltd ISBN 1-870485-32-7 ISSN 0952-6293

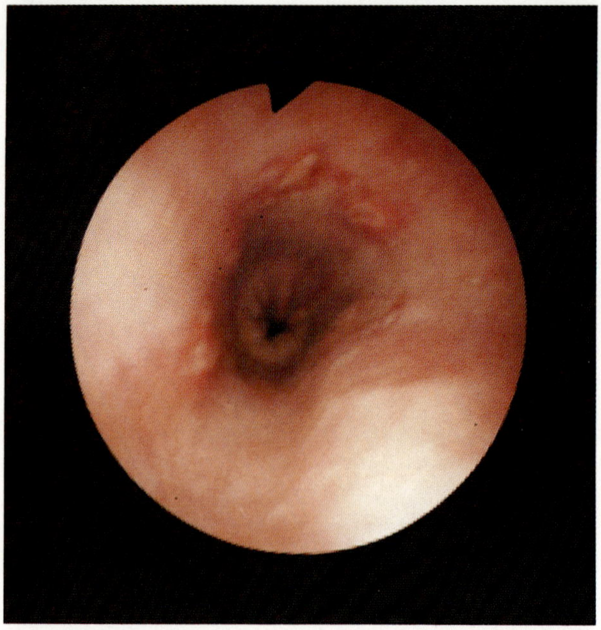

Fig. 1. Oesophageal infection with human immunodeficiency virus. The discrete lesions mimic a herpetic infection.

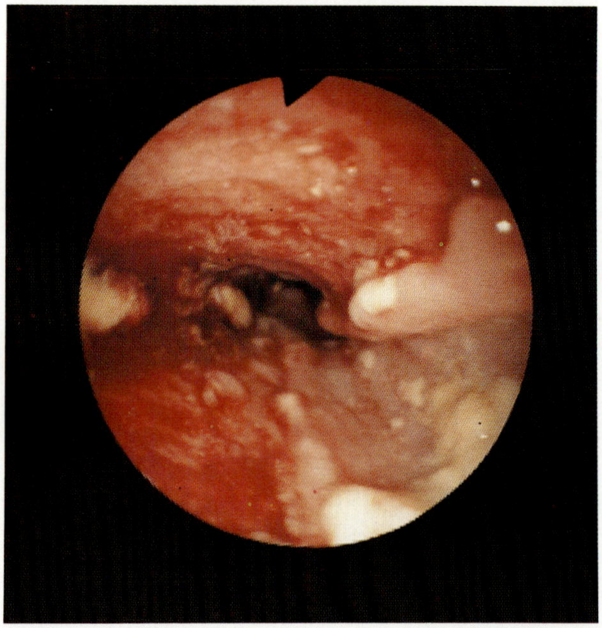

Fig. 2. Giant idiopathic oesophageal ulceration in AIDS. Almost the total circumference is ulcerated.

ing to a 'double-barrel' oesophagus [8•]. A comprehensive overview of all oesophageal infections in AIDS and of the appropriate therapy was recently published [9•].

Caustic oesophageal damage continues to be a major problem. Of all patients with a history of caustic ingestion, 20–60% have endoscopic evidence of oesophageal injury. Most investigators now agree that early endoscopy is the best means of assessing the extent and degree of injury to the oral cavity, posterior oropharynx, airways and oesophagus. Some investigators have reported that the presence of oropharyngeal injury does not correspond to the degree of oesophageal injury and have found that severe oesophageal injury can exist in the absence of any proximal burn. Others, however, have found that early evaluation of the degree of oropharyngeal injury and of oesophageal injury was a reliable indicator of prognosis. In particular, the extent of injury as judged by pharyngolaryngoscopy does correspond quite closely to the incidence of oesophageal injury. The latter is scored with respect to three zones (Fig. 3). Patients with involvement of zone III all had severe oesophageal burns, whereas those with intermediate grade injury (zone II) had only a 25% incidence of severe oesophageal injury. Patients with no oropharyngeal injury or injuries limited to the buccal mucosa, palate and uvula (zone I) had no evidence of oesophageal injury which would lead to stenosis [10]. Oesophageal injury was graded on a four-point scale: grade 0: no injury; grade 1: superficial erythema or blistering; grade 2: isolated shallow ulcerations; grade 3: deep ulcers, necrotic patches or circumferential involvement. All patients with grade 2 or 3 injury developed strictures.

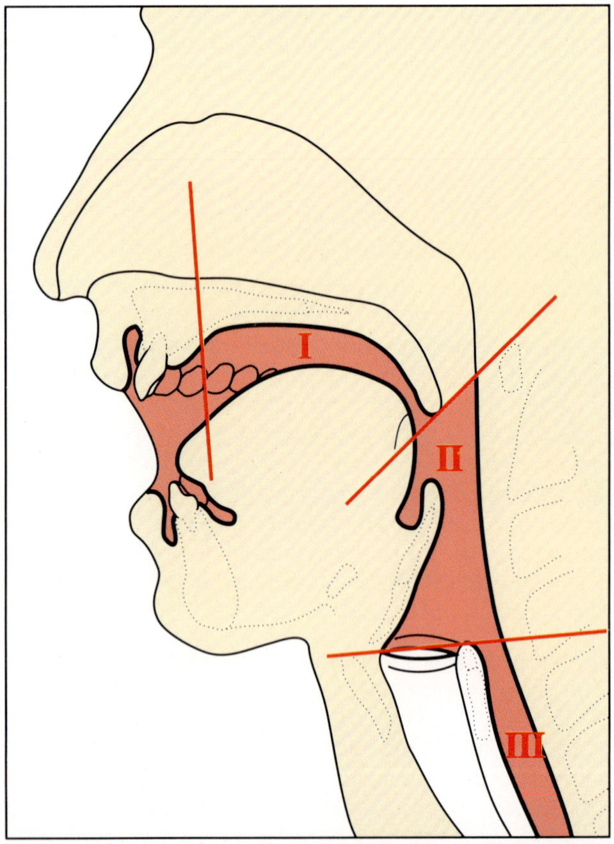

Fig. 3. Schematic representation of pharyngolaryngeal zones used to estimate risk of severe oesophageal injury. Zone I extends posteriorly from the alveolar ridge to the uvula and includes the body of the tongue, buccal mucosa, and hard and soft platlets. Zone II extends posteroinferiorly to include the posterior pharyngeal wall, tonsillar pillars, pyriform sinuses, and arytenoids. Zone III includes distal structures such as the false and true vocal cords, the trachea, and the cricopharyngeus. After Ferguson *et al.* [10].

A most comprehensive overview of drug-induced oesophageal damage has recently been published [11••].

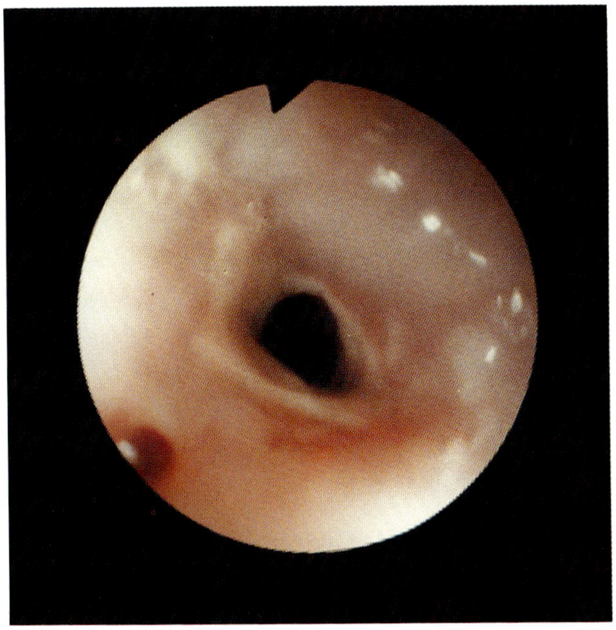

Fig. 4. Proximal oesophageal drug-induced stricture.

In addition, an overview of pill-induced oesophageal stricture has also appeared [12•] (Figs 4 and 5). The endoscopic appearance of drug-induced strictures is variable. An ulcerated mucosa overlying the stricture may be found in about half the patients. Normal-appearing mucosa distal to the stricture is typical. A circumferential membrane of exudate that easily peels away from the underlying oesophagus has been seen in several patients. The main causes of injury and stricturing are summarized in Fig. 5. Stricture development as a complication of pill-induced mucosal damage has not been comprehensively reviewed. Recognition that pill-induced injury may be responsible for a stricture has clinical importance, because conventional anti-reflux therapy may be ineffective. More than half of such strictures are in the proximal or mid-oesophagus with normal-appearing mucosa distal to the lesion. Such endoscopic findings should strongly suggest to the clinician that pill-induced damage may be responsible. Advancing age and ingestion of a sustained-release preparation were particularly important factors for pill-induced stricturing. Sustained-release preparations may also influence oesophageal injury. Only after the enteric-coated formulation for potassium chloride was changed to a wax-matrix sustained-release pill were potassium-related strictures of the oesophagus described. Impaired clearance of a potentially caustic pill by ingestion in a reclining position or by the presence of intrinsic or extrinsic oesophageal obstruction would also seem to be a logical explanation for more severe damage and stricture formation. Transit of radio-opaque pills is significantly impaired by extrinsic compression from cardiomegaly. In general, patients do well with dilatation therapy, although perforation has been described.

Many patients with oesophageal malignancy receive radiation therapy. Endoscopists should be aware of the pos-

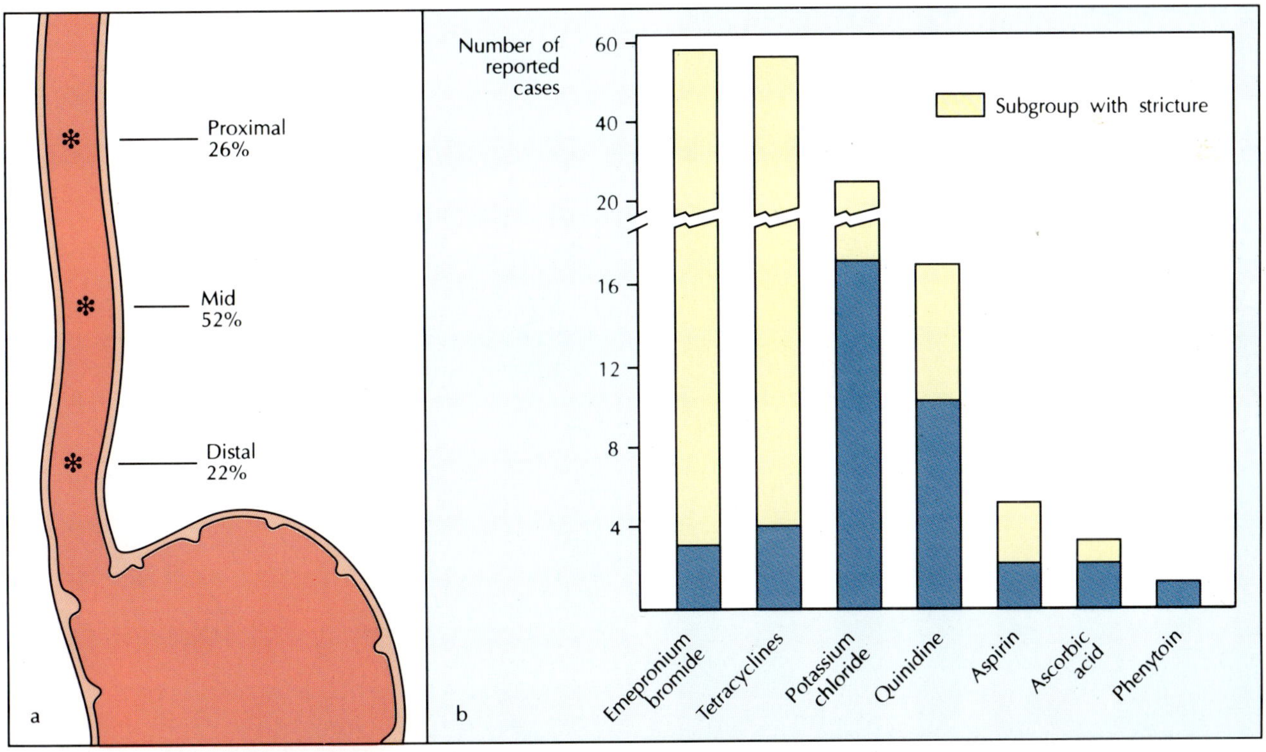

Fig. 5. (a) Distribution of pill-induced oesophageal strictures within the oesophageal regions. (b) Cases of pill-induced oesophageal injury and stricture extracted from literature review (including the five cases in this report) in relation to medication. The subset with stricture is indicated by the shaded marking for each medication. Only those medications that have been associated with stricture formation are included in this figure. The distribution of strictures is statistically different from the distribution of all cases with pill-induced damage ($P < 0.001$). After McCord and Clouse [12•].

sible radiation-induced injuries [13•]. The maximum tolerable dose is usually 60 Gy given at the rate of 10 Gy per week. The acute effects of radiation may be seen after 2 weeks and consist of mucositis, characterized by degenerative changes, and inhibition of mitosis in the germinal cells of the squamous epithelium with congestion of the microvasculature. Shortly thereafter the epithelium may slough, causing ulceration (Fig. 6). Stenosis is a common late injury, resulting from progressive fibrosis of the lamina propria and submucosa (Fig. 7). This can occur from months to years after completion of the radiation therapy. Once stricture has developed, treatment consists of careful dilatation.

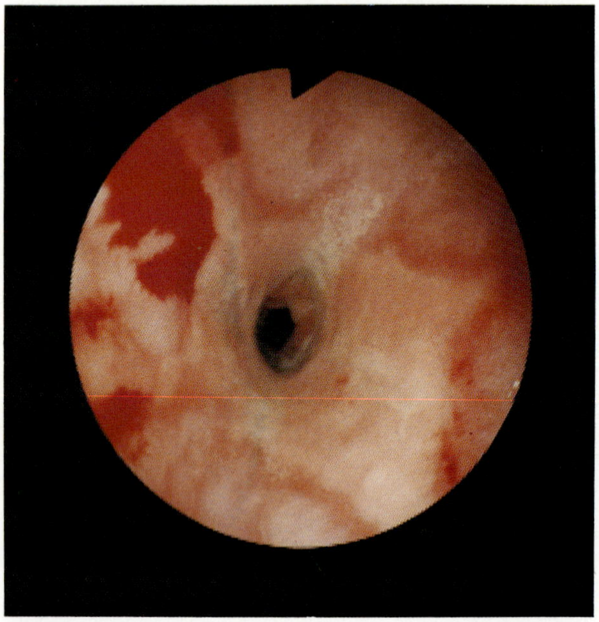

Fig. 6. Circumferential oesophageal ulceration induced by radiation therapy.

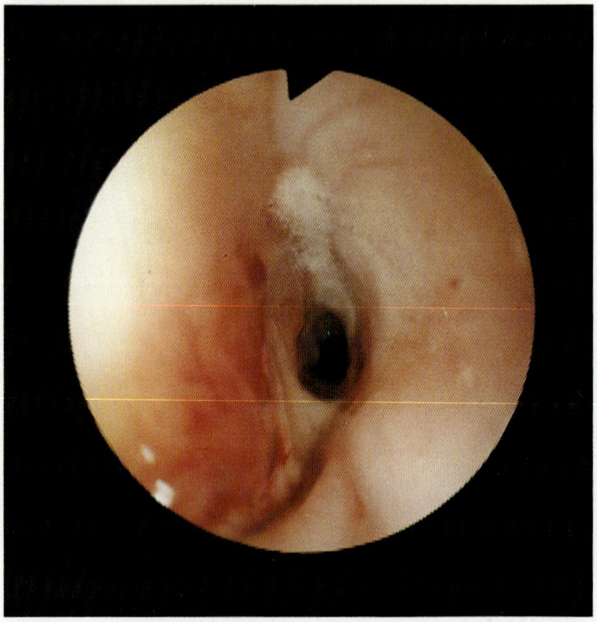

Fig. 7. Post-radiation oesophageal stricture.

Few endoscopists are aware that it might be important to examine the upper intestinal tract, especially the duodenum, using endoscopy and biopsy, to make the diagnosis of amyloidosis.

Endoscopic abnormalities may consist of a fine granular appearance, polypoid protrusions, erosions and ulcerations, together with mucosal friability. Upon biopsy, amyloid deposition may be present in 100% in the duodenum but also in 72% of oesophageal biopsies [14•].

The literature on mucosal plaques remains utterly confusing. Mucosal plaques of the oesophagus are quite common, occurring in up to 15% of patients. Despite the diverse aetiology, there is a remarkably similar endoscopic appearance in many cases. Glycogenic acanthosis is the most frequently observed oesophageal mucosal plaque. Endoscopically it is recognized as one or more rounded greyish whitish plaques, a few millimeters in size, which are usually discrete or confluent and located on the longitudinal folds of the distal oesophagus. Histologically it is characterized by thickening of the mucosa with plump squamous cells, whose clear cytoplasm imparts a mosaic appearance to adjoining cell borders. The amount of glycogen is increased. Mucosal plaques can also be caused by parakeratosis. Such lesions may be seen as whitish-blue plaques, 5–6 cm long, that easily peel off with manipulation of the biopsy forceps. There may be excessive accumulation of keratin microfilaments [14•,15•]: glycogen may be present or absent. Mucosal plaques can also be caused by hyperkeratosis. Another cause of mucosal plaques is bullous pemphygoid.

A number of vesiculobullous diseases can involve the oesophagus. These include epidermolysis bullosa, pemphigus vulgaris, toxic epidermal necrolysis, keratosis follicularis, bullous pemphygoid and benign mucous membrane pemphygoid. Benign mucous membrane pemphygoid is a chronic blistering dermatosis that shares many features with bullous pemphygoid but is distinguished by a predilection for mucous membrane involvement and a tendency to heal with scarring. Oesophageal mucosal involvement is infrequent and usually presents as dysphagia from web-like adhesions or strictures. Bullous pemphygoid can be differentiated from benign mucous membrane pemphygoid by its tendency not to heal with scarring, less predilection for mucous membrane involvement and the presence of circulating antibodies against a basement membrane component. Both diseases demonstrate the presence of immunoglobulin (Ig) G or C3 in the basement membrane zone. Oesophageal involvement is uncommon, occurring in approximately 4% of patients with benign mucous membrane pemphygoid, and even more rarely in bullous pemphygoid. Complications include the development of oesophageal webs secondary to recurrent blistering and erosions or strictures and obstruction from more chronic inflammation and scarring. The lesions most commonly occur in the upper third of the oesophagus. Bullae have been rarely reported during endoscopy, probably because this procedure is usually performed for the evaluation of dysphagia during stages of the disease when scarring and stricture formation have already occurred. Recently, a patient was described in whom bullae developed during the endoscopy, presumably as a direct consequence of pressure exerted by the endoscope, resulting in separation of the epithelium from the underlying tissue (the equivalent of Nikolsky's sign, which refers to separation of part of the epidermis from underlying tissue during application of lateral pressure to the skin). Therefore, endoscopy should be performed with utmost caution in such patients to prevent the induction of the formation of bullous lesions [17•]. Failure of benign mucous membrane pemphygoid to respond to corticosteroid therapy is rather rare. Some authors have warned against dilatation in cases of bullous oesophageal disease because of the risk of mucosal disruption. However, a recent report [18•] illustrates that careful oesophageal dilatation can be safely performed in such patients and that this therapy should be attempted first before considering resection and colon interposition.

Therapeutic endoscopic possibilities for non-malignant oesophageal obstruction

Dilatation therapy of benign oesophageal stenosis is now standard therapy. Progress has been made during the last few years with respect to dilating equipment. Increasingly the Savary Gilliard-type bougies and balloons are used in the initial approach. The development of balloons which can be passed through the instrumentation channel of the endoscope allows rapid dilatation of the majority of the strictures. For the more complex and difficult lesions it may be wise to pass the guidewire either under endoscopic control or, if that is impossible, under fluoroscopic guidance (Fig. 8) [19]. The current methods of assessing the severity of dysphagia and its response to therapy are subjective and vary enormously. In a recent study [20••], lumen diameter was measured endoscopically using an open or closed biopsy forceps as a measuring guide of the narrowest point of the stenosed area. When open, the forceps measured 6 mm in diameter and when closed it measured 2 mm in diameter. This estimate was compared with the diameter estimates obtained by watching barium capsules or tablets pass the stricture within 20 s. The diameter of the pill failing to traverse the oesophagus within 20 s correlated nicely with the endoscopically measured diameter. In contrast, a weak correlation was found between the dysphagia score and the endoscopically estimated luminal size. Changes in patient's dietary habits probably account for this discrepancy. Patients may take longer to complete a meal, they might chew their food for a long period and take small bites. For these reasons, a patient's subjective assessment of dysphagia is not reliable. The authors make a plea to use the barium pills to assess severity of dysphagia accurately and consistently but it would appear to me that one could also use the endoscopically estimated luminal diameter. The new dysphagia assessment system should allow standardization of the grading of dysphagia and should allow investigators to compare various therapies.

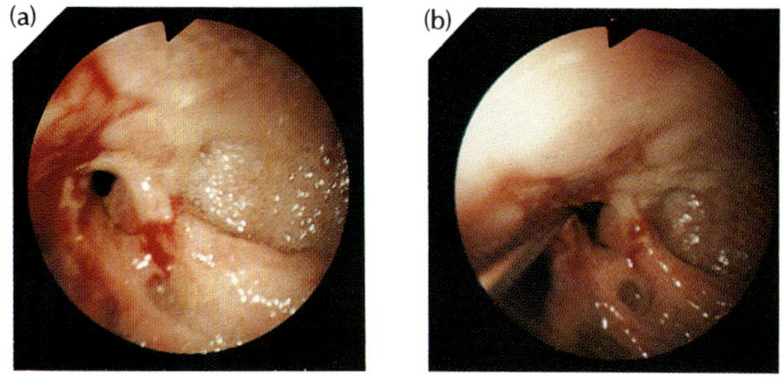

Fig. 8. Eccentric benign oesphageal stricture before (a) and after (b) insertion of a guidewire in preparation for dilatation.

Tight fibrotic strictures, especially when they resist dilatation with bougies or balloons, may also be treated with endoscopic incision with a needle-knife. A similar technique has been used for the treatment of post-surgical anastomotic membranous stenoses and for Schatzki rings. With the needle-knife, two or three longitudinal cuts are made in an upward direction along the stenosed area, avoiding the posterior wall overlying the aorta [21•]. Prospective trials comparing the various dilating modalities would be necessary to find out the proper indications for this technique in reflux-induced stricturing. Chinese authors designed a simple and effective method for retrograde dilatation of fibrotic strictures called 'gulping and pulling dilatation' with cushion retrograde dilatation (Fig. 9). A metal olive or ball of varying diameter is fixed to a nylon string and covered with a rubber cushion. After swallowing, the dilator should pass through the stenotic part. The cushion is 0.2 mm thick and elastic. Upon pulling the string, the cushion wraps around the metal dilator, increasing the width by 0.3–0.5 mm. The patient is instructed how to pull the dilator several times a day. If no further resistance is noted when the dilator passes the narrowed segment, then a larger dilator should be used or more cushions could be added to enlarge the size of the dilator. For patients with long strictures, a small dilator can be added as a guide that will easily pass through the stenosis and prevent the transversal position of the second larger dilator. The speed of dilatation depends upon the resistance. On average, a 0.5 mm larger dilator can be used every 2–5 days. Whether such a method will ever be used in units which are well equipped with all current dilating facilities is uncertain, except, perhaps, for very difficult irregular complex multifocal caustic strictures.

Controversy exists over the need for fluoroscopic guidance when performing Maloney oesophageal dilatation. This was the reason for setting up a prospective randomized study addressing this issue. Fluoroscopic guidance was shown to have a statistically significant higher success rate of dilatation than the blind technique (96 versus 80%). Three of the fluoroscopically guided dilatations were unsuccessful: one entering the trachea, one curling in the oesophagus and one curling in the hypopharynx. In contrast, 17 of the guided dilatations were unsuccessful: four entering the trachea, four curling in the oesophagus, five meeting resistance and four failing to pass through the stricture. As would be expected, use of flu-

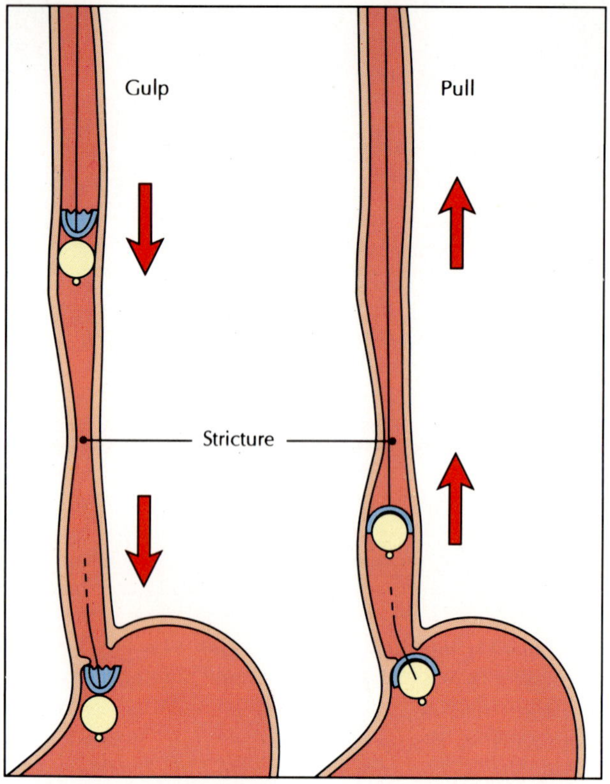

Fig. 9. Gulp and pull dilatation method. After Ka and Wu [22•].

oroscopy led to significantly greater accuracy in operator assessment of dilatation success. In 13 of the 88 blinded dilatations and in only one of the 74 fluoroscopic dilatations the operator claimed successful dilatation, while the monitor documented failure of dilator passage through the stricture. Adverse events occurred twice as often in the blinded group compared with fluoroscopy. Adverse events included the passage into the trachea, gross haematemesis and curling in a hiatal hernia pouch. Of concern was the fact the operator was aware of only two of the 10 adverse events that occurred with the blinded technique. Surprisingly of the four blinded dilatations that entered the trachea, neither the patient nor the operator was aware of and the patient failed to demonstrate any associated symptoms, such as coughing or dyspnoea. Whether Maloney users (apparently still rather popular in the USA) will change their technique and always use fluoroscopic guidance instead of blinded dilatation, even in those patients with simple benign strictures and during maintenance dilatation, remains to be seen [23••].

Dilatation of anastomotic strictures, especially when they are of small diameter and in the presence of marked tortuosity of the gut, can be notoriously difficult. Balloon dilatation was recently shown to be highly efficacious for such lesions. The balloon catheter was positioned under fluoroscopic and endoscopic control. About half the patients received only one session and a quarter needed two sessions. Relapse occurred in about 10% of the patients [24•]. For dilatation of such anastomotic strictures in the oesophagus balloons were passed over a teflon-coated guidewire, inserted under fluoroscopic control. Balloon diameters were 15, 20 mm and up to 30 mm. Dilatation was also carried out under fluoroscopic control.

There is almost universal agreement that pneumatic forceful dilatation should be the initial procedure in patients with achalasia, those except perhaps with advanced oesophageal disease. Usually pneumodilatation is carried out in inpatients, making the procedure rather expensive. In a recent study [25•] the feasibility of this technique as an out patient procedure was evaluated. The patients were dilated with Microvasive Rigiflex balloons of 30, 35 or 40 mm in diameter, guided over a floppy-tipped guidewire and fluoroscopically monitored. Subjective clinical symptoms of chest, abdominal or back pain were continuously evaluated for 4 h after the procedure. Post-procedure swallows were done first with gastrographin, and, when negative, with barium within 4 h. Eight patients complained of post-dilatation chest pain. Five had resolution of their pain within 1 h, whereas it persisted for more than 4 h in the three others who were hospitalized. Two patients had perforations (early or delayed). The authors concluded that balloon dilatation for achalasia as an out-patient procedure was safe, efficacious and cost-effective. They recommend the evaluation of post-procedure symptoms,such as pain, nausea, vomiting, hypotension, for a minimum of 4 h. In addition, patients should be followed by direct contact for a period of 2 days. Interesting in the whole discussion is the concept of delayed perforation, which in all probability is a misnomer that should be relabelled 'delayed diagnosis'. Because of oedema at the perforation site, immediate visualization of the disruption of mural integrity may be obscured.

Despite the wide use of pneumatic dilators in the treatment of achalasia there are no reports that debate the choice of high-compliance balloons versus non-expandable low-compliance balloon dilators. A theoretical advantage for the latter would be a decreased risk of perforation because the maximal diameter cannot be exceeded and excessive pressure does not increase the size of the fully inflated balloon (Fig.10). Moreover, the balloon is designed to tear longitudinally if the burst pressure is exceeded, thereby preventing a transverse blow out. In high-compliance devices, the balloon wall closely adapts its form to that of the constraining oesophagus. According to the law of Laplace, the relation between pressure p and wall tension T in an elastic cylinder with a radius R and an infinitely thin wall is $T = p \times R$. When all thickness is taken into account the approximation for tubes with a ratio of internal radius r to wall thickness δ greater than 10 is given by $T = p \times r/\delta$. As intraballoon pressure is constant, the radial forces will also be the same, whereas the oesophageal wall tension will be significantly higher in the widened part of the oesophagus compared with the strictured area. The lower compliance in the stenotic zone compared with the proximal part of the oesophagus further increases the difference in radius between these two zones and augments the differences in wall tension. The wider proximal oesophagus that is exposed to high wall tension will therefore be the more probable site of perforation. This is indeed the level where perforations in achalasia usually occur after dilatation. The newer generation of pneumatic dilators such as the Rigiflex achalasia dilator are inelastic and maintain their size and shape despite high inflation pressures. Consequently they do not fit the form of the oesophageal wall but rather apply direct radial forces only to the strictured area. These newer appliances are therefore probably safer than the high-compliance balloons and should therefore be preferred [26•].

Acute food impaction in the oesophagus remains a medical emergency. A variety of methods for removing the obstruction have been described (glucagon instillation, instillation of proteolytic enzymes, gas-forming carbonated beverages, nasogastric tubes, Foley catheters and endoscopy using snare or forceps retrieval equipment). A new approach is the use of an endoscope with a modified tip, also used for endoscopic variceal rubber band ligation [27•]. An overtube is passed over the endoscope and positioned in the oesophagus just proximal to the impaction site. The endoscope is withdrawn and the tip of the scope is replaced with a special screw-on drum tip corresponding to a hollow plastic cylinder 13 mm long, 12 mm in diameter. This converts the endoscope itself into a direct-vision suction device. Under direct vision the impacted bolus is suctioned into the drum and removed. An impacted bolus was successfully removed in all patients usually after two to three passes of the scope through the overtube. Currently snap-on drums to fit all endoscopes have been developed (Bard Interventional products, Billerica, Massachusetts, USA). A new alternative is to use the neodymium-YAG laser to vaporize the impacted meat bolus. The laser is aimed at the centre of the meat, which then shrinks rapidly and cavitates inwardly [28•].

Perforation remains the most important complication of diagnostic and therapeutic oesophageal endoscopy [29••,30•], as has repeatedly been stressed in the literature. Prevention is of the essence and so is early detection before contamination of the perforation site has occurred. The trend continues to treat many instances of oesophageal perforation conservatively instead of using the traditional management, which was emergency closure of the perforation, with possible drainage of the retro-oesophageal space. However, the number of reports is rising, showing that a conservative policy using broad-spectrum antibiotics, parenteral nutrition and nasogastric suction can lead to healing in a large proportion of patients. It should be remembered that guidewires may be dangerous. Blinded dilatation over a guidewire increases the risk of perforation when there is no control over the tip of the guidewire during dilatation. Markers on the guidewire have been used to increase control of the tip without fluoroscopy. Recently, a guidewire could not be removed after a dilatation procedure [31•], because a knotted looped guidewire was created. The wire had to be removed through a gastrotomy. This communication again stresses that the guidewire itself can present a hazard. Although the operator would wish to ensure sufficient wire distal to the site of stricture, he must be on his guard not to introduce too much to prevent knot-formation.

Benign and malignant oesophageal tumours: diagnosis and therapy

Squamous cell papilloma of the oesophagus is uncommon. Endoscopy usually reveals a small verrucous-type

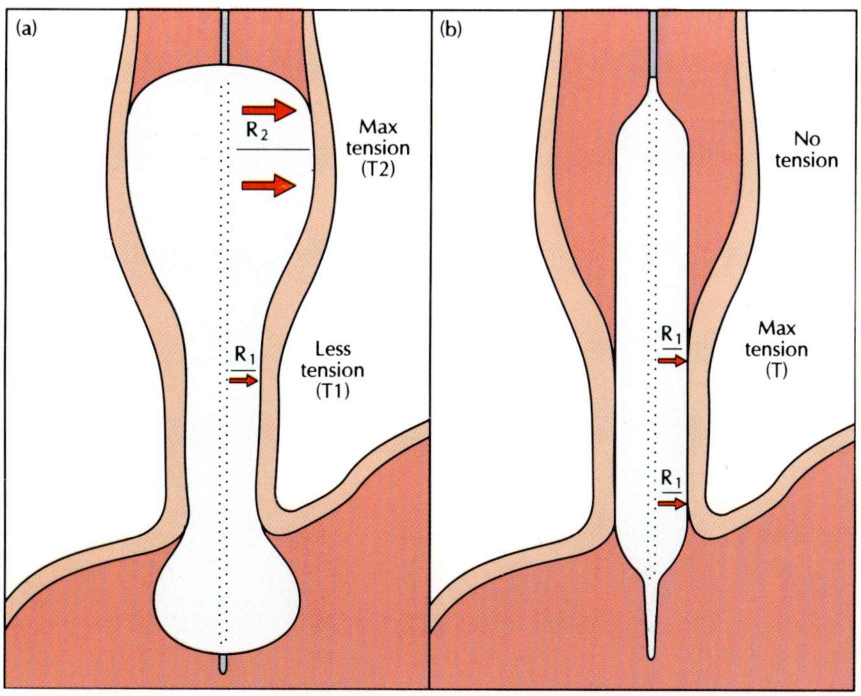

Fig. 10. (a) A high-compliance balloon, for a given pressure (P), adapts its form to that of the constraining oesophagus according to the law of Laplace; $T = (P \times R)/\delta$. Since $R_2 < R_1$ it is concluded that $T_2 < T_1$. (b) A low-compliance balloon contacts the oesophageal wall only in the stenotic area and therefore increases the suface tension in this zone only. After Rabinovici *et al.* [26•].

lesion of the middle portion of the posterior wall of the oesophagus. Histology is quite typical, with papillary structures composed of highly vascularized connective tissue and lined by spongeotic acanthotic squamous epithelium. Human papilloma virus antigens are usually absent. Most commonly the lesion is an incidental finding. Presumably chemical irritation secondary to reflux may be causal in some patients. Interestingly spontaneous disappearance secondary to auto-amputation occurred during severe vomiting in a Japanese patient [32•]. This lesion has no true malignant potential.

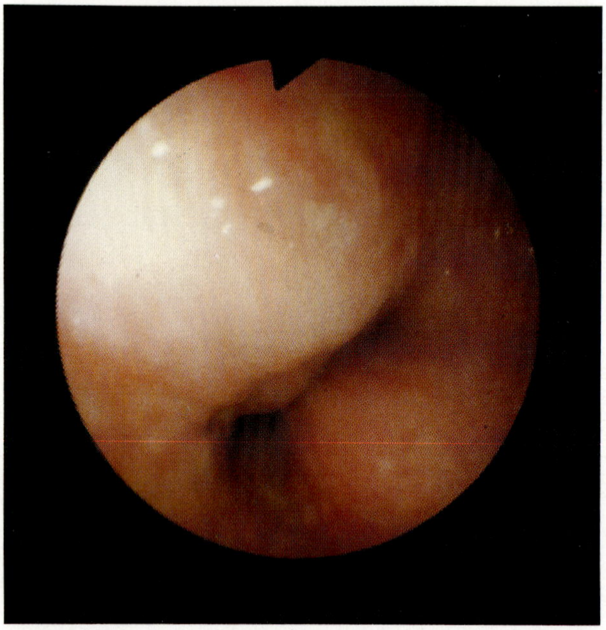

Fig. 11. Oesophageal submucosal tumour (caused by a leiomyoma).

The most common submucosal benign tumour in the oesophagus is an oesophageal leiomyoma (Fig. 11). Although about 85% of the leiomyomas are asymptomatic, they may cause dysphagia. A sharply delineated mass, apparently submucosal, that leaves the covering mucosa undamaged, it is quite characteristic. A number of endoscopic views can be misinterpreted as leiomyoma, such as extrinsic compression by mediastinal masses or aortic aneurysm. Oesophageal compression and deformity by neighbouring mediastinal tuberculous adenopathics mimicking oesophageal leiomyoma were recently described [33•]. Thus tuberculosis should also be considered in the differential diagnosis, especially if the mass lesion is located in the upper third of the oesophagus. According to many experts no attempt should be made to obtain a histological diagnosis if a leiomyoma is suspected, as disruption of the mucosal surface could unnecessarily complicate surgical enucleation. However, Japanese authors [34•] have treated 25 patients with submucosal tumours endoscopically. All patients underwent submucosography. The tumours were resected using electrocautery, usually in single sessions. Five lesions were treated with ethanol injections to necrotize the tissue after the overlying mucosa was stripped off by electrocautery. No serious complications such as perforation or bleeding occurred. Submucosography and endoscopic ultrasonography are a prerequisite to determine the extent of the tumour in relation to the thickness of the oesophageal wall.

Japanese authors in particular continue to call our attention to the occurrence of early oesophageal cancer [35•]. In up to 40% of patients such early malignancies are asymptomatic and are found incidentally. Some of these malignancies are limited to the epithelial layer, called *in situ*; others are limited to the mucosa. Minute oesophageal cancers are recognized endoscopically as shallow depression, slight elevation, redness or discolouration (Fig. 12). Dye endoscopy with Lugol's solution is considered to be very important because it allows detection and evaluation of the extent of the oesophageal mucosal cancer. A similar plea for the role of Lugol dye endoscopy was made in another Japanese publication [36•]. In order to remove the mucus, the patients were given orally or by spraying through a tube 100 ml of a solution containing 20 000 units of pronase, 1 g sodium bicarbonate and diluted dimethylpolysiloxane. Then, after conventional inspection of the mucosa, about 20 ml 1.5% Lugol solution was sprayed under direct vision and aspirated 30–60 s later. The oesophagus was then washed with 40–60 ml clean water prior to inspection. Any solution remaining in the upper alimentary tract was removed by aspiration after the examination. Ectopic mucosa, ulcer, cancer and severe dysplasia remain unstained. Lugol's staining was especially useful for the evaluation of lesions that were associated with discrete endoscopic abnormality or only colour change but still covered with epithelium. Such discoloured areas were seen as unstained, areas which greatly increases the possibility of being malignant. An unstained area by Lugol dye endoscopy is the only clue to detection of early malignancy when macroscopically visible abnormalities are lacking. It remains unclear to this reviewer when and how Lugol staining should be performed during routine endoscopy. If it is to be used only when there is a recognizable abnormality, for example discolouration, however minute the abnormality may be, then one may as well take multiple biopsies. If it is to be used when no endoscopic abnormalities are visible, then we have to find out which patients might profit from this technique.

Much attention has been given over the past year to methods for palliation of advanced obstructing oesophageal cancer, as excellently summarized in two overviews [37•,38•]. The results of a prospective randomized trial of laser therapy only and laser therapy followed by endoscopic intubation were published [39••]. Swallowing ability was assessed before and during the remainder of life on a 0–4 scale, with 0 being normal swallowing and 4 total dysphagia. There was no significant difference in dysphagia grade before or after treatment in either group. Dysphagia fluctuated more in those treated with the laser only than in those with a tube. Overall there was no significant difference in quality of life measured between the two groups. The complication rate (laser

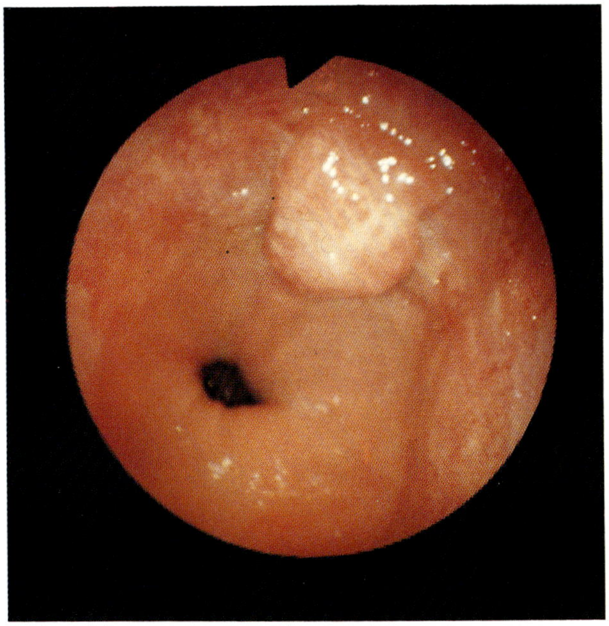

Fig. 12. Early oesophageal carcinoma.

only 10%; laser/intubation 40%) was significantly higher in intubated patients. Surprisingly the recurrent dysphagia rate (laser only 25%; laser/intubation 45%) was also higher in patients treated with intubation but these patients required fewer endoscopic procedures. According to the authors both procedures were effective in relieving dysphagia and in maintaining quality of life. There was no procedure-related mortality in either group. Ideally both techniques, laser and intubation, should be available for the management of patients with malignant dysphagia. However, this equipment is not available everywhere and the capital cost remains very high. Looking for an alternative palliative therapy which is quick, safe, painless, needs only a short in-patient stay and has a low complication rate, other British authors embarked on the use of ethanol to induce tumour necrosis [40•]. They treated 11 patients with dysphagia caused by inoperable, unresectable or recurrent cancer. The method relied on the endoscopic injection of ethanol with or without peroral dilatation to induce tumour necrosis. If occlusion of the lumen was not complete, the tumour was dilated to permit passage of the endoscope beyond the obstruction. Dehydrated ethanol was injected via the endoscope using a variceal injector needle. After one treatment session the dysphagia grade had improved from a mean of grade 3 to a mean of 1.5. An optimum dysphagia grade with a mean of 0.9 was achieved after a mean of 1.6 injection treatments. Treatments were repeated as symptoms recurred with a mean period between repeat treatments of 32 days. The needle was inserted into the tumour to its full depth. Injections were directed in 0.5 or 1 ml aliquots directly into macroscopic tumour. Satisfactory injection was recognized by blanching of the tumour mass at the injection site. Injections were sited away from macroscopically normal oesophagus to minimize the possible complication of stricture formation. The total volume injected was empirical and depended on the size of the tumour. In those patients in whom passage of the endoscope or pre-injection dilatation was impossible, circumferential ethanol injection into visible tumour was undertaken and a new attempt at dilatation was carried out one week later. In a rather similar pilot study patients with advanced cancer were injected with a solution of 5-fluorouracil and sodium morrhuate directly into the tumour to achieve debulking [41•]. Using a 25-gauge needle tip sclerotherapy catheter, a solution of 2.5% sodium morrhuate and 25 mg 5-fluorouracil per ml was injected into the tumour in 1 ml increments at 1 cm intervals on the accessible tumour surface. An average of 9 ml was injected during each session. Injections were repeated at 3–7-day intervals until luminal patency was achieved. Within the first month, however, after obtaining luminal patency all patients progressed again to luminal obstruction. Overall the therapy was not beneficial. The rapid development of luminal compromise may even have been accelerated by the scarring caused by the sodium morrhuate.

In many units insertion of a prosthesis remains the ultimate palliative step in managing malignant obstruction. The list of possible complications is well known and was recently again stressed in a series of 100 patients [42•] and consisted of haemorrhage 5%, perforation 6%, dislocation 11%, pressure necrosis 1%, tracheal obstruction 1%, cardiac insufficiency 4%, myocardial infarction 2%, pulmonary embolus 3%, pneumonia 2% and aspiration 1%, with a mortality of 16%. These figures are very high and one wonders whether some of the complications may not be secondary to the general anaesthesia which was used for insertion of the Nottingham prosthesis.

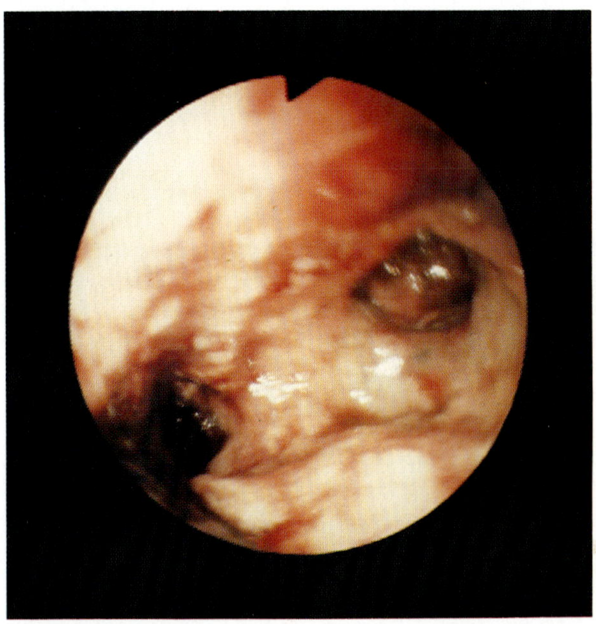

Fig. 13. Large malignant broncho-oesophageal fistula.

A particularly difficult subgroup of patients with malignant obstructions are those with oesophageal involvement by lung cancer [43••]. In 22 such patients the success of intubation was 91%, with 82% of patients discharged with a patent oesophagus. In 10 patients with malignant fistula (Fig. 13) three had the fistulous tract obliterated. This rather low success rate of closing fistulas was due to failure to seal off the space between the prosthesis and the fistula because of the absence of sufficient narrowing. Here again, in this difficult subgroup overall morbidity was 28% (18.8% perforation, 6.3% haemorrhage and 3.1% tracheal obstruction). The overall mortality rate was 18.8%, which is indeed quite impressive. The authors state that complications were more frequent than in primary oesophageal tumours but that endoscopic intubation was the only way to palliate this desperate condition and provided relief of symptoms in 66% of patients. Oesophageal involvement by lung cancer represents somewhat less than 15% of all indications for endoscopic palliation. The overall prognosis is worse than in primary oesophageal tumours. Why the risk of perforation is remarkably more frequent in primary pulmonary cancers remains poorly understood. Perhaps this might be explained partially by the fact that such extrinsic strictures are usually asymmetrical and non-circumferential. Another possible explanation may be the consistency of the extrinsic tumours, which are usually firm, making dilatation more hazardous. The success rate of closing a malignant fistula is lower when the primary tumour is pulmonary instead of oesophageal. When a fistula develops secondary to invasion of the oesophageal wall by lung cancer, there is usually no or little tumour-related oesophageal stenosis. Therefore the prosthesis cannot be adequately anchored and may fail to seal the space between the stent and the fistulous orifice. Another complication specific to extrinsic oesophageal involvement is the risk of tracheo-broncheal obstruction due to pressure of the tumour by the prosthesis. Careful bronchoscopy is therefore mandatory before oesophageal intubation is carried out to evaluate any pre-existent upper airway obstruction.

Experience with the cuffed oesophageal fistula tube (Wilson–Cook, Winston Salem North Carolina, USA) is increasing. In a recent study [44•] 10 patients with malignant oesophago-respiratory fistulas were intubated with a fistula tube. The fistula was located above the stricture in eight patients and in malignancy without narrowing into two patients. The diameter of the malignant fistula ranged from 1 to 3 cm. Adequate palliation was achieved in nine out of 10 patients. In one patient there was recurrent leakage. There mortality was attributable to the insertion procedure. These results are certainly gratifying, as they greatly contributed to the quality of life in these patients.

A new development is the introduction of a self-expanding mesh stent for oesophageal cancer. To overcome some of the disadvantages of a prosthesis, such as perforation and dislodgement, a self-expanding stainless steel mesh prosthesis, previously used for vascular and biliary strictures, was recently developed for the oesophagus. The stent may expand to a maximum diameter of 60 F when released in the stricture (Wall Stent, Metinvent SA, Lausanne, Switzerland). The stent is woven in the form of a tubular mesh from surgical grade stainless alloy filaments [45•]. The stent is pliable, self-expanding, flexible in the longitudinal axis and, when fully extended 53 mm long and 20 mm in diameter. The stent can be loaded on a small-diameter delivery catheter and constrained in its compressed form (18 French diameter) by a doubled-over plastic membrane, the outer layer of which can be progressively retracted with hydraulic assistance, thus permitting the prosthesis to expand once it has been correctly placed within the stricture. It is to be expected that many more communications will follow evaluating the usefulness of this new stent design, which, from a theoretical point of view, is very attractive.

References and recommended reading

Papers of special interest, published within the annual period of review, have been highlighted as:
- • Of interest
- •• Of outstanding interest

1. • Tytgat GNJ, Nicolai JJ, Reman FC: **Efficacy of Different Doses of Cimetidine in the Treatment of Reflux Esophagitis. A Review of Three Large, Double-Blind Controlled Trials.** *Gastroenterology* 1990, 99:629–634.

This study clearly shows that the therapeutic response to cimetidine largely depends upon the initial severity of the reflux damage. Healing in case of circumferential erosive damage is only possible in fewer than half the patients.

2. • Sartori S, Mielsen I, Trevisani L, Pazzi P, Malacarne P: **Barrett's Esophagus after Antineoplastic Chemotherapy.** *Endoscopy* 1990, 22:152.

Apparently repetitive destruction of the squamous mucosa by chemotherapeutic agents may lead to columnar metaplasia.

3. • Fennerty B, Sampliner R, Garewal H: **Esophageal Ulceration Associated with 13-*cis*-Retinoic Acid Therapy in Patients with Barrett's Esophagus.** *Gastrointest Endosc* 1989, 35, 5:442–443.

Vitamin A analogues should not be used in patients with oesophageal columnar metaplasia, in an attempt to revert the metaplastic change.

4. Wheeler RR, Peacock JE Jr, Cruz JM, *et al.*: **Esophagitis in the Immuno-Compromised Host: Role of Esophagoscopy in Diagnosis.** *Rev Infect Dis* 1987, 9:88–96.

5. • Bonacini M, Laine L, Gal AA, Lee MH, Martin SE, Strigle S: **Prospective Evaluation of Blind Brushing of the Esophagus for Candida Esophagitis in Patients with Human Immunodeficiency Virus Infection.** *Am J Gastroenterol* 1990, 85, 4:385–389.

Blind brushing had a sensitivity of 96% and a specificity of 87% for diagnosing *Candida* oesophagitis. The procedure is simple, fast and well tolerated.

6. • Bartelsman JFWM, Lange JMA, van Leeuwen R, van der Tweel JG, Tytgat GNJ: **Acute Primary HIV-Esophagitis.** *Endoscopy* 1990, 22:184–187.

Oesophageal primo-infection with human immunodeficiency virus. The discrete lesions mimicked a herpetic infection.

7. • Pedro-Botet J, Miralles R, Sauleda J, Rubiés-Prat J: **Idiopathic Ulcer of the Esophagus in the AIDS syndrome: A Potential Life-threatening Complication.** *Gastrointest Endoscopy* 1989, 35:470–476.

A large idiopathic oesophageal ulceration caused massive haemorrhage upon corticosteroid therapy.

8. STOOPACK PM, DE SILVA R, RAUFMAN J-P: **Inflammatory Double-barrelled Esophagus in Two Patients with AIDS.** *Gastrointest Endoscopy* 1990, **36**:394–396.
• Mycobacterial oesophageal infection may cause intramural sinuses and lead to a double-barrelled oesophagus.

9. RENÉ E, VERDON R, AIDS GIT GROUP: **Upper Gastrointestinal Tract Infections in AIDS.** *Baillieres Clin Gastroenterol Bailieres* 1990, 4:339–359.
• Nice overview of upper intestinal infections in patients with AIDS, including oesophageal abnormalities.

10. FERGUSON MK, MIGLIORE M, STASZAK VM, LITTLE AG: **Early Evaluation and Therapy for Caustic Esophageal Injury.** *Am J Surg* 1989, **157**:116–120.
• Interesting study that correlates the extent of oropharyngeal caustic injury with concomitant oesophageal injury.

11. BOYCE WH JR: **Drug-induced Esophageal and Gastric Damage.** *Current Topics in Gastroenterology and Hepatology*, edited by Tytgat GNJ, Van Blankenstein M. New York, Stuttgart: Thieme Verlag, 1990, pp 170–195.
•• The most comprehensive meticulously written review on drug-induced oesophageal and gastric damage.

12. MCCORD GS, CLOUSE RE: **Pill-induced Esophageal Strictures: Clinical Features and Risk Factors for Development.** *Am J Med* 1990, **88**:512–517.
• Overview of pill-induced oesophageal strictures. Potassium chloride or quinidine preparations were incriminated in 60% of patients. Older age, male sex, left atrial enlargement, ingestion of sustained-release formulations and prior structural abnormality were common.

13. CHOWHAN NM: **Injurous Effects of Radiation on the Esophagus.** *Am J Gastroenterol* 1990, **85**:115–120.
• Overview of early and late radiation-induced injury of the oesophagus. The therapeutic possibilities to relieve pain and dysphagia are discussed.

14. TADA S, *ET AL*: **Endoscopic and Biopsy Findings of Upper Digestive Tract in Patients with Amyloidosis.** *Gastrointest Endosc* 1990, **36**:10–14.
• Emphasis is given to the high frequency of endoscopic and histological abnormalities of the proximal gastrointestinal tract in patients with amyloidosis. Amyloid deposition was demonstrable in 72% of oesophageal biopsies.

15. LAM TS, LACK E, BENJAMIN SB: **Compact Parakeratosis of Esophageal Mucosa: A Non-specific Lesion Mimicking 'Leukoplakia'.** *Gastrointest Endosc* 1990, **36**:397–399.
• A patient is described with mucosal plaques caused by parakeratosis. The terminology used to described the various 'mucosal plaques' remains utterly confusing.

16. FEREY L, HERLIN P, MARNAY J, *ET AL*: **Histology and Ultrastructure of the Human Esophageal Epithelium. Normal and Parakeratotic Epithelium.** *J Submicrosc Cytol* 1985, 17:651–665.

17. WITTE JT, ICKEN JN, LLOYD ML: **Induction of Esophageal Bullae by Endoscopy in Benign Mucous Membrane Pemphigoid.** *Gastrointest Endosc* 1989, **35**:566–568.
• A patient is described with benign mucous membrane pemphigoid in whom haemorrhagic bullous lesions developed during endoscopy, presumably because of compression and shearing by the instrument.

18. ISOLAURI OF, AIRO I: **Benign Mucous Membrane Pemphigoid Involving the Esophagus: A Report of Two Cases Treated with Dilation.** *Gastrointest Endosc* 1989, **35**:569–571.
• Two patients are described with benign mucous membrane pemphigoid where careful dilatation was carried out successfully to treat oesophageal stricturing.

19. TYTGAT GNJ: **Dilatation Therapy of Benign Esophageal Stenoses.** *World J Surg* 1989, **13**:142–148.

20. GOLDSCHMID S, BOYCE HW JR, BROWN JI, BRADY PG, NORD HJ, LYMAN GH: **A New Objective Measurement of Esophageal Lumen Patency.** *Am J Gastroenterol* 1989, **84**:1245–1258.
•• Interesting study, comparing symptoms of dysphagia with endoscopically assessed luminal diameter with open or closed biopsy forceps and radiologically assessed diameter with barium pills of various diameters. There was a poor relationship between the dysphagia score and the objectively assessed luminal diameter.

21. MORETO M, ZABALLA M, IBANEZ S: **Endoscopic Incision as an Alternative to Bougienage in the Treatment of Peptic Esophageal Stricture.** *Endoscopy* 1990, **22**:105–109.
• The technique is described for incising a benign fibrotic reflux-induced stenosis with a needle-knife. Prospective trials are required to delineate the proper indications for this technique.

22. KA L, WU W-X: **A New Retrograde Dilation Method for Esophageal Cicatrical Stenosis: Gulp and Pull Dilator with Cushion.** *Dig Surg* 1990, 7:175–178.
• An interesting method is described for gradual 'self-dilatation'. Whether this method has any advantages over current techniques remains to be determined.

23. MCCLAVE SA, WRIGHT RA, BRADY PG: **Prospective Randomized Study of Maloney Esophageal Dilation — blinded Versus Fluoroscopic Guidance.** *Gastrointest Endosc* 1990, **36**:272–275.
•• The striking findings of this interesting study comparing blinded versus fluoroscopically guided dilatation with Maloney bougies are the high percentage of erroneous interpretations and adverse events (curling, entering the trachea, etc.) with the blinded technique. All endoscopists should be aware of such shortcomings.

24. FREGONESE D, DI FALCO G, DI TOMA F: **Balloon Dilatation of Anastomotic Intestinal Stenoses: Long-term Results.** *Endoscopy* 1990, **22**:153–249.
• A large group of anastomotic strictures, some seen high up in the cervical esophagus, were dilated with balloons up to 30 mm in diameter, positioned over a guidewire. The dilatation procedure was fluoroscopically monitored. No perforations occurred, which is surprising. Moreover, the early and long-term functional results were gratifying.

25. BARKIN JS, GUELRUD M, REINER DK, GOLDBERG RI, PHILLIPS RS: **Forceful Balloon Dilation: An Outpatient Procedure for Achalasia.** *Gastrointest Endosc* 1990, **36**:123–126.
• Pneumatic dilatation of achalasia as an out-patient procedure appears feasible provided the patients are carefully monitored after the procedure for 4 h for post-procedure symptoms and checked radiologically before discharge. In addition the patients should be followed by direct contact for 2 days. The only worry concerns the 'delayed perforation' which is a misnomer for delayed recognition of a perforation.

26. RABINOVICI R, KATZ E, GOLDIN E, AYALON A: **The Danger of High Compliance Balloons for Esophageal Dilatation in Achalasia.** *Endoscopy* 1990, **22**:63–64.
• According to the theoretical considerations in this study the non-expandable low-compliance balloon dilators should be preferred for pneumodilatation in achalasia.

27. SAEED ZA, MICHALETZ PA, FEINER SD, WOODS KL, GRAHAM DY: **A New Endoscopic Method for Managing Food Impaction in the Esophagus.** *Endoscopy* 1990, **22**:226–228.
• The tip of the endoscope is replaced with a screw-on drum tip, converting the instrument into a direct-vision suction device. Impacted boluses were successfully removed in all seven patients after two to three passes of the instrument through an overtube.

28. KLEIN I: **Resourceful Management of Esophageal Food Impaction.** *Gastrointest Endosc* 3680.
• Desobstruction of the oesophagus through coagulation and vaporization of an impacted meat bolus with neodymium-YAG laser energy.

29. TYTGAT GNJ: **Esophageal Perforation: Diagnosis, Prevention ●● and Therapy.** *Eur J Gastroenterol Hepatol* 1990, 2:193–202.
Detailed comprehensive review of all aspects of oesophageal perforation, including diagnosis, therapy and tips for prevention.

30. ANDERSON JR: **Oesophageal Injury. Part 1. The Changing ● Face of the Management of Instrumental Perforations.** *Gullet* 1990, 1:10–15.
Well balanced overview on incidence, diagnosis and management of esophageal perforation.

31. BHUTIAWI RP, WARRINGTON AJ: **Not a Way to do Esophageal ● Bougienage.** *Endoscopy* 1990, 22:239.
A knotted looped guidewire required gastrotomy for removal. Guidewires may be dangerous.

32. HAYASHI R, NAKAYAMA J, INOUE A, KOMATSU O, KATSUYAMA T, ● INOUE K: **Squamous Cell Papilloma of the Esophagus — A Report of Two Cases and a Review of the Literature.** *Dig Endosc* 1990, 2:377–382.
A squamous cell papilloma disappeared because of auto-amputation during an episode of severe vomiting.

33. BARCENA R, ERDOZAIN JC, LOPEZ-SAN ROMAN A, PEREZ ● HERNANDEZ F, LEDO L, BOIXEDA D: **Tuberculous Mediastinal Adenopathy Mimicking Esophageal Leiomyoma.** *Endoscopy* 1990, 22:57–58.
Tuberculous adenopathies should be added to the list of possible 'mimickers' of oesophageal leiomyoma.

34. EDA Y, ASAKI S, YAMAGATA L, SHARA S, SHIBUYA D, TOYOTA ● T: **Endoscopic Treatment for Submucosal Tumors of the Esophagus: Studies in 25 Patients.** *Gastroenterol JPN* 1990, 25, 4:411–416.
After delineating the extent of the lesions with submucosography and endoscopic ultrasonography, submucosal tumuors were endoscopically resected, usually with electrocautery. Although the results presented were gratifying, it would be wise to await further results before such therapy can be recommended on a large scale. Moreover, many such lesions may not require any therapy at all.

35. MISUMI A, HARADA K, MURAKAMI A, ARIMA K, KONDO H, AKAGI ● M, YAGI Y, IKEDA T, KABORI Y, MATSUKANE H, BABA K: **Early Diagnosis of Esophageal Cancer: Analysis of 11 Cases of Esophageal Cancer.** *Ann Surg* 1989, 210:732–739.
A beautifully illustrated series of early oesophageal malignancies is given. The main patterns are shallow depression, slight elevation, redness or discolouration. A plea is made for Lugol dye staining.

36. MISUMI A, HARADA K, MURAKAMI A, ARIMA K, KONDO H, AKAGI ● M, YAGI Y, IKEDA T, BABA K, KABORI Y, MATSUKANE H: **Role of Lugol Dye Endoscopy in the Diagnosis of Early Esophageal Cancer.** *Endoscopy* 1990, 22:12–16.
A strong plea is made for routine use of Lugol dye staining to facilitate the detection of early esophageal cancer. Findings in 17 early oesophageal cancers are illustrated.

37. TYTGAT GNJ: **Endoscopic Therapy of Esophageal Cancer: ● Possibilities and Limitations.** *Endoscopy* 1990, 22:263–267.
Detailed and comprehensive overview of the current endoscopic possibilities to palliate advanced oesophageal cancer.

38. FLEISCHER D: **Non-laser Techniques for Palliative Cancer ● Treatment.** In *Current Topics in Gastroenterology and Hepatology* edited by Tytgat GNJ, van Blankenstein M. New York, Stuttgart: Georg Thieme Verlag, 1990, pp 330–335.
Overview of non-laser possibilities to palliate oesophageal cancer with emphasis on the usefulness of tumour probes using bipolar electrophoresis.

39. BARR H, KRASNER N, RAOUF A, WALKER RJ: **Prospective Ran- ●● domized Trial of Laser Therapy Only and Laser Therapy Followed by Endoscopic Intubation for Palliation of Malignant Dysphagia.** *Gut* 1990, 31:252–257.
The roles of laser and laser plus intubation in the palliation of malignant dysphagia were compared. In the particularly difficult group with total obstruction, the laser was also shown to be effective. According to the authors, both techniques (laser and intubation) should be available for the management of malignant dysphagia.

40. PAYNE-JAMES JJ, SPILLER RC, MISIEWICZ JJ, SILK DBA: **Use of ● Ethanol-induced Tumor Necrosis to Palliate Dysphagia in Patients with Esophagogastric Cancer.** *Gastrointest Endosc* 1990, 36:43–46.
Tumour necrosis after injection of ethanol may lead to temporary improvement of malignant dysphagia caused by oesophageal malignancy. This technique is quick, safe, painless, less costly and easily repeatable. The results are encouraging.

41. WRIGHT RA, O'CONNOR KW: **A Pilot Study of Endoscopic ● Injection Chemo/Sclerotherapy of Esophageal Carcinoma.** *Gastrointest Endosc* 1990, 36:47–48.
Intramural injection of 5-fluorouracil and sodium morrhuate failed to restore luminal patency.

42. FÜGGER R, NIEDERLE B, JANTSCH H, SCHIESSEL R, SCHULTZ F: ● **Endoscopic Tube Implantation for the Palliation of Malignant Esophageal Stenosis.** *Endoscopy* 1990, 22:101–104.
A detailed account of the possible complications which one may encounter during palliation of malignant dysphagia with a prosthesis.

43. BUSET M, DES MAREZ B, CREMER M: **Endoscopic Palliative ●● Intubation of the Esophagus Invaded by Lung Cancer.** *Gastrointest Endosc* 1990, 36:357–359.
Detailed account of the results of intubation in patients with primary pulmonary cancer invading and obstructing the oesophagus or causing a malignant broncho-oesophageal fistula. Morbidity and mortality were impressive as can be expected.

44. HORDIJK ML, DEES J, VAN BLANKENSTEIN M: **The Management ● of Malignant Esophago-Respiratory Fistulas with a Cuffed Prosthesis.** *Endoscopy* 1990, 22:241–244.
Gratifying results were obtained in nine out of 10 patients with a malignant oesophagorespiratory fistula with the Wilson-Cook fistula tube carrying a foam rubber cuff.

45. DOMSCHKE W, FOERSTER ECH, MATEK W, RÖDL W: **Self-expand- ● ing Mesh Stent for Esophageal Cancer Stenosis.** *Endoscopy* 1990, 22:134–136.
The implantation of a new self-expanding mesh stent (with a diameter of 20 mm when fully extended) is reported in one patient but it is to be expected that many more communications will follow to document the usefulness of this new technique.

Endoscopy of the stomach

B.M. Schuman

Section of Gastroenterology, Medical College of Georgia, Augusta, Georgia, USA

The tenth anniversary of percutaneous endoscopic gastrostomy has been an occasion for a spate of papers that dealt with the presumptive superiority of the endoscopic technique over surgical gastrostomy, the apparent advantages of having surgical endoscopists perform percutaneous endoscopic gastrostomy, and the persistent occurrence of serious complications despite what gastrostomy procedure is done and who does it.

Introduction

Basic issues related to upper gastrointestinal endoscopy still crop up in the literature. The nagging problem of upper gastrointestinal endoscopy as the initial diagnostic study for upper abdominal symptoms was evaluated by Kerrigan *et al.* [1•], who found that about 60% of patients had positive findings whether internally referred or referred on clinical grounds by outside practitioners. The rate of disease would increase if only patients over the age of 40 underwent upper gastrointestinal endoscopy. In the USA, where radiologists are spending more time in 'high-tech' imaging studies, there is concern that gastrointestinal fluoroscopy units may be inundated if the government, in order to lower Medicare costs, insists on upper gastrointestinal series as the initial study.

The safety and necessity of pre-endoscopic sedation were evaluated in 913 endoscopic procedures, 371 of which were upper gastrointestinal endoscopy [2•]. Except for endoscopic retrograde cholangiopancreatography (ERCP), doses of meperidine combined with diazepam were comparable for all procedures. Naloxone was required to reverse oversedation in 17 of the total group (2.5%), but, overall, 85% of the patients benefited from sedation. Procedure amnesia is a pleasant boon for the patient, but I think that if open-access upper gastrointestinal endoscopy is to become a reality, we must discourage rather than encourage premedication so that after the procedure, the patient can function as well as after a barium meal.

Wrapped up in the safety issue is the need to monitor patients before, during, and after upper gastrointestinal endoscopy. Automated blood pressure and pulse recording, along with continuous oxygen saturation monitoring, are being increasingly introduced into endoscopy units. A Detroit group noted SaO_2 desaturation ($<$90%) in 12.9% of patients and systolic pressure abnormalities in 19.8% of patients undergoing upper gastrointestinal endoscopy [3•]. Desaturation occurs most prominently in the elderly and the patient with cardiopulmonary disease, two patient groups that would benefit from having little or no sedation. In my opinion it would make more sense to give all at risk-patients 2 litres of oxygen by nasal cannula and then be prepared to terminate the procedure for persistent desaturation. In 32 infants and children under 12 years old, desaturation to not greater than 90% occurred in 3.75% of patients [4•]! However, the threshold of tolerance for desaturation in children is lower, so that oxygen was not administered unless saturation fell below 80%. Children less than 1 year of age and those with cardiopulmonary compromise were most likely to show desaturation; nevertheless, the authors advise pulse oximetry for all children under 12 years of age undergoing upper gastrointestinal endoscopy. In response to a monitoring guideline [5], Berman [6] wrote a letter in which he decried waiting for 'data showing an effect on clinical outcome' by pulse oximetry that, after all, can only enhance patient safety. It is this argument that has pulse oximetry steamrollering into the endoscopy unit, and no future controlled trial demonstrating lack of improved clinical outcome will stop it.

Complications are still a fact of life for diagnostic upper gastrointestinal endoscopy, although in a review of 18 306 upper gastrointestinal endoscopies from 1982 to 1989 there was a complication rate of only 0.02%, including one death from a free perforation and another due to cardiopulmonary arrest [7•]. To prevent gastroduodenal bleeding from anticoagulant therapy for venous thromboembolism, a Barcelona group [8] advises upper gastrointestinal endoscopy at the time of hospital admission, because five patients (10%) were found to have gastric ulcers (14% duodenal ulcers) in a prospective study.

The remainder of this chapter will deal with new insights into non-steroidal anti-inflammatory drug (NSAID)-induced gastritis and an in-depth view of current percutaneous endoscopic gastrostomy literature, particularly as it pertains to innovations and complications. Unusual varieties of neoplasia of the stomach have recently been documented and, though rare, are worth knowing about. Finally, the current endoscopic management of gastric foreign bodies and gastric outlet obstruction is reviewed.

Gastritis

The effect of NSAIDs on the gastric mucosa has been traditionally assessed at gastroscopy by assigning grades of

© Current Science Ltd ISBN 1-870485-32-7 ISSN 0952-6293

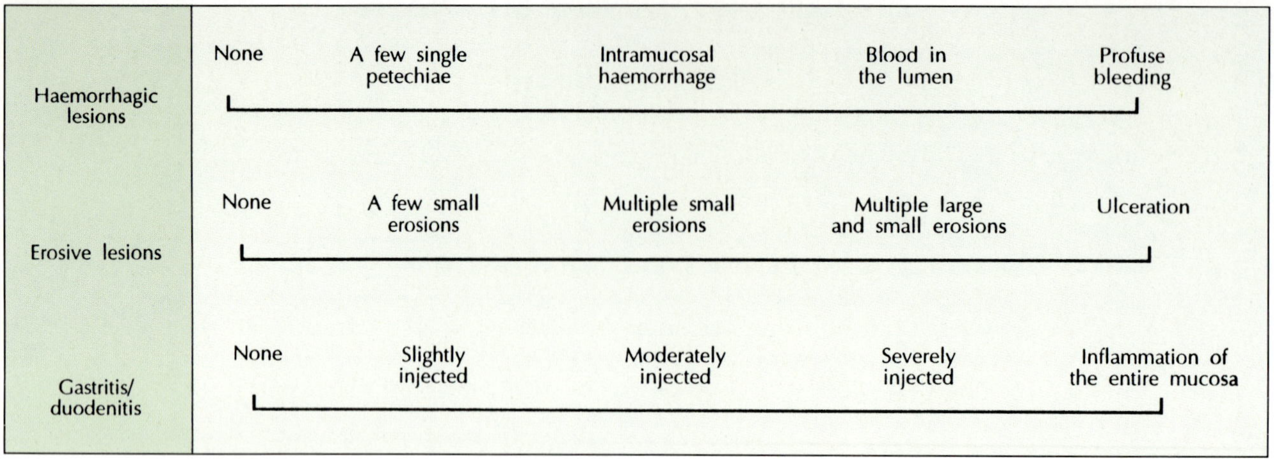

Fig. 1. Visual analogue scales for scoring of mucosal lesions. After Aabakken *et al.* [9•].

severity on a fixed point scale. From Oslo [9•] we learn that a more dependable assessment may be derived from a visual analogue system wherein three 200 mm scales with guide texts interspersed at 50 mm distances allow description along a continuum for hemorrhagic lesions, erosive lesions and gastritis/duodenitis (Fig. 1). Using the visual analogue system, two investigators with different levels of experience had similar scores, suggesting that the visual analogue scoring system will provide valid evaluation independent of endoscopic background. It seems, however, that reports of NSAID damage to the mucosa may be related to the timing of the endoscopic surveillance: Warrington *et al.* [10•] noted very little change from indomethacin or an 'oxicam' class of drug in a 28-day study. Most earlier studies in volunteers were 7-day trials that showed extensive changes of the gastric mucosa; local tolerance to NSAIDs apparently develops with sufficient time (Fig. 2).

It has been known for a number of years that patients with cirrhosis may bleed from the gastric fundus as a result of (portal) congestive gastropathy. Misra *et al.* [11•] undertook a histologic study of patients with the endoscopic appearance of congestive gastropathy: a 'scarlatine' reddening of rugae (striped) or a fine white reticular pattern (mosaic). In their largely non-alcoholic population with esophageal varices, the endoscopic and histologic features of congestive gastropathy were of low sensitivity and non-specific. However, before we throw out congestive gastropathy as a source of bleeding due to portal hypertension, a similar study in alcoholic liver disease needs to be carried out.

Not necessarily in order of degree of rarity, watermelon stomach [12•], syphilitic gastritis [13•], and collagenous gastritis [14] are reported for unique reasons. Binmoeller and Katon [12•] eliminated antral vascular ectasia in four endoscopic sessions and 188 applications of the 10-French (F) bipolar electrocoagulation probe (Fig. 3). A Japanese group found intense plasmacytosis in endoscopic biopsies of a stomach with radiographic findings of linitis plastica; serologic tests for syphilis were positive and the linitis plastica resolved with penicillin therapy. In a patient with collagenous colitis, mucosal biopsies of the gastric antrum and body revealed a collagenous layer 30–60 μm in thickness coursing through the upper part of the lamina propria rather than adjacent to the basal membrane of the epithelial cells [14].

Percutaneous endoscopic gastrostomy

The technique of percutaneous endoscopic gastrostomy was described in 1980, and so a review of 10 years' experience with the technique is appropriate. Curiously, the review appearing in the *British Journal of Surgery* [15•] was written by surgeons whose 'own experience [was limited to] 13 patients'. A previously published conclusion that percutaneous endoscopic gastrostomy 'is best performed by surgeons rather than by gastrointestinal endoscopists' because the major complications require surgical management seems to be the major thrust of the review. Another trio of surgeons compared 49 percutaneous endoscopic gastrostomies done by the surgical service with 51 done by the gastroenterology service and did not find a statistically significant difference in the number of complications occurring in each group. The patients in the non-surgical group experienced three major complications and more cases of transient fever and abdominal pain, whereas the patients in the surgical group experienced four major complications and more cases of stomal leak [16•]. Thus, no matter who performs the technique, there is a significant complication rate that is not much different from operative gastrostomy, as noted by Stiegmann *et al.* [17••], who performed a randomized prospective study comparing operative gastrostomy (under local anesthesia) with percutaneous endoscopic gastrostomy. With operative gastrostomy there was a 26% complication rate and 9% mortality rate and with percutaneous endoscopic gastrostomy there was a 25% complication rate and 12% mortality rate. Another interesting observation was that the incidence of complications in patients having previous intra-abdominal surgery, excluding partial gastrectomy, was much lower with per-

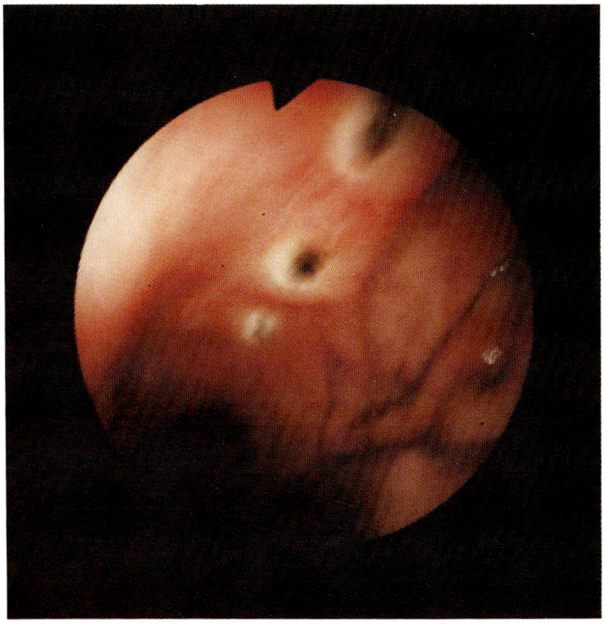

Fig. 2. NSAID-induced erosions of the stomach. By courtesy of G.N.J Tytgat, Academic Medical Center, Amsterdam, The Netherlands.

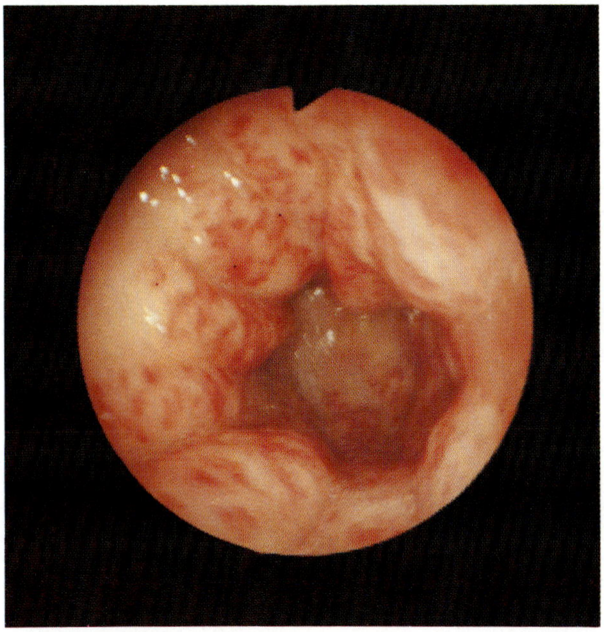

Fig. 3. A 'watermelon' stomach—angiomatosis of the antrum. By courtesy of G.N.J Tytgat, Academic Medical Center, Amsterdam, The Netherlands.

cutaneous endoscopic gastrostomy than with operative gastrostomy. Although percutaneous endoscopic gastrostomy did not substantially save lives, an economic analysis revealed that it did save money.

If there is a turf battle between surgeons and gastrointestinal endoscopists over who should perform percutaneous endoscopic gastrostomy, both sides should be aware that there is a third contestant to be reckoned with. Radiologically guided percutaneous tube gastrostomy employing percutaneously placed T-fasteners that are non-surgically sutured to the anterior abdominal wall was successfully performed in 124 out of 125 patients with only one major complication [18••]. Included in the series were patients with partial gastrectomy who had failed percutaneous endoscopic gastrostomy. Wolfsen *et al.* [19•], however, caution that diagnostic upper gastrointestinal endoscopy is essential before any type of gastrostomy tube placement to recognize pre-existing conditions that may contraindicate gastrostomy or require major changes in medical management to ensure the success of the gastrostomy procedure.

Where percutaneous endoscopic gastrostomy is contraindicated, a combined endoscopic and operative gastrostomy will aviod the risks of general anesthesia and laparotomy and ensure adhesion of the gastric serosa to the anterior abdominal wall [20•]. Moreover, when a respect percutaneous endoscopic gastrostomy is required it can be carried out simply as an outpatient procedure using the original site [21].

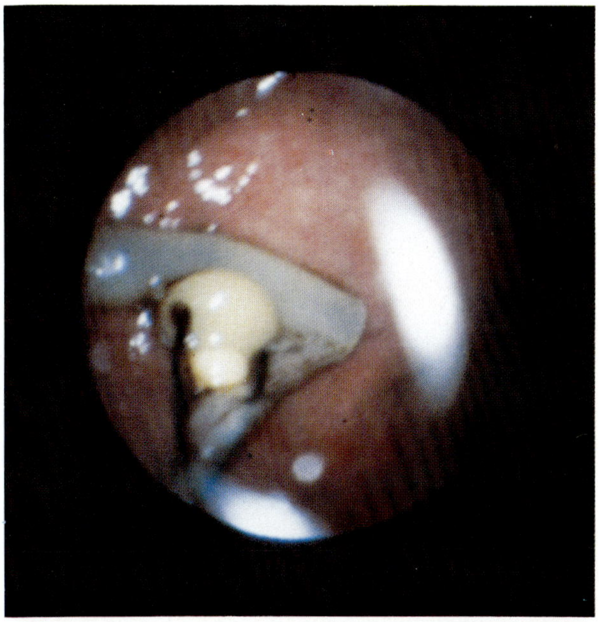

Fig. 4. The bumper is positioned so that it glides freely over the gastric mucosa.

Complications, and what to do about them, dominate the literature. A comparison of percutaneous endoscopic gastrostomy patients who had had judicious traction on the gastrostomy tube with patients who had had no traction applied convinced Chung and Schertzer [22•] that the complications of peristomal drainage, cellulitis, fasciitis, catheter extrusion and bleeding could be reduced if no effort was made to bring the gastric serosa to the abdominal wall (Fig. 4). It is evident now that after several weeks a fibrous sheath forms around the tube and effectively seals the gastrocutaneous fistula. We have not put traction on the tube for the last 2–3 years and, in fact, go to some trouble to ensure that the bumper moves freely over the gastric mucosa. Indeed, the bumper has extruded into the abdominal wall often enough to earn the sobriquet of the 'buried bumper syndrome'. The buried bumper has initiated several ingenious methods of extraction: Savary dilators advanced over a guidewire placed through the bumper [23], replacing the extruded tube by pushing it out with a new percutaneous endoscopic gastrostomy tube [24], or simply removing it with a rat tooth forceps [25•].

It is better to replace a percutaneous endoscopic gastrostomy tube with the gastrostomy button [26] than a Foley-type catheter. The catheter balloon can deflate, allowing the catheter to fall out [27], or the balloon may migrate into the small bowel and cause a bowel obstruction [28•].

Neoplasm

The gastric stump is slowly disappearing in the USA and concern for the development of cancer in the stomach remnant is diminishing with it. This concern still exists, however, on the other side of the Atlantic. A London group [29•] enlisted 87 subjects who had had gastric surgery 20 years earlier into a screening program and found epithelial dysplasia and intestinal metaplasia primarily at the stoma and mostly in patients who had had Billroth II operations (Fig. 5). Therefore, a rational surveillance program would involve only patients with gastrojejunostomy and biopsy would be restricted to the stoma, reducing the number of patients to be followed and the histological workload. This study supports the view that endoscopic screening for stump cancer *per se* is not worthwhile, but screening to identify the subgroup at high risk for developing stump cancer is meaningful because it allows endoscopic follow-up for the detection of early gastric cancer.

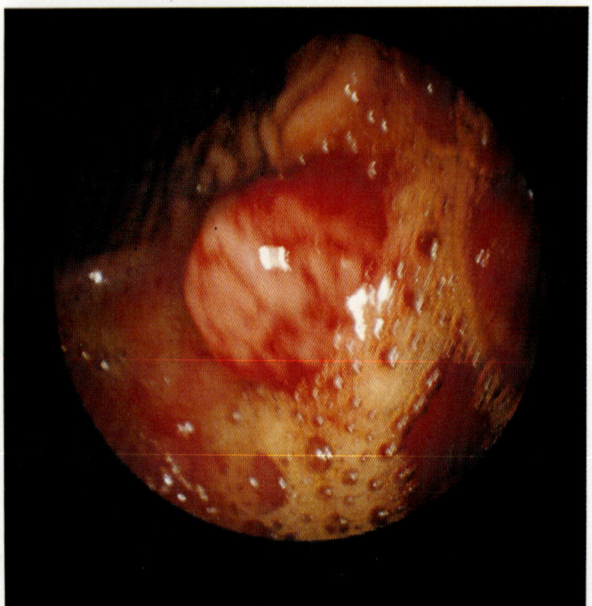

Fig. 5. Stump cancer in a patient with a subtotal gastrectomy. By courtesy of G.N.J Tytgat, Academic Medical Center, Amsterdam, The Netherlands.

A recent approach [30•] to early gastric cancer involves the use of videoendoscopy, which is purported to give better image resolution than fiberoptic endoscopy. Eighteen patients with early gastric cancer were randomized to fiberoptic endoscopy and videoendoscopy with and without indigo dye spraying. The advantage of videoendoscopy lies not so much in the detection of the lesion, but rather in its ability to define the limits of the early gastric cancer. For those patients with early gastric cancer who are not candidates for surgery, endoscopic polypectomy or strip biopsy, a method whereby snare excision is performed after elevating a flat or depressed lesion with a submucosal injection of 5–10 ml saline, constitutes the initial therapeutic approach [31•]. When this approach was not possible or failed to remove the lesion completely, laser therapy or injection of the antineoplastic, OK–432, followed. All lesions under 20 mm in diameter were successfully treated and in this group of 33 patients there was no evidence of recurrence or metastasis after a mean of 37 months follow-up.

Multiple endoscopic biopsies, usually six to eight, are considered adequate to establish a histological diagnosis of gastric cancer. Routine uses of cytology have been generally abandoned. However, Waldron *et al.* [32•] achieved a 95% reliability rate with combined biopsy and cytology for gastric malignancy. They attribute their high return (78%) of positive cytology to the fact that they carried out brush cytology before the biopsy.

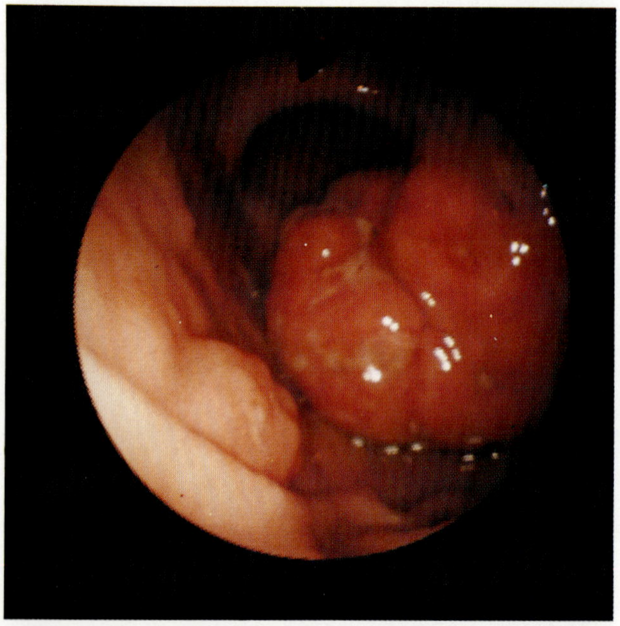

Fig. 6. Gastric lymphoma presenting as umbilicated submucosal nodules with overlying glistening mucosa. By courtesy of G.N.J Tytgat, Academic Medical Center, Amsterdam, The Netherlands.

The reason for failure of gastric biopsy to detect all cancers was investigated by Awad *et al.* [33]. A retrospective study was carried out to determine whether mucosal thickening adjacent to gastric cancer interfered with obtaining malignant tissue. The authors showed that ulcerative or infiltrating lesions had a lower positive rate because mucosal thickening did not allow a good approach to the tumor rim by the forceps.

In a study by Hedenbro *et al.* [34], two Swedish patients presented with rare submucosal tumors pathologically identified as parietal cell carcinoma after surgical resection; both of these cancers were diagnosed endoscopically as leiomyomas. In Japan, a gastric lesion with the endoscopic appearance of an early gastric cancer proved to be a manifestation of adult T-cell leukemia previously diagnosed by node biopsy [35].

The difficulties of establishing an endoscopic diagnosis of gastric lymphoma are reviewed by Amano *et al.* [36•]. Endoscopic features of early gastric lymphoma were the presence of a shallow ulcer and glistening nodules ('lustrous granules'). Repeated and deep biopsies are essential to obtain a tissue diagnosis, which eludes the endoscopist in over 50% of cases (Fig. 6). In my experience, biopsy of the base of the ulcer will enhance the possibility of obtaining submucosal tissue that will provide a diagnosis of gastric lymphoma.

Forty-six patients with hyperplastic gastric polyps and 21 with adenomas of the stomach had endoscopic Congo red tests followed by four-point biopsies [37•]. Patients with hyperplastic polyps tended to have atrophic gastritis of the body predominantly and those with adenomas had intestinal metaplasia of the antrum as the most common associated feature. Cancer within gastric adenomas has been found almost as frequently as in the surrounding mucosa and it must be emphasized that after polypectomy patients be entered in a gastroscopic surveillance program (Fig. 7).

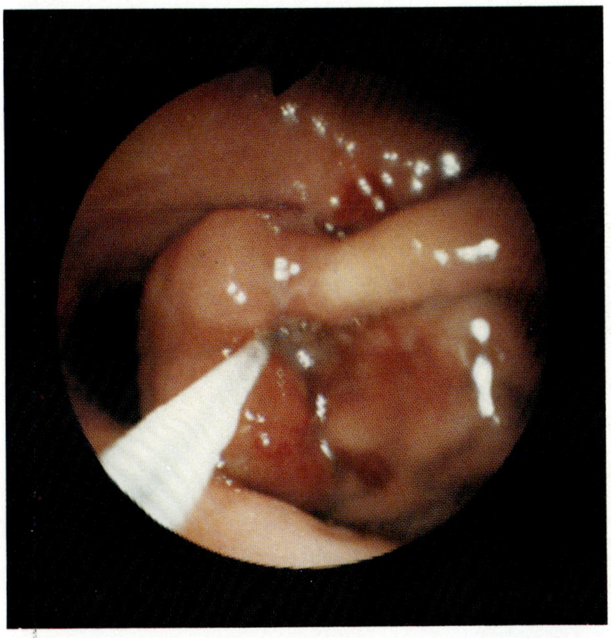

Fig. 7. Pedunculated adenoma of the stomach. By courtesy of G.N.J Tytgat, Academic Medical Center, Amsterdam, The Netherlands.

The problem with submucosal tumors for endoscopists is the inability to obtain tissue diagnosis, even using special large-particle forceps or a snare. A guillotine needle was employed by Spandre *et al.* [38•] to retrieve core tissue 2–10 mm long. The group was able to get histological proof of seven leiomyomas, one Schwannoma and one lipoma of the stomach. This technique should be particularly valuable for a tissue diagnosis of gastric lymphoma. Fukumoto *et al.* [39] carried out snare polypectomy of two pedunculate ectopic gastric mucosa lesions of the body of the stomach; this is usually a flat submucosal lesion identified in resected gastric specimens. Another unusual lesion was a 6 cm polypoid mass composed of ectatic submucosal vessels noted endoscopically around the cardia in a 41-year-old man with a family history of Osler–Weber–Rendu disease [40]. A unique vascular lesion in the antrum was described by Chawla *et al.* [41•], who noted a dense collection of angiodysplastic lesions, presumably a variant of the 'watermelon' stomach (Fig. 3).

Foreign bodies and outlet obstruction

A body-packer ingested 80 four gram packets of cocaine and passed them all except for one that remained in the stomach. Having demonstrated that a retrieved packet would resist breaking open when snared, Sherman and Zingler [42•] extracted the retained packet uneventfully when the body-packer refused surgery. New packet construction reduces the risk of disruption and acute cocaine toxicity, making gastroscopic retrieval safer.

Removal of an Angelchick prosthesis that had eroded intact into the stomach 6 years after insertion was accomplished endoscopically by first cutting the tie of the prosthesis and then using a rat tooth forceps, snare and double-channel endoscope for withdrawal [43]. Removing toothbrushes from the stomach endoscopically is not so easy, as Chinitz and Bertrand [44] learned from their experience with three patients and 25 toothbrushes. A snare does not work because of the difficulty of putting the toothbrush in the axis of the overtube and so the bristles, which may come loose, have to be grasped with a forceps. A toothbrush with a bent handle is virtually impossible to extract.

Kozarek *et al.* [45•] carried out a retrospective review of 23 patients who had undergone balloon dilatation of outlet obstruction because of peptic ulcer disease (12), anastomotic stricture (seven) and NSAID therapy (four). Five patients required surgery, one for perforation by the tip of the balloon catheter, but the remainder were asymptomatic, six of whom maintained H_2 blockade for a follow-up of 16–23 months. It is generally acknowledged that balloon dilatation of surgical anastomoses gives better results than dilatation for post-ulcer pyloric stenosis. This was certainly the case for 15 out of 16 patients treated by balloon dilatation for postgastrectomy anastomotic stricture reported by Kadota *et al.* [46•].

Stricture of the stoma after gastric surgery for morbid obesity occurs in up to 20% of patients and relief of obstruction can be expected in about two thirds of patients by endoscopic dilatation techniques: endoscope tip, Savary dilators or balloon. Twenty-seven out of 40 patients were relieved of obstruction endoscopically, and the 13 failures were mostly attributed to a horizontal angulation of the stoma making intubation or even guidewire passage almost hopeless [47•]. In another group of morbidly obese patients treated by means of gastric stapling and loop gastrojejunostomy, anastomotic strictures developed in eight, seven of whom underwent successfully balloon dilatation [48].

Miscellanea

A new mechanical device was constructed to achieve definitive endoscopic hemostasis [49•]. The apparatus is a 1.5 cm long helical steel wire (Fig. 8a). The helix suture is attached to the end of an endoscope and by means of a cable inserted through the biopsy channel the wire is rotated into gastric mucosa (Fig. 8b). The device was successfully used in two patients after animal trials demonstrated its safety and efficacy.

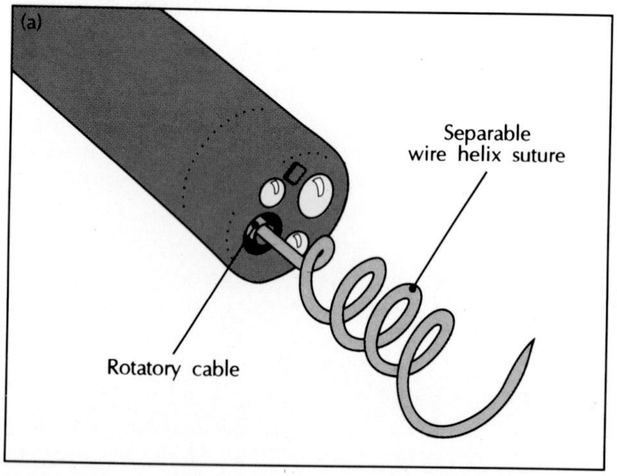

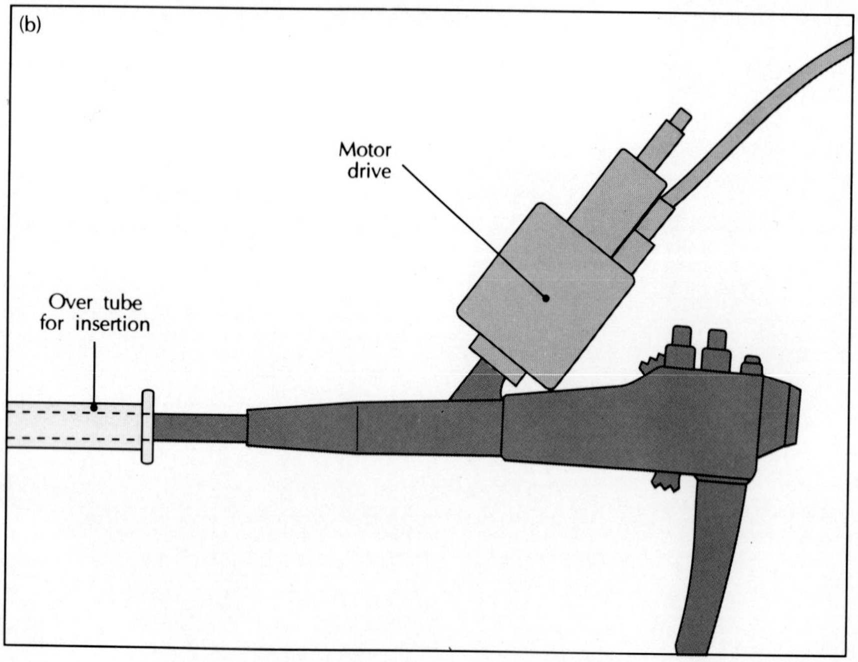

Fig. 8. (a) The conical helicoidal steel suture placed at the tip of the fiberscope. It is twisted into the bleeding point, then pull-separated from its rotatory cable. (b) A view of the endoscope with the outer tube and the rotatory cable passed through the biopsy channel.

In an experimental canine model, 5% sodium morrhuate was injected into the submucosa of the gastric cardia at six sites [50•]. The sclerosis prevented high-dose atropine-induced gastroesophageal reflux, although the lower esophageal sphincter pressure was unaffected. Fibrotic thickening of the gastric cardia apparently behaves in a fashion similar to fundoplication.

Chronic organoaxial volvulus of the stomach, rotation through the cardiopyloric axis greater than 180°, was treated endoscopically in seven patients [51•]. Derotation is accomplished by fixing the tip of the endoscope in the duodenal bulb and then rotating the endoscope through 180° in a counterclockwise direction before withdrawal. Success can be documented by easy passage of the endoscope through the lumen of stomach and into the second portion of the duodenum. A barium meal needed to establish the diagnosis also confirms the correction of the volvulus.

A rather elaborate classification of gastric varices was assembled by a Japanese group, who evaluated 124 patients with bleeding gastric varices [52•]. Varices were classified into three groups based on form, and five groups based on location and color. Bleeding correlated with protruding varices that had a red color spot and were located at the anterior or greater curvature of the cardia.

One hundred and three out of 900 runners in the 1988 Chicago Marathon volunteered to have endoscopy to determine the cause of occult gastrointestinal bleeding, a phenomenon well described in long-distance runners [53•]. Fecal occult blood was positive in nine of the 41 runners who completed the race. Of the seven volunteers undergoing endoscopy, two who were examined within 48 hours had oozing gastric antral erosions, but the others, examined several days after the race, had a negative endoscopic study. It is presumed that, as blood flow to the gut is reduced by as much as 80% with strenuous exercise, the lesions were a result of ischemia.

References and recommended reading

Papers of special interest, published within the annual period of review, have been highlighted as:
• Of interest
•• Of outstanding interest

1. • KERRIGAN DD, BROWN SR, HUTCHINSON GH: **Open Access Gastroscopy: Too Much To Swallow?** *Br Med J* 1990, **300**:374–376.

To reduce the workload and increase the diagnostic yield would require denying access to patients under the age of 40.

2. • ANDRUS CH, DEAN PA, PONSKY JL: **Evaluation of Safe, Effective Intravenous Sedation for Utilization in Endoscopic Procedures.** *Surg Endosc* 1990, **4**:179–183.

The thrust of this article suggests that intravenous sedation with meperidine and diazepam/midazolam has become a standard for gastrointestinal endoscopy. For routine, elective diagnostic upper gastrointestinal endoscopy, however, we might take a lesson from countries where no premedication is the rule.

3. • STEFFES CP, SUGAWA C, WILSON RF, HAYWARD SR: **Oxygen Saturation Monitoring During Endoscopy.** *Surg Endosc* 1990, **4**:175–178.

Although 12.9% of patients undergoing upper gastrointestinal endoscopy showed arterial oxygen desaturation, no serious complications occurred. Cardiopulmonary disease and age over 60 are risk factors during upper gastrointestinal endoscopy.

4. • CASTEEL HB, FIEDOREK SC, KIEL EA: **Arterial Blood Oxygen Desaturation in Infants and Children During Upper Gastrointestinal Endoscopy.** *Gastrointest Endosc* 1990, **36**:489–493.

Desaturation in children did not correlate with medication, tolerance to procedure, weight or age.

5. FLEISCHER D: **Monitoring the Patient Receiving Conscious Sedation for Gastrointestinal Endoscopy: Issues and Guidelines.** *Gastrointest Endosc* 1989, **35**:262–266.

6. BERMAN IR: **Monitoring and Patient Safety [letter].** *Gastrointest Endosc* 1990, **36**:160.

7. • FRUHMORGEN P, PFAHLER A: **Komplikationen bei 39397 Endoskopischen Untersuchungen — eine 7-jährige Prospektive Dokumentation uber Art und Haufigkeit.** *Leber Magen Darm* 1990, 1:20–32.

Would monitoring the 18306 diagnostic upper gastrointestinal endoscopies in this 1982–1989 series for oxygen desaturation have prevented the one cardiopulmonary death?

8. MONREAL M, BOIX J, HUMBERT P, LAFOZ E, AGUADO A, REY-JOLY C: **Gastroduodenal Ulcer Incidence in Patients with Venous Thromboembolism.** *Gastrointest Endosc* 1989, **35**:386–388.

9. • AABAKKEN L, LARSSEN S, OSNES M: **Visual Analogue Scales for Endoscopic Evaluation of Nonsteroidal Anti-Inflammatory Drug-induced Mucosal Damage in the Stomach and Duodenum.** *Scand J Gastroenterol* 1990, **25**:443–448.

This system apparently makes it possible for the endoscopic neophyte to interpret the extent of mucosal damage, as well as the endoscopic master.

10. • WARRINGTON SJ, DEBBAS NMG, FARTHING M, *ET AL.*: **Lornoxicam, Indomethacin and Placebo: Comparison of Effects of Faecal Blood Loss and Healthy Upper Gastrointestinal Endoscopic Appearances in Healthy Men.** *Postgrad Med J* 1990, **66**:622–626.

The implication from this 28-day study is that the gastric mucosa adapts to NSAID effects if given sufficient time to do so.

11. • MISRA SP, DWIVEDI M, MISRA V, AGARWAL SK, GUPTA R, GUPTA SC, MITAL VP: **Endoscopic and Histologic Appearance of the Gastric Mucosa in Patients with Portal Hypertension.** *Gastrointest Endosc* 1990, **36**:575–579.

In essence, portal congestive gastropathy does not exist — at least in non-alcoholic patients.

12. • BINMOELLER KF, KATON RM: **Bipolar Electrocoagulation for Watermelon Stomach.** *Gastrointest Endosc* 1990, **36**:399–402.

The watermelon stomach comes in three varieties: striped, diffuse, and patchy.

13. • ANAI H, OKADA Y, OKUBO K, KORENAGA D, MAEHARA Y SUGIMACHI K, OHI Y: **Gastric Syphilis Simulating Linitis Plastica Type of Gastric Cancer.** *Gastrointest Endosc* 1990, **36**:624–626.

Gastric syphilis also comes in three varieties: ulcerative, infiltrative, and nodular.

14. STOLTE M, RITTER M, BORCHARD F, KOCH-SCHERRER G: **Collagenous Gastroduodenitis on Collagenous Colitis.** *Endoscopy* 1990, **22**:186–187.

15. • MORAN BJ, TAYLOR MB, JOHNSON CD: **Percutaneous Endoscopic Gastrostomy.** *Br J Surg* 1990, 77:858–862.

This review covers the gamut of percutaneous endoscopic gastrostomy experience. The authors are concerned that this 'surgical technique' is being performed by non-surgical gastrointestinal endoscopists.

16. • DAVIS JB JR, BOWDEN TA JR, RIVES DA: **Percutaneous Endoscopic Gastrostomy. Do Surgeons and Gastroenterologists Get the Same Results?** *Am Surg* 1990, **56**:47–51.

Surgeons and gastroenterologists obtained the same results with percutaneous endoscopic gastrostomy or, at least, there was no statistically significant difference in success and complication rates.

17. •• STIEGMANN GV, GOFF JS, SILAS D, PEARLMAN N, SUN J, NORTON L: **Endoscopic Versus Operative Gastrostomy: Final Results of a Prospective Randomized Trial.** *Gastrointest Endosc* 1991, **36**:1–5.

A prospective randomized study of operative gastrostomy with local anesthesia compared with percutaneous endoscopic gastrostomy showed similar complication and mortality rates. Percutaneous endoscopic gastrostomy cost much less so long as the tube did not need to be replaced.

18. •• SAINI S, MUELLER PR, GAA J, *ET AL.*: **Percutaneous Gastrostomy with Gastropexy: Experience in 125 Patients.** *AJR* 1990, **154**:1003–1006.

This radiologically guided percutaneous endoscopic gastrostomy technique, which includes gastropexy, had a complication rate of 11.1%, no deaths and no tube extrusions in 124 cases. In the group of 121 patients reported above [17], the overall mortality was 10.5% and the complication rate 25.5%. Eliminating the endoscope and staying out of the abdomen seems to confer a real advantage on the radiologic method.

19. • WOLFSEN HC, KOZAREK RA, BALL TJ, PATTERSON DJ, BOTOMAN VA, RYAN JA: **Value of Diagnostic Upper Endoscopy Preceding Percutaneous Gastrostomy.** *Am J Gastroenterol* 1990, **85**:249–251.

Upper gastrointestinal endoscopy may identify conditions that contraindicate the procedure or require ongoing new therapy. However, the endoscopist cannot identify colon overlying the stomach whereas fluoroscopic guidance allows selection of a needle site that avoids the colon.

20. • MANSBERGER JA, KAVOUKLIS JH: **Combined Endoscopic and Surgical Gastrostomy When Percutaneous Endoscopic Gastrostomy is Contraindicated.** *Am Surg* 1990, **56**:138–140.

This combined technique is recommended for cases where percutaneous endoscopic gastrostomy is contraindicated. Unfortunately it combines the two features that increase morbidity: the endoscope and incision into the abdominal cavity.

21. CULLADO MJ, SLEZAK FA, PORTER JA: **Repeat Percutaneous Endoscopic Gastrostomy (PEG): An Outpatient Procedure.** *Surg Endosc* 1990, **4**:173–174.

22. • CHUNG RS, SCHERTZER M: **Pathogenesis of Complications of Percutaneous Endoscopic Gastrostomy. A Lesson in Surgical Principles.** *Am Surg* 1990, **56**:134–137.

Traction on the gastrostomy tube is the culprit!

23. KLEIN S, HEARE BR, SOLOWAY RD: **The 'Buried Bumper Syndrome': a Complication of Percutaneous Endoscopic Gastrostomy.** *Am J Gastroenterol* 1990, **85**:448–451.

24. Fay DE, Luther R, Gruber M: **A Single Procedure Endoscopic Technique for Replacing Partially Extruded Percutaneous Endoscopic Gastrostomy Tubes.** *Gastrointest Endosc* 1990, 36:298–300.

25. Pfeil S, Blades E, Yang P: **Complications of Percutaneous • Endoscopic Gastrostomy Removal.** *Gastrointest Endosc* 1990, 36:316.

Case reports [23,24,25] prove the point made by Chung and Schertzer [22].

26. Foutch PG, Talbert GA, Gaines JA, Sanowski RA: **The Gastrostomy Button: a Prospective Assessment of Safety, Success and Spectrum of Use.** *Gastrointest Endosc* 1989, 35:41–44.

27. Esker AH, Hall CH Jr: **Replacement of the Damaged Percutaneous Endoscopic Gastrostomy Feeding Tube in the Immature Tract.** *Gastrointest Endosc* 1990, 36:380–391.

28. McGovern R, Barkin JS, Goldberg RI, Phillips RS: **Duo- • denal Obstruction: A Complication of Percutaneous Endoscopic Gastrostomy Tube Migration.** *Am J Gastroenterol* 1990, 85:1037–1038.

Patients who require replacement of the percutaneous endoscopic gastrostomy tube are better served by a gastrostomy button than a Foley catheter.

29. Savalgi RS, Corbishley CM, Caygilkl C, Hill M, Cook MG, • Kirkham JS, Northfield TC: **Relation Between Severity and Extent of Precancerous Lesions in the Postoperative Stomach.** *Lancet* 1990, 336:413–416.

Endoscopic surveillance of the gastric stump should not be just a cancer-finding expedition but a hunt for mucosal dysplasia that identifies the patient at high risk for cancer.

30. Demirci S, Gohchi A: **A Comparative Study for Fiberoptic • and Video Endoscope Determination of the Extent in Minimal Changes of Gastric Mucosa Using Indigo Dye Spraying.** *Surg Endosc* 1990, 4:80–82.

The limits of early gastric cancer were best defined by videoendoscopy using indigo dye spray. This may have some practical value for the surgeon carrying out gastric resection.

31. Haruma K, Sumii K, Inoue K, Teshima H, Kajiyama G: **Endo- • scopic Therapy in Patients with Inoperable Early Gastric Cancer.** *Am J Gastroenterol* 1990, 85:522–526.

Aggressive endoscopic therapy can eradicate early gastric cancer if the lesion is less than 2 cm in diameter.

32. Waldron R, Kerin M, Ali A, McAnena OJ, McGuire M, • McCarthy CH, Given HF: **Evaluation of the Role of Endoscopic Biopsies and Cytology in the Detection of Gastric Malignancy.** *Br J Surg* 1990, 77:62–63.

A high rate of positivity for brush cytology in gastric cancer may depend on carrying out the brushing before the biopsy.

33. Awad JA, Lee EY, Wang TC, Deschryver-Kecskemeti K, Clouse RE: **Effect of Mucosal Thickening Near Gastric Carcinoma on the Endoscopic Diagnosis of Malignancy.** *Dig Dis Sci* 1990, 35:317–320.

34. Hedenbro JL, Hägerstand I, Rychterova V: **Parietal Cell Carcinoma — A New Differential Diagnosis for Submucosal Gastric Tumours.** *Endoscopy* 1990, 22:47–48.

35. Obata S, Tsukamoto A, Kimura K, Maeda K, Kawamura R: **Adult T-cell Leukemia Presenting as IIa + 11c-like Lesions in the Stomach on Endoscopic Examination.** *Endoscopy* 1990, 22:81–82.

36. Amano Y, Ishihara S, Takatori Y, Imaoka T, Watanabe M, • Fukumoto S: **Endoscopic Retrospective Study on Gastric Malignant Lymphoma — With Special Reference to the Appearance of the Initial Lesion.** *Dig Endosc* 1990, 2:396–401.

Early endoscopic signs of gastric lymphoma are shallow ulcer, areas of macular redness, and lustrous granules (perhaps better described as glistening nodules). Biopsies have a low yield but in my experience biopsying the base of the gastric ulcer may improve the positivity rate in lymphoma.

37. Nakano H, Persson B, Slezak P: **Study of the Gastric Mu- • cosal Background in Patients with Gastric Polyps.** *Gastrointest Endosc* 1990, 36:39–42.

Type A gastritis is associated with hyperplastic polyps and intestinal metaplasia with adenomas.

38. Spandre M, Cavallero M, Pennazio M, *et al.*: **Needle Biopsy • of Submucosal Lesions of the Gastrointestinal Tract.** *Surg Endosc* 1990, 4:161–163.

A special guillotine needle made submucosal biopsy successful in 20 out of 22 cases.

39. Fukumoto S, Adachi K, Ohtsu K, *et al.*: **Pedunculated Submucosal Ectopic Mucosa of the Stomach Treated by Endoscopic Polypectomy: Report of Two Cases.** *Dig Endosc* 1990, 2:434–438.

40. Yakshe PN, Albert F, Ragsdale B, Travers R, Benjamin S: **An Unusual Vascular Lesion in a Patient with Hereditary Hemorrhagic Telangiectasia.** *Gastrointest Endosc* 1990, 36:513–516.

41. Chawla SK, Ramani K, Presti PL: **The Honeycomb Stomach: • Coalesced Gastric Angiodysplasia.** *Gastrointest Endosc* 1990, 36:516–518.

This antral angiodysplatic lesion, called the 'honeycomb' stomach, presented as submucosal cherry-red lesions and probably represents another variant of the watermelon stomach.

42. Sherman A, Zingler BM: **Successful Endoscopic Retrieval of • a Cocaine Packet from the Stomach.** *Gastrointest Endosc* 1990, 36:152–154.

Cocaine packet wrapping is now so elaborately constructed that body-packers do not fear spontaneous rupture nor disruption by a retrieval snare.

43. Moussa SE, Tunuguntla K, Chan CH, Sedarat A, Rybnicek K: **Endoscopic Removal of an Intact Anti-reflux Prosthesis 6 Years After Implantation.** *Gastrointest Endosc* 1990, 36:525–527.

44. Chinitz MA, Bertrand G: **Endoscopic Removal of Toothbrushes.** *Gastrointest Endosc* 1990, 36:527–530.

45. Kozarek RA, Botoman VA, Patterson DJ: **Long-term Follow- • up in Patients Who Have Undergone Balloon Dilatation for Gastric Outlet Obstruction.** *Gastrointest Endosc* 1990, 36:558–561.

Seventy per cent of 23 patients who underwent balloon dilatation for gastric outlet obstruction were asymptomatic after a mean of 2.5 years follow-up. My long-term results of dilatation of pyloric stenosis due to ulcer disease have not been so good as with anastomotic stricture, the reverse of what these authors have found.

46. Kadota T, Hiraide H, Imai J, Tamakuma S: **An Easy and • Safe Modified Method of Endoscopic Balloon Dilation for Postgastrectomy Anastomotic Stricture.** *Surgery Gyn Obstet* 1990, 170:445–447.

One hundred per cent success was achieved in 16 patients with post-gastrectomy anastomotic stricture.

47. Sataloff DM, Lieber CP, Seinige UL: **Strictures Following • Gastric Stapling for Morbid Obesity. Results of Endoscopic Dilatation.** *Am Surg* 1990, 56:167–174.

Two-thirds of 40 patients had successful dilatation of strictures associated with vertical band gastroplasty. An angulated channel was the major factor interfering with dilatation.

48. Rajdeo H, Bhuta K, Ackerman NB: **Endoscopic Management of Gastric Outlet Obstruction Following Surgery for Morbid Obesity.** *Am Surg* 1989, 55:724–727.

49. Escourrou J, Delvaux M, Buscail L, Darmana R, Frexinos J, • Morucci JP, Ribet A: **First Clinical Evaluation and Experimental Study of a New Mechanical Suture Device for Endoscopic Hemostasis.** *Gastrointest Endosc* 1990, 36:494–497.

This unique steel helix is inserted into gastric mucosa with a rotation of 600 rounds/min delivered by a motor at the handle of the endoscope.

50. DONAHUE PE, CARVALHO PJPC, DAVIS PE, SHEN Y-JE, MIIDLA I,
• BOMBECK T, NYHUS LM: **Endoscopic Sclerosis of the Gastric Cardia for Prevention of Experimental Gastroesophageal Reflux.** *Gastrointest Endosc* 1990, **36**:253–256.

Over 300 injections of 5% sodium morrhuate were made into the gastric cardia of 14 dogs without evidence of perforation. Nevertheless, I think collagen injections are preferable if a choice is to be made.

51. BHASIN DK, NAGI B, KOCHHAR R, SINGH L, GUPTA NM,
• MEHTA SK: **Endoscopic Management of Chronic Organo-axonial Volvulus of the Stomach.** *Am J Gastroenterol* 1990, **85**:1486–1488.

Endoscopic rotation 180° counterclockwise worked in six out of seven cases of primary volvulus.

52. HASHIZUME M, KITANO S, YAMAGA H, KOYANAGI N, SUGIMACHI
• K: **Endoscopic Classification of Gastric Varices.** *Gastrointest Endosc* 1990, **36**:276–280.

One-fourth of the patients with gastric varices had had sclerotherapy for esophageal varices and another fourth had hepatoma.

53. SCHWARTZ AE, VANAGUNAS A, KAMEL PL: **Endoscopy to Evaluate**
• **Gastrointestinal Bleeding in Marathon Runners.** *Ann Intern Med* 1990, **113**:632–633.

In addition to erosive gastritis, ischemic colitis has also been identified in marathon runners.

Endoscopy of the small bowel and duodenum

A.J. Lobo and A.T.R. Axon

Gastroenterology Unit, The General Infirmary, Leeds, UK

Endoscopic visualization of the small bowel has resulted in publications in 1990 on gastrointestinal bleeding, small intestinal polyps and neoplasms, inflammatory bowel disease, enteral feeding, small-bowel involvement in systemic diseases, and a number of more esoteric case reports and small series.

Introduction

Most of the small bowel is inaccessible by conventional endoscopic techniques but, despite this, a number of interesting and varied contributions have been made to the field of small-bowel endoscopy. The problem of access to the more distal small bowel is a particular difficulty, but several authors, in different contexts, call for the more widespread application of those techniques that are available.

The recognition of upper gastrointestinal malignancy as a feature of the familial adenomatous polyposis syndrome is of considerable importance, and has therefore been included for discussion in this review, although the papers quoted were published in 1989.

Gastrointestinal bleeding

Perhaps the most common reason to seek endoscopic visualization of the small bowel, if it were widely available, would be in the diagnosis of gastrointestinal bleeding of unknown cause. There are patients in whom upper gastrointestinal endoscopy, colonoscopy and barium studies of the small bowel are negative. Approximately 5% of cases remain undiagnosed.

A number of endoscopic techniques have been described to improve the rate of diagnosis of bleeding small-bowel lesions. Vascular malformations are the major cause and may be difficult to diagnose on arteriography. The role of endoscopy is to make the diagnosis, localize lesions as accurately as possible, and, where possible, allow endoscopic treatment of bleeding lesions.

The main techniques under evaluation and in limited clinical use are push enteroscopy (in which an endoscope, usually a paediatric colonsocope, is passed orally and advanced into the proximal small bowel); peroperative enteroscopy (in which the small bowel is telescoped over an endoscope during laparotomy); and thirdly, the Sonde-type instrument (a long, narrow, flexible instrument with a balloon at the distal tip that is allowed to pass spontaneously through the small bowel; the intestine is visualized on withdrawal).

Push enteroscopy has been described using paediatric colonoscopes and also a modified instrument, as reported by Shimuzu *et al.* [1]. The first of these approaches is generally well tolerated but has the advantage of a short working length. The second requires special equipment, two endoscopists, radiographic screening and an overtube to prevent looping in the stomach.

Foutch *et al.* [2•] have described a technique that may be more generally applicable. It allows preoperative assessment and also the option of endoscopic therapy. The authors used a conventional 160 cm colonoscope, advanced by pushing, and using changes in the patient position to aid steering. This allowed passage of the instrument to 45–60 cm beyond the ligament of Treitz (taking, on average, 50 min). The authors found a cause for bleeding in the distal duodenum or proximal jejunum in 38% of their patients. Use of an overtube with this technique may allow deeper passage and therefore increase the diagnostic yield.

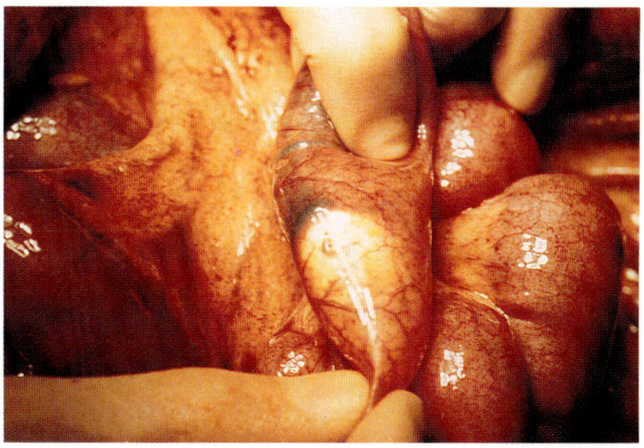

Fig. 1. Peroperative endoscopy demonstrating small intestinal vascular malformation, transilluminated and viewed from serosal aspect. By courstesy of Dr R.J. Dickinson, Hinchingbrooke Hospital, Huntingdon, UK.

Peroperative enteroscopy involves the passage of an endoscope into the small bowel by the oral or anal route. The tip of the endoscope is guided into the small intestine by the abdominal surgeon, who then telescopes the bowel over the endoscope 'like rolling a stocking over a golf-club' [3•]. The lumen is inspected by the endoscopist whilst the transilluminated serosal surface is in-

© Current Science Ltd ISBN 1-870485-32-7 ISSN 0952-6293

spected by the abdominal surgeon (Fig. 1). Care must be taken to avoid excess insufflation of air. The small bowel should be decompressed at the end of the procedure. Alternatively, a segmental approach can be employed, using a non-crushing intestinal clamp applied immediately distal to the length of bowel under inspection. It has been suggested that the combination of laparotomy and intraoperative enteroscopy or angiography should reduce the rate of undiagnosed gastrointestinal bleeding to below 5% [4].

Lesions in the small bowel are much harder to localize at surgery even if detected preoperatively, because the bowel is not anatomically fixed. The advantage of accurate localization of lesions and synchronous lesions is that it enables limited segmental resections of small bowel to be performed [5], thereby reducing the length of bowel removed. Lau [6•] has reviewed 9 years' experience of this procedure and lists the reasons for its use in gastrointestinal bleeding. In summary, these are to detect occult bleeding lesions, to localize lesions precisely, to confirm bleeding from these lesions, to help in deciding the appropriate length of gut resection, and as a first-line investigation when emergency intervention precludes a thorough preoperative work-up.

A different technique involves the Sonde-type enteroscope, which has been illustrated in a previous annual [7]. This can provide quite beautiful pictures of otherwise inaccessible bleeding lesions in the small bowel (Figs 2 and 3), and is clearly an important technical advance, but at present the instruments remain limited to a few centres and lack an instrument channel for therapeutic work.

Polyps and neoplasms

Familial adenomatous polyposis

Recent publications have highlighted the almost universal risk that patients with familial adenomatous polyposis have of developing gastroduodenal adenomatous polyps (Fig. 4) and dysplasia (Fig. 5). The distribution of these, especially concentrated around the ampulla, suggests that their occurrence is related to mucosal exposure to bile.

Spigelman *et al.* [8], from St Mark's Hospital, London, described 102 patients with familial adenomatous polyposis who underwent upper gastrointestinal endoscopy, and commented on the higher rate of duodenal dysplasia compared with gastric dysplasia. In their series, 100 out of 102 patients had duodenal abnormalities, usually in the second or third part of the duodenum, and the periampullary area showed dysplasia in 72 out of 97 patients.

Similar findings were reported in the USA by Gahtan *et al.* [9]. Both groups called for close surveillance of these patients by upper gastrointestinal endoscopy and biopsy. This should be performed with both an end-viewing gastroscope and a side-viewing duodenoscope, and the examination should extend into the third part of the duodenum. Gahtan's group make the further point that small lesions should be carefully monitored, but larger ones, especially when periampullary, require surgery.

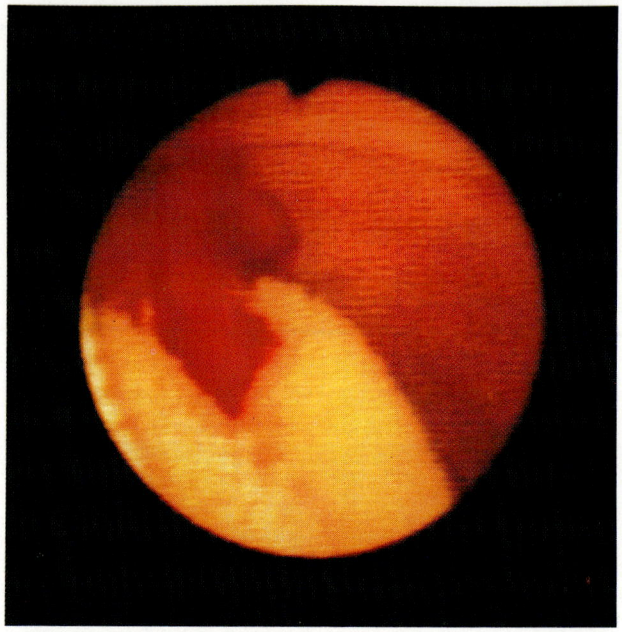

Fig. 2. Actively bleeding jejunal ulcer observed at enteroscopy with Sonde-type enteroscope. By courtesy of Dr J.F. Mackenzie, Royal Infirmary, Glasgow, UK.

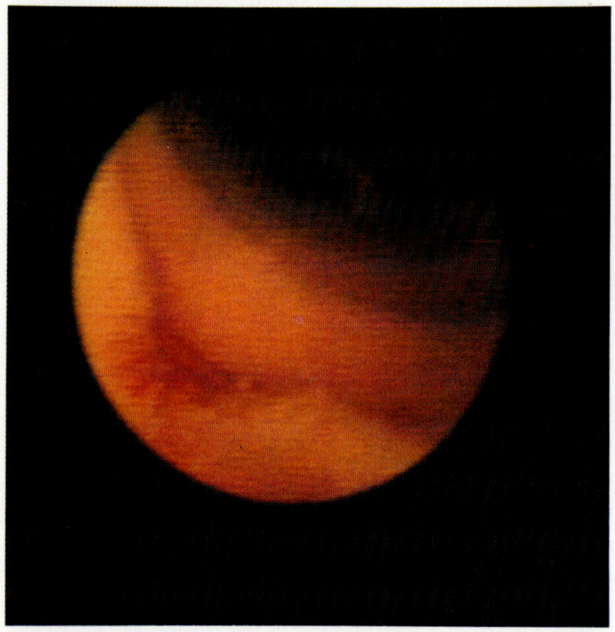

Fig. 3. Jejunal erosion seen at enteroscopy with Sonde-type enteroscope. By courtesy of Dr J.F. Mackenzie, Royal Infirmary, Glasgow, UK.

Careful histological examination of duodenal biopsies from patients with familial adenomatous polyposis has revealed that 98% of adenomas are of tubular type, and there is also a previously unrecognized endocrine hyperplasia associated with the adenomata [10].

Peutz–Jeghers syndrome

This syndrome, inherited as an autosomal dominant trait, comprises gastrointestinal hamartomatous polyps in association with mucocutaneous pigmentation. Problems arise as a result of intussusception, obstruction and bleeding. Regular laparotomy is therefore often necessary, and a number of authors have advocated peroperative endoscopy to reduce this relaparotomy rate.

Petroianu and Garcia de Carvalho [11] described a single case in which several polyps were snared via an endoscope. This was introduced through a jejunostomy, advanced retrogradely into the duodenum and then antegradely into the distal jejunum and ileum by rucking the small bowel over the endoscope.

The conventional method of detecting polyps at laparotomy is by palpation. Polyps are then removed via an enterotomy. Panos *et al.* [3•] described a single case (with the endoscope introduced perorally) to illustrate that palpation may be misleading, by missing polyps, or by incorrectly identifying the site of origin of a polyp because of a long stalk. This results in an enterotomy at a distance from the required site. Further, scars from previous enterotomies may be misconstrued as polyps and result in unnecessary enterotomies.

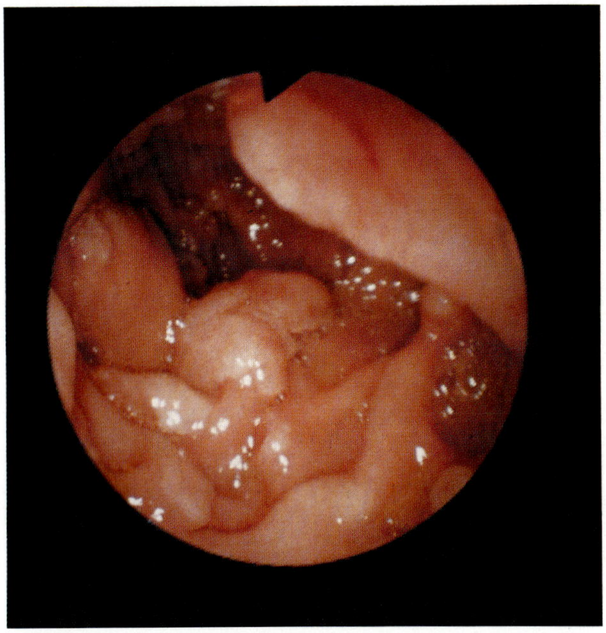

Fig. 4. Duodenal adenomatous polyps in a patient with polyposis coli. By courtesy of G.N.J Tytgat, Academic Medical Centre, Amsterdam, The Netherlands.

The vast St Mark's experience has also been used to collect a series of patients with this unusual condition [12••]. Again the message is that, at laparotomy, palpation, even with small-bowel transillumination, missed 38% of hamartomas. The majority of these were large enough to snare, illustrating the other advantage of peroperative enteroscopy: that polyps can be treated endoscopically, reducing the enterotomy rate as well as the subsequent relaparotomy rate.

Duodenal gastrinomas

Duodenal gastrinomas occur in 6–23% of patients with the Zollinger–Ellison syndrome. It is hoped that improved detection of small primary tumours, which may be frequently missed, will lead to an improvement in the cure rate for this condition.

Frucht *et al.* [13•] describe operative endoscopic transillumination in the diagnosis of duodenal gastrinomas. In their series, this technique had a higher sensitivity than both preoperative imaging (with upper gastrointestinal endoscopy, magnetic resonance imaging of the abdomen, abdominal computed tomography and ultrasound scans, and selective abdominal angiography) and intraoperative ultrasound and palpation. Gastrinomas show up as areas that fail to transilluminate and the sensitivity quoted refers to this finding rather than appearances through the endoscope.

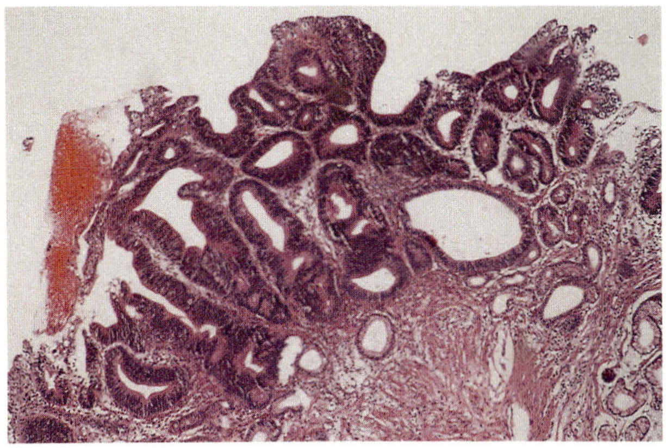

Fig. 5. Periampullary biopsy with microadenoma showing moderate dysplasia in a patient with familial adenomatous polyposis (haematoxylin and eosin stain). By courtesy of Dr P. Quirke, University Department of Pathology, Leeds General Infirmary, UK.

Occasionally, these tumours may be diagnosed by endoscopy and biopsy. One such tumour [14] was diagnosed by biopsy of a sessile, hemispheric, periampullary polyp, and although only six cases diagnosed at endoscopy had previously been described, the authors suggest that endoscopists are familiar with the appearance of this tumour. In the previous cases the tumours had a central depression, but it seems unlikely that this is characteristic.

Other neoplasms

Submucosal tumours of the terminal ileum are rare but three cases have been reported this year, all treated by endoscopic polypectomy [15,16]. Two cases were lipomas, which are most commonly seen in the colon, followed by the small bowel, and one of which was a lymphangioma. Whilst commending the skill of the endoscopists involved, it should be emphasized that great care must be taken in attempting to snare large, sessile, submucosal lesions.

A positive diagnosis of intestinal lipoma (wherever the site) is of value, in that observation or, if necessary, local excision or endoscopic removal is all that is required. Endoscopic clues to the diagnosis are the yellowish colour, the 'squeeze' sign (changes in contour and configuration as a result of peristalsis), the 'tenting' sign (easy retractability of mucosa overlying the lipoma), and the 'cushion' sign (sponge-like impression made when biopsy forceps pressed into the lipoma).

Computed tomography may help towards a positive diagnosis, and a homogeneous, unseptated lesion of low density is suggestive of lipoma [15].

Inflammatory bowel disease

Crohn's disease

The relationship between the endoscopic appearance of the mucosa (especially of the small bowel) and disease activity is often unclear. Assessment of disease activity in Crohn's disease is notoriously difficult. Both clinical indices and laboratory tests may be misleading.

There may be a discrepancy between improvement in symptoms and the appearance of the terminal ileum at colonoscopy [17•]. The authors of this paper noted that ileal erythema and aphthous ulceration persisted after treatment with systemic steroids despite significant improvement in a clinical index. Interestingly, these same endoscopic features do not appear to correlate with a global assessment of disease severity in the colon [18•].

However, retrograde ileoscopy and biopsy of the terminal ileum at the time of colonoscopy may be extremely useful in children with suspected Crohn's disease [19]. Comparing barium follow-through, ileoscopy and histological appearances, no single test was completely reliable in diagnosis, because of difficulty in obtaining optimal views and the patchy nature of the disease. Nevertheless, the combination of macroscopic appearances and biopsy result was completely accurate.

A valiant attempt has been made to develop an endoscopic index for assessing Crohn's disease [18•]. Although based on the appearance in Crohn's colitis, ileal appearances were included in the construction of the index. The study identified swollen mucosa and superficial and deep ulceration as correlating with an overall assessment of disease severity. However, no attempt was made to correlate the endoscopic appearance with the clinical Crohn's disease activity index.

Future advances in enteroscope technology will no doubt add further information about the small bowel mucosal appearances in Crohn's disease and their relationship to symptoms and laboratory indices of disease activity. New prototype enteroscopes are under evaluation [20], but have the limitations of unpredictable depth of insertion, restricted views and the inability to obtain biopsies.

Ulcerative colitis

It may seen perverse to discuss ulcerative colitis in a review of small-bowel endoscopy. However, the widespread use of an ileal pouch in the surgical treatment of patients with ulcerative colitis has led to the emergence of a fascinating complication, pouchitis, which may shed light on the pathogenesis of ulcerative colitis itself. Small-bowel epithelium in the pouch undergoes metaplasia to colonic type epithelium (Fig. 6), and this 'colon-ized' pouch becomes susceptible to recurrent inflammation almost identical to ulcerative colitis. Stasis in the pouch and bacterial overgrowth are likely contributory factors, but the complication is virtually unknown in those undergoing the same operation for familial adenomatous polyposis. The subject has been well reviewed by Madden *et al.* [21•], although more questions than answers remain.

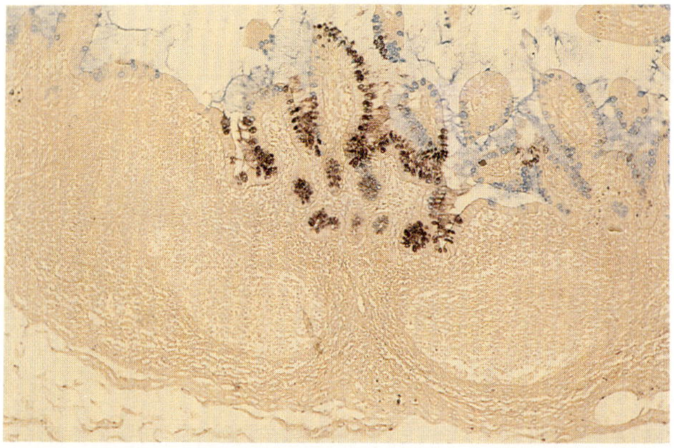

Fig. 6. Section from terminal ileum in a patient undergoing pan-proctocolectomy for ulcerative colitis, demonstrating metaplasia to colonic type epithelium. With this high iron diamine HIDL/Alcian blue stain, areas of colonic metaplasia show up as brown, and normal small bowel mucins appear blue. These changes are also commonly seen in ileal pouches constructed in patients with ulcerative colitis. By courtesy of Dr M.F. Dixon, University Department of Pathology, Leeds General Infirmary, UK.

The endoscopic appearances of pouchitis have been described as polymorphic [22], with congestion, petechiae, oozing areas, mucus hypersecretion, and multiple superficial ulcers being most common, but deeper, round or irregular ulcers also occur.

Coeliac disease

Biopsy of the distal duodenum may be useful in the diagnosis of coeliac disease. A number of patients undergo upper gastrointestinal endoscopy for the investigation of iron-deficiency anaemia. It should therefore be automatic to biopsy the second part of the duodenum, preferably with large or 'jumbo' biopsy forceps, when no other cause for anaemia is seen at endoscopy. This may lead to an unexpectedly high diagnostic yield of coeliac disease, usually in younger patients [23].

Jejunal feeding tubes

Percutaneous endoscopic jejunostomy

Percutaneous endoscopic gastrostomy for the positioning of a feeding tube is now so widely practised that, in the USA, it is said to be the second commonest indication for upper gastrointestinal endoscopy in hospitalized patients [24•].

One troublesome complication is aspiration of the feed, and percutaneous endoscopic jejunostomy may be preferable in such patients. Conversion of percutaneous endoscopic gastrostomy to percutaneous endoscopic jejunostomy has been shown to reduce the rate of aspiration, but a paper by DiSario *et al.* [25•] was less encouraging, reporting an aspiration rate of 67%. This was discussed in a detailed and informative editorial [24•], pointing out that adequate positioning of the jejunal tube beyond the ligament of Treitz is the most reliable way of reducing aspiration. The high rate of aspiration in DiSario's patients may have been due to a number of tubes placed in the duodenum.

(a)

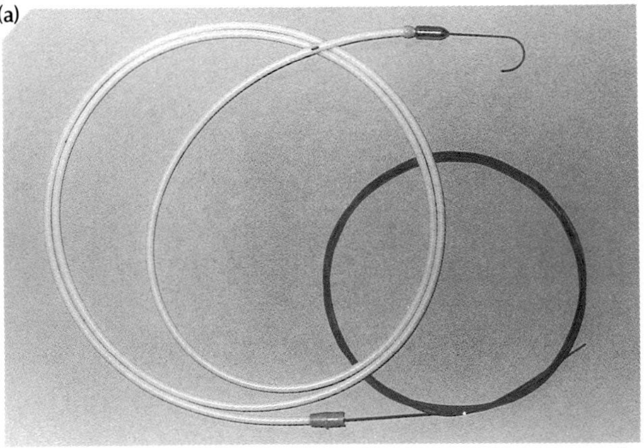

(b)

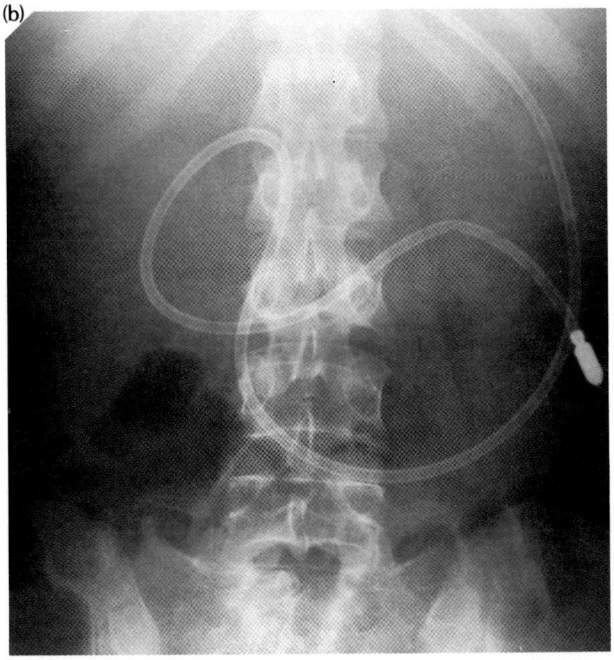

Fig. 7. Jejunal feeding tube (a) with a 'J' wire through its lumen and (b) in position with tip well beyond ligament of Treitz (plain abdominal radiograph). By courtesy of Dr Blair S. Lewis, Mount Sinai Medical Center, New York,USA.

Jejunal feeding tubes can be placed in three ways. First, a long feeding tube can be passed through a percutaneous endoscopic gastrostomy, and pulled down into the duodenum with a push enteroscope (an orally passed paediatric colonoscope). Second, direct percutaneous jejunostomy can be performed. Finally a jejunal tube can be passed over a previously positioned guidewire.

Lewis [26•] described a rapid Seldinger-based technique for placement of a jejunal tube by the oral route (Fig. 7). An endoscope (gastroscope or paediatric colonoscope) is advanced as far as possible into the small intestine. A 'J'-tip wire is advanced through the endoscope and thence into the small-bowel lumen and beyond the ligament of Treitz. The endoscope is slowly removed and the wire advanced under fluoroscopic control. The wire is then transferred from the patient's mouth to the nose by a short transfer tube similar to that used in the positioning of nasobiliary tubes. The feeding tube is passed over the taut wire. If looping occurs as the tube comes up against the pylorus, wire and tube can be advanced together until the pylorus is traversed.

Other topics

Non-steroidal anti-inflammatory drugs and the duodenum

The effect of non-steroidal anti-inflammatory drugs on the gastric and duodenal mucosa is well known, but the precise relevance of minor mucosal changes is not known. Objective assessment of such changes forms an important part of clinical trials assessing the adverse effects of individual drugs, or the beneficial effect of drugs designed to protect from or treat such damage. Most current assessments use a fixed-point scale such as that devised by Lanza [27], but a carefully evaluated visual analogue scale has been described [28•], which may reduce the sample size requirements in trials requiring endoscopic evaluation.

Whipple's disease

Upper gastrointestinal endoscopy extending into the duodenum may aid in the diagnosis of Whipple's disease. The typical endoscopic finding is of yellow-white plaques caused by villous distension with characteristic periodic acid schiff (PAS)-positive macrophages. Even in the absence of typical macroscopic appearances, all the duodenal biopsies (even from the bulb) in one series contained PAS-positive macrophages, suggesting that more distal biopsies are not necessary [29•]. Confusion may be caused by aquired immunodeficiency syndrome-associated *Mycobacterium. avium intracellulare* infection, small-bowel histoplasmosis and intestinal involvement in Waldenstrom's macroglobulinaemia, which may cause similar white-yellow plaques. In *M. avium intracellulare* infection, biopsies also show accumulation of large foamy cells, but these are PAS-negative.

Amyloidosis

Amyloid is frequently deposited in the gastrointestinal tract, and rectal biopsy is widely used in its diagnosis.

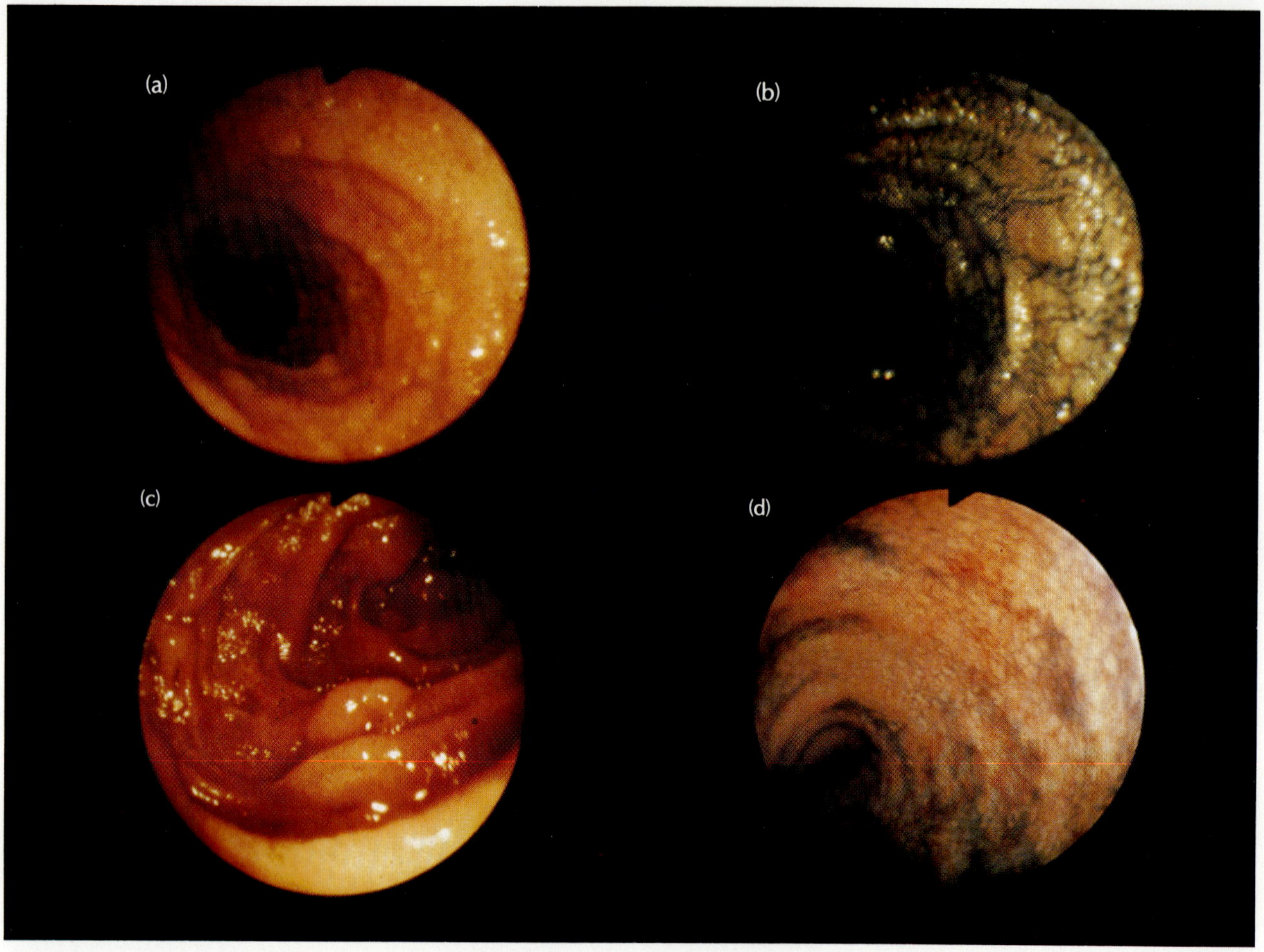

Fig. 8. Endoscopic appearances of amyloidosis affecting the second part of the duodenum. (a) Coarse mucosal appearance with multiple granules. (b) Granularity enhanced by dye-spray technique. (c) Multiple yellow-white protrusions. (d) Granular appearance in colon. By courtesy of Dr Shuji Tada, Fukuoka, Japan.

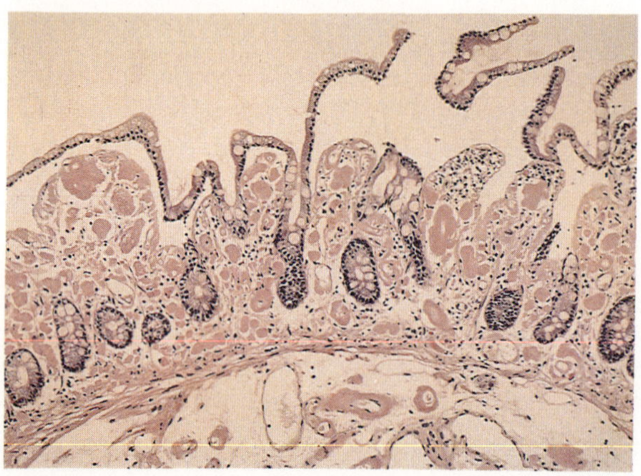

Fig. 9. Biopsy from second part of duodenum demonstrating marked amyloid deposition in the mucosa and submucosa (H&E, original magnification ×230). By courtesy of Dr Shuji Tada, Fukuoka, Japan.

The endoscopic appearance and biopsy findings of a Japanese group [30•] in a large series have been descried (Figs 8 and 9). Amyloid deposition in the duodenum was seen in all patients, compared with 95% of patients in the stomach, 72% in the oesophagus and 91% in the colorectum. This fits with the recognized post-mortem finding that amyloid deposition in the small bowel is more common than in the large bowel.

The most common endoscopic appearance in the duodenum was a fine granular appearance, most marked in the second part of the duodenum. Multiple polyps, erosions, ulceration and mucosal friability were also seen. The appearances at others sites were similar.

Functional lymphangiectasia of the duodenal mucosa

Intestinal lymphangiectasia may be primary and associated with malabsorption and protein loss, or secondary to a number of other small bowel conditions. The endoscopic appearances are of tiny white-tipped villi in the duodenum. Patel and DeRidder [31] have described a small series in which this abnormality was an incidental finding in patients being investigated for abdominal pain and who remained well over a mean period of 30 months. The implication from this study is that lymphangiectasia of the small bowel may therefore be asymptomatic and a chance finding in some patients, and is not always pathological.

Duodenal nodules

Duodenal nodules may occur in around 5% of patients undergoing upper gastrointestinal endoscopy [32]. Multiple nodules appear to be associated with peptic ulcer disease (26%) and chronic renal disease (8%). Single duodenal nodules are less common. A quarter of those that were biopsied in this series were neoplastic, the majority being malignant.

Hydrogen peroxide enteritis

Residual hydrogen peroxide in the water channel of gastroscopes and colonoscopes resulted in an outbreak of hydrogen peroxide colitis and enteritis at a renowned New York institution [33•]. The authors noted that on busy days, some patients 'had patches of absolute white mucosa extending over multiple mucosal crests and valleys, creating a scene reminiscent of new fallen snow in the mountains': the snow-white sign, in perhaps the most lyrical endoscopic description of the year.

References and recommended reading

Papers of special interest, published within the annual period of review, have been highlighted as:
- • Of interest
- •• Of outstanding interest

1. Shimuzu S, Tada M, Kawai K: **Development of a New Insertion Technique in Push-Type Enteroscopy.** *Am J Gastroenterol* 1987, **82**:844–847.

2. Foutch PG, Sawyer R, Sanowski RA: **Push-enteroscopy for**
• **Diagnosis of Patients with Gastrointestinal Bleeding of Obscure Origin.** *Gastrointest Endosc* 1990, **36**:337–341.
Use of a conventional adult colonoscope to visualize proximal small bowel. Potential for more widespread use of this technique compared with other ways of visualizing the small bowel.

3. Panos RG, Opelka FG, Nogueras JJ: **Peutz-Jeghers Syn-**
• **drome: A Call for Intraoperative Enteroscopy.** *Am Surg* 1990, **56**:331–333.
Case report of intraoperatic enteroscopy in this condition. A number of important lessons from a single case report.

4. Moncure AC, Tompkins RG, Athanasoulis CA, Welch CE: **Occult Gastrointestinal Bleeding: Newer Techniques and Diagnosis and Therapy.** *Adv Surg* 1989, **22**:141–147.

5. Lau WY, Wong SY, Yuen WK, Wong KK: **Intraoperative Enteroscopy for Bleeding Angiodysplasia of Small Intestine.** *Surg Gynecol Obstet* 1989, **168**:341–344.

6. Lau WY: **Intraoperative Enteroscopy — Indications and Lim-**
• **itations.** *Gastrointest Endosc* 1990, **36**:268–271.
Indication for intraoperative enteroscopy defined on the basis of 9 years' experience. The only limitations are in patients with adhesions or where extensive neoplasia obstructs passage or enteroscope.

7. Axon ATR: **Endoscopy of the Small Bowel and Duodenum.** In *Annual of Gastrointestinal Endoscopy* edited by Cotton PB, Tytgat GNJ, Williams CB. London: Current Science, 1989, pp 33–40.

8. Spigelman AD, Williams CB, Talbot IC, Domizio T, Phillips RKS: **Upper Gastrointestinal Cancer in Patients with Familial Adenomatous Polyposis.** *Lancet* 1989, ii:783–785.

9. Gahtan V, Nochomovitz LE, Robinson AM, Garcia VF, Smith LE: **Gastroduodenal Polyps in Familial Polyposis Coli.** *Am Surg* 1989, **55**:278–280.

10. Mogensen AM, Bulow S, Hage E: **Duodenal Adenomas in Familial Adenomatous Polyposis: Their Structure and Cellular Composition with Particular Reference to Endocrine Hyperplasia.** *Virchows Arch [A]* 1989, **414**:315–319.

11. Petroianu A, Garcia de Carvalho D: **Peroperative Endoscopy in Peutz-Jeghers Syndrome.** *Lancet* 1989, ii:1403.

12. Spigelman AD, Thomson JP, Phillips RK: **Towards Decreasing**
•• **the Relaparotomy Rate in the Peutz–Jeghers Syndrome: the Role of Peroperative Small Bowel Endoscopy.** *Br J Surg* 1990, **77**:301–302.
A large series of an unusual condition used to illustrate an important message. Peroperative endoscopy has the potential to reduce the relaparotomy rate for Peutz–Jeghers syndrome.

13. Frucht H, Norton JA, London JF, *et al.*: **Detection of**
• **Duodenal Gastrinomas by Operative Endoscopic Transillumination.** *Gastroenterology* 1990, **99**:1622–1627.
Well illustrated series. Detection of small duodenal gastrinomas should increase the cure rate for these patients, and the technique described seems the most sensitive at present.

14. Rolny P, Ekman R, Sjolund K, Wickbom G, Ohrn PG: **Endoscopic Diagnosis and Treatment of Duodenal Gastrinoma.** *Gastrointest Endosc* 1990, **36**:511–513.

15. Kang JY, Chan-Wilde C, Wee A, Chew R, Ti TK: **Role of Computed Tomography and Endoscopy in the Management of Alimentary Tract Lipomas.** *Gut* 1990, **31**:550–553.

16. Matsumoto T, Lida M, Matsui T, *et al.*: **Submucosal Tumours of the Terminal Ileum Managed by Endoscopic Polypectomy.** *Gastrointest Endosc* 1990, **36**:505–508.

17. Olaison G, Sjodhl R, Tagesson C: **Glucocorticoid Treatment**
• **in Ileal Crohn's Disease: Relief of Symptoms but not of Endoscopically Viewed Inflammation.** *Gut* 1990, **31**:325–328.
Interesting observation that colonic appearances may improve on steroids, but ileal changes may not. The relationship between mucosal appearances and symptoms is still uncertain.

18. Group d'Etudes Therapeutiques des Affections Inflamma-
• toires du Tube Digestif (GETAID) presented by Mary JY, Modigliani R: **Development and Validation of an Endoscopic Index of the Severity for Crohn's Disease: a Prospective Multicentre Study.** *Gut* 1989, **30**:983–989.
This group has undertaken the difficult task of standardizing endoscopic appearances and then attempting to correlate them with disease severity. The index requires a period of training before it can be accurately used and may be too cumbersome for widespread clinical use. Nevertheless, useful data are presented and attempts to tackle this problem should be welcomed.

19. Lipson A, Bartram CI, Williams CB, Slavin G, Walker-Smith J: **Barium Studies and Ileoscopy Compared in Children with Suspected Crohn's Disease.** *Clin Radiol* 1990, **41**:5–8.

20. Bozdech JM, Farmer RG: **Diagnosis of Crohn's Disease.** *Hepatogastroenterol* 1990, **37**:8–17.

21. Madden MV, Farthing MJG, Nicholls RJ: **Inflammation in**
• **Ileal Reservoirs: 'Pouchitis'.** *Gut* 1990, **31**:247–249.
Timely review of a fascinating subject. Definition, prevalence, aetiology, pathology and treatment are discussed.

22. Di Febo G, Miglioli M, Lauri A, *et al.*: **Endoscopic Assessment of Acute Inflammation of the Ileal Reservoir after Restorative Ileo-anal Anastomosis.** *Gastrointest Endosc* 1990, **36**:6–9.

23. Dumas O, Etaix JP, Barthelemy C, Boucheron S, Audigier JC: **Intérêt des Biopsies Duodénales Endoscopiques System-**

atiques lors d'un Bilan d'Ánemie Isolée [letter]. *Gastroenterol Clin Biol* 1989, 13:944.

24. Lewis BS: **Perform PEJ, not PED [editorial].** *Gastrointest Endosc* 1990, 36:311–312.
• Practical and informative comments on the use and placement of jejunal feeding tubes.

25. DiSario JA, Foutch PG, Sanowski RA: **Poor Results with Percutaneous Endoscopic Jejunostomy.** *Gastrointest Endosc* 1990, 36:257–260.
• Note of caution on the use of percutaneous endoscopic jejunostomy, which seems otherwise to be a useful alternative when percutaneous endoscopic gastrostomy is complicated by aspiration.

26. Lewis BS: **The Rapid Placement of Jejunal Feeding Tubes: the Seldinger Technique Applied to the Gut.** *Gastrointest Endosc* 1990, 36:139–141.
• An alternative jejunal feeding tube that is appealingly simple and non-invasive.

27. Lanza FL: **Endoscopic Studies of Gastric and Duodenal Injury After the Use of Ibuprofen, Aspirin, and Other Non-steroidal Anti-inflammatory Agents.** *Am J Med* 1984, 77:19–24.

28. Aabakken L, Larsen S, Osnes M: **Visual Analogue Scales for Endoscopic Evaluation of Nonsteroidal Anti-inflammatory Drug-induced Mucosal Damage in the Stomach and Duodenum.** *Scand J Gastroenterol* 1990, 25:443–448.
• Important contribution to the area of gastric and mucosal damage by non-steroidal anti-inflammatory drugs. These scales should be useful in drug trials, looking at both the non-steroidal anti-inflammatory drugs and the protective effects of other drugs.

29. Geboes K, Ectors N, Heidbuchel H, Rutgeerts P, Desmet V, Vantrappen G: **Whipple's Disease: Endoscopic Aspects Before and After Therapy.** *Gastrointest Endosc* 1990, 36:247–251.
• Interesting account of endoscopy in Whipple's disease. Biopsies from the second part of the duodenum are likely to be adequate in the diagnosis of this disease.

30. Tada S, Lida M, Iwashita A, *et al.*: **Endoscopic and Biopsy Findings of the Upper Digestive Tract in Patients with Amyloidosis.** *Gastrointest Endosc* 1990, 36:10–14.
• Delightfully illustrated account of endoscopy in amyloidosis. Endoscopy and biopsy are used to demonstrate that the duodenum is the commonest site of amyloid deposition in the gastrointestinal tract.

31. Patel AS, DeRidder PH: **Endoscopic Appearance and Significance of Functional Lymphangiectasia of the Duodenal Mucosa.** *Gastrointest Endosc* 1990, 36:376–378.

32. Fernandez-Melone JH, Triadafilopoulos G, Chandler JG: **Nodular Duodenitis and Single Duodenal Nodules.** *Am Surg* 1990, 56:175–177.

33. Bilotta JJ, Waye JD: **Hydrogen Peroxide Enteritis: the 'Snow White' Sign.** *Gastrointest Endosc* 1989, 35:428–430.
• Graphic description of a very unusual complication of endoscopy.

Endoscopy of upper gastrointestinal bleeding

B.H. Laurence

Gastroenterology/Liver Unit, Sir Charles Gairdner Hospital, Perth, Western Australia

Support for therapeutic endoscopy in both variceal and non-variceal bleeding continues to grow, particularly for the high-risk cirrhotic or the sick, elderly patient with an ulcer.

Introduction

Endoscopy maintained its pre-eminent place in the management of upper gastrointestinal bleeding in 1990, and the literature again focused mainly on its therapeutic potential. The need for early recognition and endoscopic treatment of the high-risk ulcer patient with a high-risk lesion was further emphasized. The best haemostatic method — electrothermal or chemical sclerosis — is still to be decided. Rebleeding remains a problem and, when this occurs, there is growing support for repeated endoscopic therapy. A method for reliably determining the effectiveness of endoscopic treatment is required; an early, 'second look' endoscopy has been suggested and, it is hoped, developments in Doppler ultrasound may be able to indicate whether the vessel in an ulcer base has been adequately occluded.

Sclerotherapy remains the treatment of choice for the emergency control of variceal bleeding, even if the results of its long-term use are less than ideal. As the literature suggests, there is a need to re-examine how the technique is deployed and to explore new strategies in its use combined with drug therapy and surgery. Substantial advantages from modifications in the basic technique or application of new methods, such as variceal ligation, remain to be demonstrated.

Variceal bleeding

Few comprehensive reviews were published on variceal haemorrhage in 1990. That of Salena and Sivak [1•] is devoted to the role of endoscopic therapy. They critically examine the evidence for emergency, selective and prophylactic variceal sclerosis and are in favour of the first two but not the last.

In another review [2•] Grace, a hepatologist, gives his personal approach to the management of variceal bleeding based on a consideration of the published trials. One-third of patients with cirrhosis and portal hypertension face the risk of bleeding from varices; once this occurs there is a 70% chance of rebleeding with a mortality of up to 50%. Although non-selective β-adrenergic blocking drugs (propranolol and nadolol) significantly reduce the chance of an initial variceal bleed, Grace advocates caution in their widespread use because of their side effects, the unknown duration of treatment and potential problems with medication compliance. For a patient with a minor variceal bleed, he recommends a combination of vasopressin and nitroglycerin with sclerotherapy (using any of the common sclerosants) reserved for major haemorrhage. If these measures fail, staple transection of the oesophagus rather than a porto-systemic shunt is indicated. To prevent recurrent variceal bleeding in patients with good liver function (Child's class A and B), the author feels that there is sufficient evidence to support the long-term use of β-blocking drugs. In poor-risk (Child's class C) patients with alcoholic cirrhosis, the varices should be eradicated by repeated sclerotherapy.

Endoscopic diagnosis

Oesophageal varices, erosive gastritis and peptic ulceration are all important causes of gastrointestinal bleeding in patients with alcoholic cirrhosis. The prevalence of these conditions in patients with non-bleeding alcoholic cirrhosis or other types of cirrhosis is uncertain. Rabinovitz *et al.* [3•] carried out a prospective study on the presence of these and other endoscopic findings in 510 individuals with cirrhosis of varying causes. Oesophagitis occurred in 4.9% of the entire group, oesophageal varices in 82.7%, gastric varices in 7.8%, gastritis (gastropathy) in 42.7%, gastric ulcer in 3.7%, duodenitis in 12.7% and duodenal ulcer in 5%. Oesophagitis and gastric ulceration were significantly more frequent in patients with alcoholic cirrhosis than in those with other forms of non-viral cirrhosis. The prevalence of gastritis was significantly greater in patients with parenchymal liver disease than in those with cholestatic liver disease (49.8% compared with 30.9%). The reason for these differences was not apparent.

Large varices, and those with overlying cherry-red spots (Fig. 2; see also Fig. 1), are more likely to bleed. These features are being used more frequently to select patients for prophylactic treatment and it is therefore essential that they can be accurately and reliably identified. Cales *et al.* [4•], in a prospective study of the endoscopic features of portal hypertension in 100 consecutive cirrhotic patients, have examined the level of observer variability, the intra-association between these features and their relationship to the severity of hepatic dysfunction. The endoscopic findings were recorded on video tape and independently reviewed by four experienced endoscopists according to an agreed classification of the relevant signs: size, extent, colour and red signs of oesophageal varices,

© Current Science Ltd ISBN 1-870485-32-7 ISSN 0952-6293

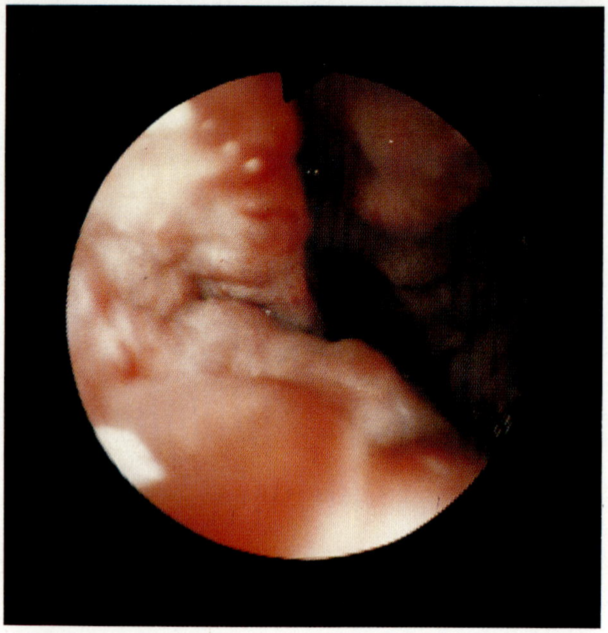

Fig. 1. Very pronounced varices with surface red dots. By courtesy of G.N.J Tytgat, Academic Medical Centre, Amsterdam, The Netherlands.

Fundamental colour	
Blue	
Red	Colour
	Red-wale marking
	Cherry-red spot
	Haematocystic spot

Fig. 2. High-risk varices according to the Japanese Research Society for Portal Hypertension [74].

the mosaic pattern, congestive gastropathy, fundal varices and associated gastric lesions. The level of agreement was evaluated by κ statistics. Good agreement was noted between the observers (κ index between 0.75 and 0.4) on variceal size (grade 0–3), the presence of a red sign, the severity of gastropathy and the presence of other gastric lesions. These findings, in relation to variceal size and red signs, are in accordance with those of the Italian Liver Cirrhosis Project [5]. The size of the varices was significantly associated with both their extent and the presence of a red sign, and a direct correlation was found between increasing variceal size and deteriorating hepatic function. The gastric pattern appeared not to be related to either the oesophageal features or the level of hepatic dysfunction.

Another study on observer variability in the diagnosis of varices and their size has been carried out by Bendtsen *et al.* [6•]. The video-taped endoscopic findings in 28 patients with cirrhosis were shown to 22 endoscopists, who graded variceal size on a scale from 0 to 3. Overall agreement on the presence of varices (grade 0 versus grades 1–3) was 70%. There was good agreement in discriminating between small (grades 0–1) and large varices (grades 2–3), with a κ value of 0.52 — a result similar to that found by Cales *et al.* [4•]. The extent of previous endoscopic experience did not seem significantly to affect the degree of observer variation. However, the overall level of disagreement between the endoscopists highlighted the importance of standardizing observations for any trial based on variceal size. Video-taped documentation of findings under equivalent conditions and review by the same panel of expert observers is probably essential for such trials.

	Rebleeding		
Authors	Sclerotherapy (%)	Control (%)	*P* value
Terblanche *et al.* [75]	58	77	<0.10
Westaby *et al.* [76]	56	82	<0.01
Korula *et al.* [77]	50	80	<0.10
Copenhage Esophageal Varices Sclerosis Project [78]	48	54	>0.10
Soderlund *et al.* [79]	56	66	>0.10

Fig. 3. Results of five controlled trials of long-term injection sclerotherapy Published by permission [76].

Sclerotherapy

The current status of sclerotherapy for variceal bleeding has been reviewed by Westaby and Williams [7••]. Endoscopic sclerosis of oesophageal varices is of value both in stopping bleeding and in preventing its recurrence. Immediate sclerotherapy for active bleeding is feasible at the time of the initial endoscopy and has a high success rate (90%). It results in significantly better control of bleeding and a lower incidence of rebleeding than the use of balloon tamponade or the administration of vasopressin and nitroglycerin. If this approach is not possible because of inadequate access to the bleeding varix, initial control of bleeding by tamponade with delayed sclerotherapy is also highly successful. Gastric varices along the lesser curve can usually be managed by sclerotherapy but the results for treating fundal varices by this method are poor. Repeated injections of sclerosant until the varices are obliterated significantly reduce the number of rebleeding episodes and prolongs survival (Fig. 3). Nevertheless, with this approach there is still a high incidence of rebleeding and further trials are necessary to define the most appropriate use of this technique. Bleeding from sclerotherapy-induced mucosal ulceration may account for 40% of rebleeding episodes (Fig. 4). The authors recommend that this be reduced by the administration of sucralfate. As almost 50% of patients with cirrhosis die from their initial variceal bleed, prevention by sclerotherapy seems attractive. However, recent trials have failed to show any significant benefit from prophylactic sclerotherapy and the authors conclude that this is no longer justified.

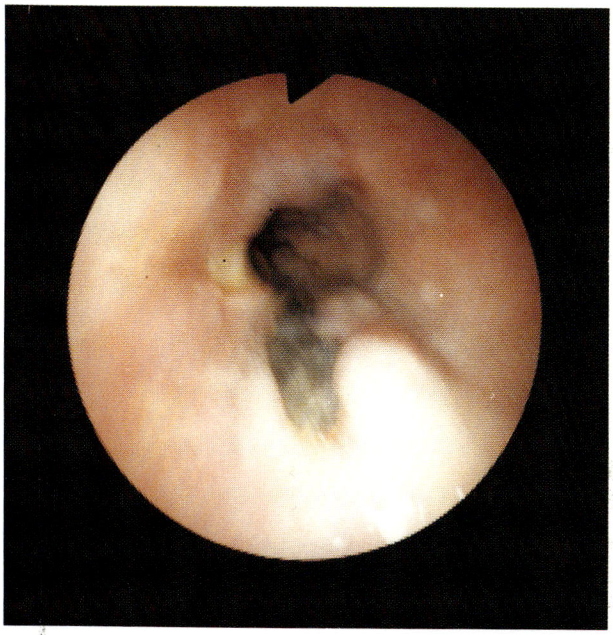

Fig. 4. Post-sclerotherapy ulceration. By courtesy of G.N.J Tytgat, Academic Medical Centre, Amsterdam, The Netherlands.

Agent	
Sodium morrhuate	Cefazolin
Sodium tetradecyl sulphate	Linoleic acid
Ethanolamine oleate	Urea
Polidocanol	Sterile paraffin
Hypertonic glucose	Phenol-almond oil
Ethanol	Guinine
Thrombin (bovine)	Bucrylate (tissue glue)

Fig. 5. Agents used in variceal sclerosis [1].

Terblanche [8•], in a recent review, also supports the immediate use of sclerotherapy for varices which are actively bleeding or have stopped bleeding at the time of the initial endoscopy; using this approach, his group successfully controlled bleeding in 90–95% of cases. When bleeding continues or recurs soon after immediate sclerotherapy, or after the administration of vasopressin with sublingual nitroglycerin, balloon tamponade should be instituted. This situation carries a very high mortality in poor-risk patients (Child's class C) and consideration should be given to immediate surgical rescue. Long-term management with repeated sclerotherapy can eradicate varices and reduce the risk of rebleeding. Patients in whom this is unsuccessful should be identified early and treated surgically by a porto-systemic shunt, a transection and devascularization procedure, or, where appropriate, liver transplantation.

Which sclerosant?

Although variceal sclerosis has been in wide use for a decade, the choice of sclerosant (Fig. 5) is still largely determined by personal preference and availability rather than any detailed data on its efficacy and safety. In a comprehensive review, Sarin *et al.* [9••] examined the chemistry of sclerosants, the mechanism of their action and the results of the experimental and clinical studies on each agent. As they pointed out, the results of these studies have often been conflicting and there is a pressing need to identify the ideal sclerosant — with high thrombogenic activity and minimal necrotic effects.

Kochhar *et al.* [10•] have compared three sclerosants — 5% ethanolamine oleate, 3% sodium tetradecyl sulphate and absolute alcohol — in a randomized trial involving 64 patients with both cirrhotic and non-cirrhotic portal hypertension. Between one and three injections of the sclerosant, in 1–2 ml amounts, were made into the varices at sites 2 cm apart; this was repeated at 3-weekly intervals until the varices were obliterated. The success rate (variceal obliteration or ≥ 50% downgrading of the variceal score) was similar for each agent: ethanolamine 86.4%, sodium tetradecyl sulphate 73.7%, absolute alcohol 82.6%. There was no significant difference in the complication rates: 18–22% for ulceration, 16–18% for strictures, 16–23% for rebleeding. Significantly smaller volumes of alcohol were used in significantly fewer treatment sessions to achieve variceal eradication (4.8 compared with 10.1 for ethanolamine, 9.2 for sodium tetradecyl sulphate). These results suggest that absolute alcohol is more effective than the other two agents in inducing vascular sclerosis, a view supported by Sarin *et al.* [11]. Comparative information on other sclerosants is limited [12–14] (Fig. 6) and further studies involving both intravariceal and paravariceal injections are required.

Emergency sclerotherapy

A comparison between emergency and delayed sclerotherapy in bleeding varices has been reported by Shemesh *et al.* [15•]. One hundred and thirty-four patients, 90% of whom had portal hypertension secondary to non-alcoholic cirrhosis, were studied. Emergency sclerotherapy was carried out with both intravariceal and paravariceal injections of ethanolamine within 6 h of presentation and active bleeding was controlled in all 43 patients. In 41 patients, initial treatment consisted of tamponade, vasopressin and transfusion, with sclerotherapy being delayed for 24–48 h after admission. Rebleeding during the index admission occurred less frequently in the patients treated with emergency sclerotherapy (4.7 compared with 17.1%). Although sclerotherapy was repeated in both groups until the varices were obliterated, a lower mortality rate was seen in the group undergoing emergency therapy (9.3 compared with 14.6%). The only significant difference between the groups, however, was a lower rebleeding rate within the first 12 months in those undergoing emergency sclerosis. This was attributed to the use of larger volumes of sclerosant (26 compared with 13 ml) at the initial procedure.

Authors (year)	Sclerosant (%)	Schedule (weeks)	Success (%)	Time to varix obliteration (weeks)	Rebleeding (%)	Ulceration (%)
Kitano [12] (1987)	Polidocanol (1%)	1	80	5.4	8	44
	Ethanolamine (5%)	1	100	4.7	nil	nil
Kitano [14] (1988)	STD (2%)	1	75	4.4	24	43
	Ethanolamine (5%)	1	100	4.9	nil	9
Sarin [73] (1987)	Alcohol (50%)	3	54	20.1	28	10
	Alcohol (100%)	3	93	14.3	21	13
Sarin [11] (1988)	Ethanolamine (5%)	3	40	22.3	30	13
	Alcohol (100%)	3	100	12.9	21	16
Kochhar [10] (1990)	Alcohol (10%)	3	82.6	4.8 Sessn	17.4	21.7
	Ethanolamine (5%)	3	86.4	10.1 Sessn	22.7	18.2
	STD (3%)	3	73.7	9.2 Sessn	15.8	21.0

Fig. 6. Randomized trials comparing different sclerosants (modified from Sarin *et al.* [9]).

Beta adrenergic blocking drugs and sclerotherapy

The role of β-adrenergic blockade in the overall management of variceal bleeding continues to be debated and researched. Westaby *et al.* [16••] recently reported the results of a randomized trial comparing oral propranolol with sclerotherapy in a group of 108 patients whose varices had stopped bleeding spontaneously before the initial endoscopy. Propranolol was administered in a dose sufficient to reduce the resting pulse rate by 25%. Sclerotherapy was carried out at weekly intervals until the varices were obliterated. Rebleeding in the sclerotherapy group was managed by repeat variceal sclerosis. Patients who rebled in the propranolol group, if still bleeding at endoscopy, had a single sclerotherapy treatment; if bleeding had ceased, propranolol was continued. Follow-up ranged from 12 to 64 months. In the propranolol group, 28 out of 52 (54%) patients rebled compared with 25 out of 56 (45%) patients in the sclerotherapy group. On an intention-to-treat basis there was no significant difference in the risk of bleeding per patient month of follow-up (0.05 and 0.037, respectively); survival in both groups was similar. Patients taking propranolol who had a high pretreatment pulse rate (>90 beats/min) or a reduction in pulse rate of less than 25% on medication were significantly more likely to rebleed. This study supports the use of propranolol as an alternative to chronic sclerotherapy providing the patient has an adequate pulse response to the drug.

Jensen and Krarup [17] demonstrated a significant reduction in rebleeding in patients undergoing sclerotherapy and taking propranolol up to the time of variceal eradication. Conversely, Bertoni *et al.* [18•], in a study using nadolol rather than propranolol, were unable to confirm any benefit from this combined approach. Patients were randomly allocated at the time of the initial variceal injection to having sclerotherapy either alone or with nadolol; one-third were excluded from the trial because of the possibility of β blockade aggravating a pre-existing condition. No significant difference occurred in the outcome of the two groups, particularly with respect to rebleeding or mortality. Although this finding is in keeping with the experience of others [19], the relevance of the study is uncertain because of the small number of trial patients (28) and the inclusion in the final analysis of four patients who had ceased taking nadolol because of side effects.

In a recent paper, Jensen and Krarup [20•] extended their previous observations on the early benefits of combining sclerotherapy and propranolol to include their long-term results. Propranolol was given for the first 6 months and, in both the drug-treated and control groups, sclero-
therapy was repeated until the varices were eradicated (a mean period of 5 months). In the 18-month period after eradication, recurrence of varices in patients having combined therapy was significantly reduced compared with the rate in those having sclerotherapy alone (2 compared with 73%); of the patients in whom varices recurred, 69% rebled.

The apparent clinical benefit of combined sclerotherapy and propranolol is supported by the study of Okano *et al.* [21•] on changes in variceal blood flow in cirrhosis. A laser Doppler velocimeter was used endoscopically to measure blood flow in varices before and after sclerosis (50% glucose, thrombin and Aethoxyskerol) and after the administration of propranolol alone or in combination with sclerosis. The Doppler flow signal fell significantly after variceal sclerosis from 6.86 to 2.41 V, an effect which lasted about 1 month. Variceal blood flow decreased by 30% after oral propranolol but fell by 80% when propranolol was combined with sclerotherapy.

Complications

Septicaemia and peritonitis

Bacteriaemia after endoscopic variceal sclerosis is well documented, occurring in up to 50% of patients [22,23]. In most instances, it is transient and clinically insignificant. Serious sepsis such as infective endocarditis or brain abscess can result, however [24,25]. Recent reports have incriminated sclerotherapy in causing bacterial peritonitis and both meningococcal and *Streptococcus pneumoniae* septicaemia.

Tam *et al.* [26•] examined the ascitic fluid in 11 patients with cirrhosis and upper gastrointestinal bleeding before and after emergency endoscopy with or without sclerotherapy. Three of the five patients undergoing variceal sclerosis initially had no laboratory evidence of bacterial peritonitis but developed clinical signs of sepsis between 9 and 48 h after the procedure; each had an increase in the ascitic white cell count characteristic of bacterial peritonitis and organisms — *Enterococcus* and *Staphylococcus aureus* — were cultured from the fluid in two patients. Post-sclerotherapy oesophageal ulceration was considered to be the possible source of infection in one of the patients. Bacterial peritonitis did not develop in any of the patients undergoing upper gastrointestinal endoscopy alone. Although the authors do not recommend the use of prophylactic antibiotics, they suggest that the ascitic fluid should be examined routinely after sclerotherapy.

Another case of post-sclerotherapy peritonitis and septicaemia has been reported in a letter by Van Zaanen *et al.* [27•]. A 51-year-old man with alcoholic cirrhosis and portal hypertension became febrile and hypotensive 30 h after variceal injection. *Diplococci* were demonstrated in the ascitic fluid and *Neisseria meningitidis* was cultured from the blood. The infection responded rapidly to antibiotics.

Aguado *et al.* [28•] also described a case of septicaemia with symptoms occurring 10 h after emergency sclerotherapy. The patient with cirrhosis (and an intact spleen) developed a high fever and chills and *Streptococcus pneumoniae* was cultured from the blood; unfortunately no pharyngeal cultures were taken. Clearly patients undergoing sclerotherapy as a day-case procedure should be made aware of the possibility of delayed fever and its implications.

Normal oropharyngeal flora such as α haemolytic *Streptococci* are the most common isolates in post-sclerotherapy bacteriaemia. Contamination of the endoscope with these organisms during its insertion is almost impossible to prevent. Antibiotic prophylaxis is obviously indicated immediately before and after the procedure in patients with congenital or valvular heart disease or known immunodeficiency. Flick [29•] has also drawn attention to the increased risk of infection in children undergoing sclerotherapy for extrahepatic portal hypertension who have had a previous splenectomy.

Pericarditis

Retrosternal pain is a common and usually short-lived complication of variceal sclerosis. When severe pain persists, oesophageal perforation, mediastinitis or pleurisy must be excluded. Rarely, it can also indicate the presence of pericarditis, as a recent report by Caletti *et al.* [30•] emphasizes. The two patients developed persistent chest pain and fever within 3 days of intravariceal injections of standard volumes of 5% ethanolamine; both had a pericardial friction rub with electrocardiographic and echocardiographic evidence of pericarditis with a small pericardial effusion. Both settled with conservative management and no signs of pericardial disease had appeared 16 months later. Five other cases of pericarditis after sclerotherapy have been described [31–33]. Review of all these cases fails to demonstrate any correlation between the development of clinical pericarditis and the number of sclerotherapy sessions, the nature or volume of sclerosant or the length of needle used.

Portal thrombosis

Extensive thrombosis of the portal venous system after endoscopic variceal sclerosis is rare and usually fatal. Terada *et al.* [34•] reported the twelfth recorded case of this occurrence in a 60-year-old woman with cirrhosis undergoing prophylactic sclerotherapy with standard volumes of intravariceal ethanolamine. The patient developed severe abdominal pain shortly after the fourth course of injections and died of hepatic failure and massive gastrointestinal bleeding 10 days later; autopsy revealed occlusion of the portal vein and its tributaries, with red thrombi and haemorrhagic infarction of the small bowel. If thrombolytic therapy is to have any chance of success, the possibility of this complication must be considered early in any patient developing severe abdominal pain and rapid deterioration of liver function after sclerotherapy.

Oesophageal ulceration

Superficial mucosal ulceration is almost universal after sclerosis of oesophageal varices, but, unlike deep ulceration, it usually heals rapidly without the need for specific treatment. Singal *et al.* [35•] evaluated the symptoms associated with this ulceration in a prospective study of 40 patients who had intravariceal injections of absolute alcohol (0.5–2 ml). All the patients were found to have mucosal ulceration when examined the day after sclerotherapy, but only two-thirds were symptomatic, with mild dysphagia (53%), mild to moderate retrosternal pain (28%) and low-grade fever (15%). The dysphagia and chest pain usually improved rapidly and had resolved within 3–4 days — even though in most patients ulcer healing took several days or weeks. The size of the ulcers was directly related to the volumes of alcohol injected and patients with the largest ulcers (> 1 cm in diameter) were more likely to be symptomatic. The ulcers healed significantly more slowly in patients with a low serum albumin (< 3 g/dl), this being attributed to poor nutritional status.

Madonia *et al.* [36•] have also shown that deep ulceration after variceal sclerosis is related to the volume of sclerosant used. Forty patients were re-examined endoscopically 1 week after sclerotherapy with sodium tetradecyl sulphate or if they rebled. Six patients (15%) who developed deep ulcers had been injected with significantly more sodium tetradecyl sulphate than those with shallow ulceration (12.8 compared with 9.3 ml). The incidence of deep ulceration was also increased by the use of balloon tamponade.

These two studies beg the question of the optimal volume of sclerosant that should be used. Sarin *et al.* [37,38] consider the appearance of a circumscribed area of whitening around the needle — 'blanching' — as the end point for intravariceal injections of alcohol or ethanolamine. The minimum effective volume probably depends not only on the potency of the sclerosing agent but also on factors such as variceal size and blood flow that would determine the concentration of the agent in the varix and the endothelial contact time. There is certainly room for more work in understanding the action of sclerosants.

Oesophageal carcinoma

Dysphagia is a not-uncommon symptom after variceal sclerosis. That this is not always due to a motility disturbance or a benign oesophageal stricture [39,40] is highlighted in a report by Kokudo *et al.* [41•]. Two males (47 and 52 years old) developed dysphagia due to squamous cell carcinoma of the oesophagus 2 years after sclerotherapy (with 5% sodium morrhuate paravariceally in one and 5% ethanolamine intravariceally in the other). Both tumours occurred in the lower one-third of the oesophagus, extending almost to the oesophagogastric junction. One patient died after resection, the other 1 year after chemotherapy. Although the association between variceal sclerosis and subsequent development of oesophageal carcinoma is likely to be fortuitous, a causal relationship must be considered. Six other cases have been reported and are reviewed by the authors. There seems to be no consistent association with the type or volume of sclerosant, the site of the tumours or the interval between sclerotherapy and onset of dysphagia.

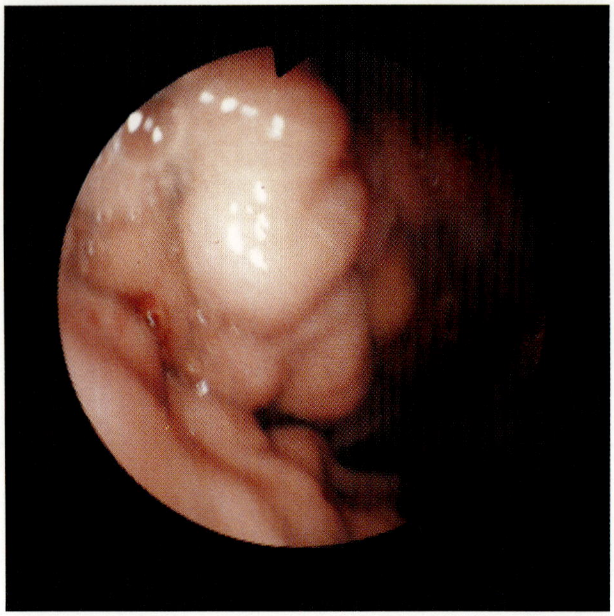

Fig. 7. Large gastric varix.

Gastric varices

Gastric varices are widely believed to be much less common than those in the oesophagus, even though the reported incidence in portal hypertension varies from 6 to 100% [42,43] (Fig. 7). A recent study by Mathur *et al.* [44•] indicates that they occur almost as frequently as oesophageal varices. In 104 patients undergoing sclerosis for oesophageal varices, gastric varices were demonstrated in 81 (78%) by endoscopy and in 69 (66%) by splenoportography. In 31 patients, varices only became apparent in the stomach 1–56 weeks after oesophageal sclerotherapy. In the majority (75%) the varices occurred along the lesser curve of the stomach, and the main feeding vein shown at portography was the left gastric (75%); in only 9% were the varices localized to the fundus. Only nine (11%) patients bled from their gastric varices and in six the bleeding originated in the fundus.

Hashizume *et al.* [45•] have proposed a new endoscopic classification of gastric varices based on their observations in 124 patients with portal hypertension. The patients were grouped according to the form, location and colour of the varices. Almost half the varices were tortuous and winding (F1), 38.7% were small to moderate in size and nodular (F2) and 12.1% were tumorous and large (F3); 33.9% were located on the posterior wall of the cardia (Lp), with 16.9% on the anterior wall (La), 14.5% on the lesser curve (Ll) and 9.7% on the greater curve (Lg). Glossy, thin-walled focal redness was found in 19.4% (red colour spot). Forty-three of the patients subsequently bled from their gastric varices and four factors that independently affected the risk of bleeding were identified by regression analysis. These, in descending order of relative risk, were the presence of a red colour spot, anterior location, nodular form and location on the greater curve.

An obscure cause for bleeding gastric varices has been reported by Heseltine *et al.* [46•]. The patient was a 48-year old woman with ureteric obstruction and splenic vein occlusion secondary to intra-abdominal fibrosis — proven histologically to be Weber–Christian disease. The varices were obliterated by endoscopic sclerotherapy with no further bleeding. This raises a potential diagnostic dilemma: should retroperitoneal fibrosis be considered in patients who continue to have variceal bleeding while on long-term β blockers!

Extrahepatic portal obstruction

The value of endoscopic sclerotherapy in the management of variceal bleeding secondary to extrahepatic portal obstruction has again been highlighted, this time in a large series from India by Chawla *et al.* [47•]. Sodium tetradecyl sulphate was used and injections were repeated every 3 weeks until the varices were obliterated. One hundred and four patients were studied for a mean period of 24 months. Eradication of varices was achieved in 95 (91.3%) in a median of five sessions. Rebleeding during the course of injections occurred in 15 patients (15.8%), but this was from oesophageal ulceration in seven and from varices in only three. Five patients rebled after variceal obliteration — two from gastric and one from oesophageal varices. Sclerotherapy resulted in a significant reduction in the number of bleeds per patient per month, from 0.208 before treatment to 0.028 after. Varices recurred in 15 patients (15.8%) after a mean interval of 8 months. There were few serious complications: three out of 26 children less than 12 years of age, developed a perforation and 25.3% of patients had oesophageal ulceration which eventually healed. Only six (5.7%) died as a result of bleeding: five before the varices were totally obliterated and one, a year later. Sclerotherapy is a safe and effective method for preventing variceal bleeding in extrahepatic portal hypertension and gives results that are seemingly comparable to shunt surgery. A controlled trial is required to establish the relative clinical roles of these two treatment modalities.

Surgery for portal hypertension secondary to schistosomiasis was followed by further variceal bleeding in 15% [48] and many of these patients were then treated by sclerotherapy. Sakai *et al.* [49•] compared the value of variceal sclerosis in 75 patients who rebled after surgery with 22 patients having endoscopic treatment without prior surgery. Two-thirds of the post-surgical patients had undergone either splenectomy alone or oesophagogastric devascularization with splenectomy. Ethanolamine was injected either into (40 patients) or adjacent to the varix (57 patients). Overall, 38 (39%) of the patients rebled after sclerotherapy but significantly fewer of these were in the post-surgical group (36% compared with 50%). Intravariceal sclerosis was more effective in eradicating the varices and was associated with less rebleeding than paravariceal injections. These results suggest that splenectomy improves the effectiveness of sclerotherapy, possibly by reducing portal blood flow.

Elastic band ligation

Endoscopic ligation of oesophageal varices (EVL) using elastic 'O' rings was first described by Stiegmann *et al.* in 1988 and has been previously reported in this Annual (1989, 1990). These workers [50••] have now updated their earlier experience with this technique. One hundred consecutive patients with bleeding oesophageal varices have been treated. Twenty-one were bleeding at endoscopy and this was successfully controlled by EVL in 18 (86%); two of the three failures had uncontrollable bleeding from sclerotherapy-induced ulceration. EVL requires less precision than sclerotherapy, which may prove to be an advantage when the varix is partly obscured by blood. Bleeding had ceased in 79 patients and none rebled during the initial admission after EVL. The 88 survivors had repeat EVL at 7–14-day intervals until the varices were eradicated. This was achieved in 60 (68%) after a median of five treatments; nine patients required alternative forms of treatment for recurrent bleeding. Over a mean follow-up period of 15 months, there were only three non-bleeding complications related to EVL: oesophageal bolus obstruction in one patient and strictures requiring a single dilatation in two others. EVL certainly seems to be as effective as sclerotherapy in controlling active bleeding and eradicating varices. A major advantage is the low incidence of early and late side effects and the results of comparative studies are awaited with interest.

Sclerosis of varices and feeder vein

The advantage of sclerosing oesophageal varices together with the main feeder vein has been evaluated by Takase *et al.* [51•]. Their technique involves compressing the varix with a balloon, craniad to the injection site, to prevent sclerosant from flowing into the systemic circulation. A mixture of 5% ethanolamine and iopamidol was used and sclerosant was injected under fluoroscopic control until the feeder veins filled (requiring up to 30 ml of sclerosant). The injection site was compressed by an inflated balloon catheter for up to 3 h. Two to four treatment sessions were necessary to eliminate the varices. A group of 26 patients who had undergone percutaneous transhepatic portography, both before and after sclerotherapy, were studied for 2 years after treatment. In 16 patients, both the varices and the feeder veins were obliterated and in these, varices recurred in only one out of 16 (6.3%). The recurrence rate in 10 patients in whom only the varices had been eradicated was 70%. The authors feel that occlusion of the varix and its feeder vein is essential to minimize the chance of recurrent varices. No complications were reported following this technique but the risk of extensive thrombosis of the portal system is likely to be higher than with conventional sclerotherapy.

Sclerotherapy and shunt surgery

Henderson *et al.* [52••] in a randomized study compared chronic sclerotherapy with the distal splenorenal shunt for preventing recurrent variceal bleeding. Thirty-seven patients were allocated to endoscopic treatment and 35 to surgery; the groups were well matched for aetiology and the severity of liver disease — 60%, overall having alcoholic cirrhosis with 58% Child's class A or B. There was a distinct survival advantage for patients undergoing sclerotherapy with an estimated 4-year survival of 65% compared with 43% for those having a shunt; this advantage was maintained when both good-risk (Child's class A or B) and poor-risk (Child's class C) patients were compared. Rebleeding was significantly less frequent after surgical management (3%) than with chronic sclerotherapy (59%). Uncontrolled rebleeding occurred in 13 (35%) of patients in the endoscopy-treated group and in 12, bleeding necessitated surgery for its control. This combined therapy gave a survival advantage to patients with alcoholic cirrhosis but not to those with non-alcoholic cirrhosis. Patients with alcoholic cirrhosis who were treated by sclerotherapy, in contrast to those having a distal splenorenal shunt, maintained portal perfusion and showed improvement in hepatocyte function. The authors conclude that the optimum treatment for variceal bleeding in patients with alcoholic cirrhosis is sclerotherapy with surgical rescue for uncontrolled bleeding. Spina *et al.* [53•] have also reported the results of a trial comparing sclerotherapy with distal splenorenal shunt in preventing variceal bleeding. Forty patients, all Child's class A or B, were randomly allocated to two equal groups for endoscopic or surgical treatment. As in the studies of Henderson and others [54–56], there was significantly less variceal rebleeding in the patients undergoing distal splenorenal shunt. The 2-year survival rates for the shunt (95%) and sclerotherapy (90%) treated groups were similar.

The value of continued sclerotherapy has been prospectively compared [57•] with the results of a surgical shunt procedure in 173 good-risk patients (Child's class A and B) in whom chronic sclerotherapy was followed by bleeding from oesophageal varices, sclerosis-induced mucosal ulceration or gastric varices. The two treatment groups were similar in their demographic characteristics and the severity and cause of cirrhosis. The type of surgery was based on specific selection criteria, 54 patients undergoing a narrow lumen mesocaval interposition shunt and 32 a distal splenorenal shunt. There was no significant difference in the early, 30-day mortality, but after a mean follow-up period of 52 months, there was a significantly lower mortality in the shunt-treated group (17% compared with 36%).

Should sclerotherapy with surgical rescue for rebleeding now be the treatment of choice for oesophageal variceal haemorrhage? As Grace [58•] points out in an editorial, this needs to be substantiated by a trial deliberately incorporating surgical rescue as part of the design (Fig. 8). Certainly, initial therapy with either variceal sclerosis or β blocker drugs has the advantage of preserving the patient for transplantation should this become necessary. If rebleeding occurs in patients with alcoholic cirrhosis, a shunt may be the next best treatment, as suggested by Henderson *et al.* For the non-alcoholic cirrhotic, liver transplantation may be more appropriate.

Non-variceal bleeding

In the past year there have been two excellent reviews on endoscopic therapy in non-variceal bleeding. Salena and Sivak [1•] evaluate the various injected agents, alone or in combination, for control of ulcer bleeding and emphasize that the optimal agent remains to be determined. The review by Kovacs and Jensen [59••] examines the role of electrothermal methods of treatment. They consider that all the studies to date support the use of the heater or multipolar probe for safe and effective haemostasis.

Rebleeding risk

Branicki *et al.* [60••], in a prospective study of 701 patients, have re-examined the factors associated with

Authors	Alcoholics (%)	Child's class (%)	Index bleed to incln (days)	Treatment (%)	Rebleed (%)	Surgical rescue (%)	Deaths (%)
Teres *et al.* [56], 1987	71	A/B, 100	10–15	SCT	18/48 (38)	3	27
				DSRS	6/42 (14)	NA	19
Rikkers *et al.* [54], 1987	86	A/B, 67	NA	SCT	17/29 (59)	4	40
				DSRS	5/26 (19)	NA	37
Cello *et al.* [55], 1987	98	C, 100	NA	SCT	12/16 (75)	7	28
				PSS	0/14 (0)	NA	12.5
Henderson *et al.* [52], 1987	60	A/B, 57	3–5	SCT	22/37 (59)	12	34
		C, 43		DSRS	1/35 (3)	NA	57

Fig. 8. Prospective trials comparing shunt surgery (DSRS/PSS) with chronic sclerotherapy (SCT) for the prevention of recurrent variceal haemorrhage (Grace [58]).

a poor outcome following ulcer bleeding. Endoscopy was carried out within 24 hours of hospital admission and almost 50% had endoscopic signs of recent haemorrhage (ESRH). Five hundred and thirty-three patients (76%) were managed conservatively with a mortality of 2.6%. The overall rebleeding rate was 16.1% and 134 patients underwent emergency surgery because of either continuing hypovolaemia (9.3%) or rebleeding (9.8%), with a mortality of 14.9%. The 'high-risk patients' once again proved to be elderly, sick from another illness or in shock. Patients over the age of 60 years were twice as likely to rebleed (22.1% compared with 10.9%) and twenty times more likely to succumb. Both concomitant medical illness and shock on admission had an adverse effect on outcome with a greater risk of rebleeding and a doubling of mortality (9.5% compared with 3.7%). The 'high-risk lesions' were large ulcers with ESRH. Ulcers greater than 1 cm in diameter rebled twice as frequently as smaller ulcers (23.9% compared with 12.4%) and were associated with an almost eightfold increase in mortality. The risk of rebleeding tripled when ESRH were demonstrated (6.7% compared with 2.6%).

The rebleeding rate in ulcers with a visible vessel varies between 33 and 100%. There is no reliable way at present to predict which of these will rebleed and which are likely to benefit from endoscopic therapy. Lin *et al.* [61•], in a prospective study, followed the outcome of 57 patients with non-bleeding visible vessels, initially treated conservatively. Twenty-two (38%) bled again within a week and a further three within the first month. Eight of these patients (25%) stopped bleeding permanently with conservative management alone; four were successfully controlled with either adrenaline injections three or heat probe coagulation one and 10 required surgical intervention. Patients over the age of 60 years, in shock or requiring more than 500 ml of blood, had a two to threefold increased risk of rebleeding. Advanced age, and coffee-ground material in the stomach were independent factors for predicting failure of conservative management. The authors suggest that such high-risk patients with non-bleeding visible vessels should be treated aggressively by either surgery or therapeutic endoscopy.

Sclerotherapy for bleeding ulcers

Since demonstrating in a randomized trial the benefits of adrenaline and polidocanol injections in controlling ulcer bleeding [62], Panes and colleagues [63•] have applied this treatment to a further 50 ulcer patients with both bleeding (18) and non-bleeding visible vessels (32). Arterial bleeding was controlled in all 18; in nine of the others, arterial bleeding was induced by puncturing the vessel but was controlled by further adrenaline injections. Fourteen patients (28%) had a minor rebleed necessitating repeat sclerotherapy and only five patients (10%) had a major rebleed requiring surgical intervention. The overall mortality rate was 10%, two out of the five deaths being directly due to rebleeding. This study provides additional support for sclerotherapy and emphasizes the need to repeat the injection if rebleeding occurs. Such rebleeding is often minor in nature and further therapy can be carried out without a significant increase in the risk of complications.

Balanzo *et al.* [64•] take this approach a step further. They suggest that routine re-examination of the ulcer a few days after treatment with repeat injection of a visible vessel if still present, may improve the overall outcome. In a randomized trial involving 64 patients with either active ulcer bleeding or a visible vessel, they compared the effects of adrenaline and thrombin injections with adrenaline injections alone. Four to seven injections of 1–2 ml of 1 : 10 000 adrenaline were injected around the bleeding site or visible vessel in both groups of patients; one group had additional injections of 5 to 10 ml thrombin (30 IU/ml) into similar sites. There was no significant difference in outcome — permanent hemostasis (81.3% versus 84.4%), rebleeding (18.6% versus 15.6%), transfusion requirements or need for emergency surgery — in the two groups. None of the patients died.

Forty-nine of the patients (25 from one group and 24 from the other) had a follow-up endoscopy between the third and fifth day after treatment and seven, still with a visible vessel, had repeated injections; none of these patients rebled. This approach may well have merit but needs to be proven in a randomized trial. It is unlikely that every visible vessel on repeat endoscopy represents a patent artery and high-frequency endoscopic Doppler ultrasound might indicate which of these should be retreated.

Heat probe

Lin *et al.* [65•] compared the effects of the endoscopic heat probe with alcohol injection and non-endoscopic therapy in 137 patients with ulcer bleeding. The three groups were compatible in terms of both patient and ulcer risk factors; there was a high incidence of active bleeding from arterial (26–33%) and oozing (26–33%) in all three. An Olympus heat probe was used and four to eight 15–30 J pulses were applied around the bleeding site; the procedure was repeated until no further bleeding was observed over a 5 min period. Absolute alcohol in 0.3–0.5 ml amounts to a total volume of 1–2 ml was used in the other treatment group; if bleeding continued for 5 min after treatment, the heat probe was applied and the patients withdrawn from the study. The initial and long-term haemostatic effects of the heat probe (97.8 and 91.1%) were significantly better than those achieved with the injection of alcohol (67.4 and 67.4%). These differences were attributed to difficulty in adequately injecting alcohol where access to the ulcer was limited and to the failure of alcohol to control arterial bleeding. Both forms of treatment significantly reduced the need for emergency surgery, the period of hospitalization and the mortality rate. The authors conclude that heat probe coagulation should be the treatment of first choice in ulcer bleeding. The haemostatic rate with alcohol injection was significantly lower than that reported by others [66] and better results might have been obtained using larger volumes of alcohol and a longer period of observation before declaring the treatment unsuccessful.

The effect of introducing endoscopy therapy (heater probe) on the need for surgery and mortality in gastrointestinal bleeding has been studied by Fullarton *et al.* [67•]. The outcome of 826 patients having conventional surgical management over a 5-year period was assessed retrospectively and compared with that of 263 patients treated after the introduction of the heater probe. The mean age of the two groups was similar but there were significantly more patients with duodenal ulcer in the earlier group and more with gastric ulceration in the heater probe group. Patients with 'high-risk' stigmata — continuing haemorrhage or a visible vessel in the ulcer base — were considered suitable for endoscopic therapy. Treatment of bleeding gastric ulcers with the heater probe resulted in a significant reduction in the need for surgery (7% compared with 16%) and the overall mortality (8.9% compared with 2.6%); there was a similar but non-significant trend for the treatment of duodenal ulcers. In all patients with a visible vessel, the reduction in the surgery rate after endoscopic therapy (4.5% compared with 71.4%) was striking.

Further evidence supporting the value of endoscopic therapy in the high-risk patient with ulcer bleeding has been provided in another study by Lin *et al.* [68•]. In a randomized prospective control trial of patients with non-bleeding visible vessels, they compared the value of the heat probe in 30 patients with conventional management in 31. The heater probe was applied in 15–30 J pulses with an average of 498 ± 62 J; bleeding was induced by treatment in five (16.7%) out of 30 patients, but was controlled by further heater probe coagulation. There was a significant reduction in the need for emergency surgery in the treated patients (6.7%) compared with the controls (29%), with no significant difference in the rebleeding rate, transfusion requirements, length of hospitalization or mortality (1.8 versus 9.7%). In a subgroup of high-risk patients who were elderly (greater than 60 years of age), shocked, with blood in their stomach and requiring more than 500 ml of blood, the heater probe did, however, provide significantly more effective long-term haemostasis.

Sclerotherapy with early surgery

Emergency surgery for the control of ulcer bleeding has a significantly higher mortality than elective ulcer surgery, particularly in the elderly or poor-risk patient. In a prospective study, Winkeltau *et al.* [69•] examined the value of combining therapeutic endoscopy with early elective surgery. Sixty-three patients with endoscopic signs of recent haemorrhage were treated endoscopically by the injection of adrenaline followed by 1% polidocanol. Initial control of haemorrhage was achieved in 98% of cases. Thirty-two of these patients (48%), all with Forrest type 1a to IIvv lesions, were considered to be especially at risk because of their age, associated medical problems or a posterior wall duodenal ulcer; all underwent early elective surgery without mortality. Two further patients required emergency surgery and died after the operation — an overall surgical mortality of 6%. All of the patients treated by endoscopic therapy alone, survived. Although the authors claim that this approach has major advantages — low mortality, elimination of rebleeding in the follow-up period, optimal conditions for surgery and a reduced need for transfusion — it does increase the morbidity from an unnecessary operation in a significant number of high-risk patients who would otherwise be safely managed by therapeutic endoscopy alone.

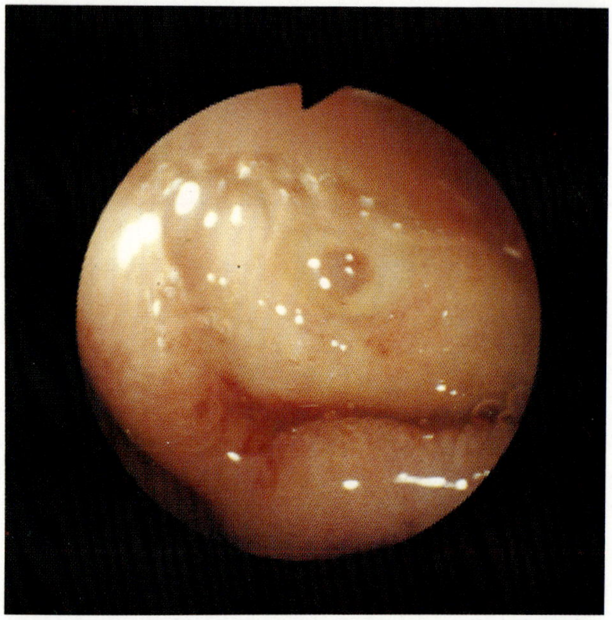

Fig. 9. Duodenal ulcer with visible vessel. By courtesy of G.N.J Tytgat, Academic Medical Centre, Amsterdam, The Netherlands.

Endoscopic Doppler ultrasound

Beckley *et al.* [70,71] were the first to describe the use of an endoscopic Doppler ultrasound probe to detect patent arteries in the base of ulcers. In 49 patients bleeding from peptic ulceration, the chance of rebleeding in those with overlying clot was 30% and in those with a visible vessel, 44% (Fig. 9); if there was a positive Doppler signal, this increased to 67 and 89%, respectively. The outcome was correctly predicted on the basis of the Doppler results in 44 out of 49 patients (90%) with a sensitivity of 73% and specificity of 95%.

The value of endoscopic Doppler ultrasound in determining the risk of rebleeding has recently been re-examined by Fullarton and Murray [72•]. They used a continuous wave Doppler probe (Transendoscopic Vascular Detector, TVD1, Key-Med Ltd, Southend on Sea, UK) passed through the endoscope channel; recordings were taken from each quadrant and the centre of the ulcer (Fig. 10). Twenty-two patients with active haemorrhage, a visible vessel or clot adherent to the ulcer were studied. Nine patients (eight with a visible vessel) rebled, seven of whom had a positive Doppler signal; overall seven out of the eight patients who were Doppler-positive rebled, giving an 87% sensitivity and 86% specificity for rebleeding. Not surprisingly, the technique had a significant failure rate

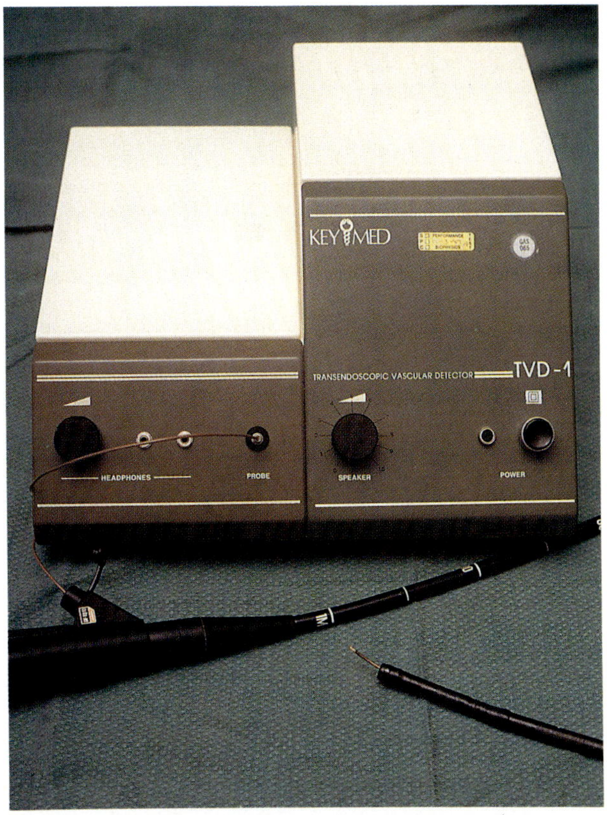

Fig. 10. Transendoscopic Doppler vascular detector.

— six of the initial 56 patients considered for the study were excluded because of inaccessibility to the ulcer or torrential haemorrhage.

These results suggest that endoscopic Doppler ultrasound gives essentially the same prognostic information as the endoscopic demonstration of a visible vessel. However, the number of patients in this study was small and the rebleeding rate from visible vessels was particularly high. Larger studies, preferably with high-frequency (20 mHz) pulsed Doppler probes that eliminate artefact owing to detection of large vessels deep to the ulcer base, are obviously required. This technique may yet have a role in determining the adequacy of endoscopic therapy.

References and recommended reading

• Of interest
•• Of outstanding interest

1. SALENA BJ, SIVAK MV: **Injection Therapy in the Treatment of Upper Gastrointestinal Hemorrhage.** *Eur J Gastroenterol Hepatol* 1990, **2**:79–86.
•
A critical review of the evidence supporting the role of endoscopic sclerotherapy in both variceal and non-variceal bleeding.

2. GRACE ND: **A Hepatologist's View of Variceal Bleeding.** *Am J Surg* 1990, **160**:26–31.
•
Recommends β blockers (with caution) to prevent the initial variceal bleed; vasopressin and nitroglycerine for minor bleeds and sclerotherapy for major bleeds; oesophageal staple transection if these fail. Long-term β blockers should be used to prevent recurrent bleeding in good-risk patients and chronic sclerotherapy in poor-risk patients; surgical rescue with a shunt is recommended if bleeding continues to recur.

3. RABINOVITZ M, YOO YK, SCHADE RR, DINDZANS VJ, VAN THIEL DH, GAVALER JS: **Prevalence of Endoscopic Findings in 510 Consecutive Individuals with Cirrhosis Evaluated Prospectively.** *Dig Dis Sci* 1990, **35**:705–710.
•
The most frequent findings were oesophageal varices in 82.7%, gastritis (gastropathy) in 42.7%, and duodenitis in 12.7%; gastric varices occurred in 7.8%. Oesophagitis and gastric ulceration were more commonly associated with alcoholic cirrhosis than with other forms of chronic liver disease.

4. CALES P, ZABOTTO B, MESKENS C, CAUCANAS JP, VINEL JP, DESMORAT H, FERMANIAN J, PASCAL JP: **Gastro-esophageal Endoscopic Features in Cirrhosis. Observer Variability, Interassociations, and Relationship to Hepatic Dysfunction.** *Gastroenterology* 1990, **98**:156–162.
•
There was good observer agreement on variceal size (grade 0–3), the presence of red sign, the severity of gastropathy and the presence of associated lesions; increasing variceal size correlated with increasing hepatic dysfunction.

5. THE ITALIAN LIVER CIRRHOSIS PROJECT: **Reliability of Endoscopy in the Assessment of Variceal Features.** *J Hepatol* 1987, 4:93–98.

6. BENDTSEN F, SKOVGAARD LT, SORENSEN TIA, MATZEN P: **Agreement Among Multiple Observers on Endoscopic Diagnosis of Esophageal Varices Before Bleeding.** *Hepatology* 1990, **11**:341–347.
•
Overall agreement on the presence of varices (grade 0 versus grade 1–3) in 70%. Agreement on distinguishing small and large varices was also good. The need for standardized observations in trials based on variceal size was stressed.

7. WESTABY D, WILLIAMS R: **Status of Sclerotherapy for Variceal Bleeding in 1990.** *Am J Surg* 1990, **160**:32–35.
••
Endoscopic sclerotherapy is effective in both controlling active variceal bleeding and preventing early rebleeding. Its repeated use until varices are obliterated significantly reduces the overall rebleeding rate and prolongs survival. Even with chronic sclerotherapy there is still a high incidence of rebleeding and the most appropriate use of this technique is still to be defined. Prophylactic sclerotherapy is not justified at present.

8. TERBLANCHE J: **Has Sclerotherapy Altered the Management of Patients with Variceal Bleeding?** *Am J Surg* 1990, **160**:37–42.
•
Support given to both immediate and long-term sclerotherapy. A plea for early recognition of those patients in whom this management has failed so that they can be considered for a porto-systemic shunt, oesophageal transection and devascularization procedure or where appropriate, liver transplantation.

9. SARIN SK, KUMAR A: **Sclerosants for Variceal Sclerotherapy: a Critical Appraisal.** *Am J Gastroenterol* 1990, **85**:641–649.
••
Examines the chemistry of sclerosants, the mechanism of their action and the results of both experimental and clinical studies for each agent.

10. KOCHHAR R, GOENKA MK, MEHTA S, MEHTA SK: **A Comparative Evaluation of Sclerosants for Esophageal Varices: a Prospective Randomized Controlled Study.** *Gastrointest Endosc* 1990, **36**:127–130.
•
Compares the effectiveness of ethanolamine oleate, sodium tetradecyl sulphate and absolute alcohol in variceal sclerosis. There was no significant difference in their ability to obliterate varices and the complication rates were similar. However, smaller volumes and fewer treatment sessions favour the use of absolute alcohol.

11. SARIN SK, MISRA SP, SACHDEV GK, THORAT V, DALAL L, BROOR SL : **Ethanolamine Oleate Versus Absolute Alcohol as Variceal Sclerosant: a Prospective Randomized Controlled Trial.** *Am J Gastroenterol* 1988, **83**:526–530.

12. KITANO S, ISO Y, KOYANAGI N, HIGASHI H, SUGIMACHI K: **Ethanolamine Oleate is Superior to Polidocanol (Aethoxysklerol) for Endoscopic Injection Sclerotherapy of Esophageal Varices: a Prospective Randomized Trial.** *Hepatogastroenterololgy* 1987, **34**:19–23.

13. ATAMKURI SP, BHARGAVA DK, SHARMA MP: **Endoscopic Sclerotherapy for Esophageal Varices: a Prospective Randomized**

Trial of Absolute Alcohol Versus Polidocanol. *Indian J Gastroenterol* 1988, 7:87–89.

14. KITANO S, ISO Y, YAMAGA H, HASHIZUME N, HIGASHI H, SUGIMACHI K: **Trial of Sclerosing Agents in Patients with Esophageal Varices.** *Br J Surg* 1988, 75:751–753.

15. • SHEMESH E, CZERNIAK A, KLEIN E, PINES A, BAT L: **A Comparison Between Emergency and Delayed Endoscopic Injection Sclerotherapy of Bleeding Esophageal Varices in Nonalcoholic Portal Hypertension.** *J Clin Gastroenterol* 1990, 12:5–9.
Rebleeding during the index admission occurred less frequently in those patients treated by emergency sclerotherapy. Although both groups were subsequently treated by chronic sclerotherapy, the beneficial effects of emergency endoscopic treatment were carried through to a lower rebleeding rate at 12 months.

16. •• WESTABY D, POLSON RJ, GIMSON AES, HAYES PC, HAYLLAR K, WILLIAMS R: **A Controlled Trial of Oral Propranolol Compared with Injection Sclerotherapy for the Long-Term Management of Variceal Bleeding.** *Hepatology* 1990, 11:353–359.
Oral propranolol (sufficient to reduce the pulse rate by 25%) was as effective as chronic sclerotherapy in preventing variceal rebleeding (rebleed rate 45–50%). Patients with high pretreatment pulse rates were less likely to have a good response.

17. JENSEN LS, KRARUP N: **Propranolol in Prevention of Rebleeding from Esophageal Varices During the Course of Endoscopic Therapy.** *Scand J Gastroenterol* 1989, 24:339–345.

18. • BERTONI G, FORNACIARI G, BELTRAMI M, CONIGLIARO R, MORTILLA MG, RICCI E, CASTAGNETTI E, BEDOGNI G, PLANCHER AC: **Nadolol for Prevention of Variceal Rebleeding During the Course of Endoscopic Injection Sclerotherapy: a Randomized Pilot Study.** *J Clin Gastroenterol* 1990, 12:364–365.
Unable to demonstrate any benefit from sclerotherapy combined with non-selective β-adrenergic blockade. A pilot study only with a small number of patients: its significance is doubtful.

19. WESTABY D, MELIA W, HEGARTY J, GIMSON AES, STELLON AJ, WILLIAMS R: **Use of Propranolol to Reduce the Rebleeding Rate During Injection Sclerotherapy Prior to Variceal Obliteration.** *Hepatology* 1986, 6:673–675.

20. • JENSEN LS, KRARUP N: **Propranolol may Prevent Recurrence of Esophageal Varices after Obliteration by Endoscopic Sclerotherapy.** *Scand J Gastroenterol* 1990, 25:352–356.
Treatment with propranolol for 6 months while varices are being eradicated by sclerotherapy, seems to be worthwhile. It not only reduces the risk of rebleeding until the varices are obliterated, but also diminishes the varix recurrence rate over the next 18 months (2% compared with sclerosis only at 73%).

21. • OKANO H, TSUJI H, KODAMA T, TAKINO T, MURAKAMI M: **Effect of Endoscopic Sclerotherapy and Propranolol on the Blood Flow of Esophageal Varices.** *Am J Gastroenterol* 1990, 85:30–33.
The blood flow in oesophageal varices is significantly reduced by propranolol or sclerotherapy alone (lasting up to 1 month) and most of all by combined sclerotherapy and β-blocker treatment (an 86% fall).

22. COHEN LB, KORSTEN MA, SCHERL EJ, *ET AL.*: **Bacteremia after Endoscopic Injection Sclerosis.** *Gastrointest Endosc* 1983, 29:198–200.

23. BRAYKO CM, KOZAREK RA, SANOWSKI RA, *ET AL.*: **Bacteremia During Esophageal Variceal Sclerotherapy: its Cause and Prevention.** *Gastrointest Endosc* 1985, 31:10–12.

24. BASKIN G: **Prosthetic Endocarditis after Endoscopic Variceal Sclerotherapy: a Failure of Antibiotic Prophylaxis.** *Am J Gastroenterol* 1989, 84:311–312.

25. COHEN FL, KOERNER RS, TAUB SJ: **Solitary Brain Abscess Following Endoscopic Injection Sclerosis of Esophageal Varices.** *Gastrointest Endosc* 1985, 31:331–332.

26. • TAM F, CHOW H, PRINDIVILLE T, CORNISH D, HAULK T, TRUDEAU W, HOEPRICH P: **Bacterial Peritonitis Following Esophageal Injection Sclerotherapy for Variceal Hemorrhage.** *Gastrointest Endosc* 1990, 36:131–133.
Three patients developed bacterial peritonitis up to 2 days after variceal sclerosis. All had normal ascitic fluid before the procedure and organisms were subsequently cultured from the peritoneal fluid in two. Sclerotherapy-induced mucosal ulceration was considered the portal of entry in one.

27. • VAN ZAANEN HCT, SCHOTBORGH RH, CHAMULEAU RAFM: **Meningococcus Septicemia: a Complication of Endoscopic Injection Sclerotherapy [letter].** *Am J Gastroenterol* 1990, 85:631–632.
Another case with delayed symptoms of septicaemia and evidence of peritonitis 30 h after sclerotherapy. *Diplococci* demonstrated in the ascites and *Neisseria meningitidis* were recovered from the blood.

28. • AGUADO J, NAPAL J, ALSAR MJ: **Pneumococcal Bacteremia: a Late Complication Following Endoscopic Variceal Sclerotherapy.** *Postgrad Med J* 1990, 66:790–791.
Another case of delayed septicemia following variceal sclerosis.

29. • FLICK JA: **Antibody Prophylaxis During Sclerotherapy for Esophageal Varices.** *J Paediatrics* 1990, 116:156–157.
Antibiotic prophylaxis during sclerotherapy is recommended not only for children with valvular heart disease and known immunodeficiency, but also for those who have had a splenectomy.

30. • CALETTI GC, BROCCHI E, LABRIOLA E, GASBARRINI G, BARBAR L: **Pericarditis: a Probably Overlooked Complication of Endoscopic Variceal Sclerotherapy.** *Endoscopy* 1990, 22:144–145.
A report of two patients with persistent chest pain after sclerotherapy due to pericarditis. Characteristic electrocardiographic and echocardiographic signs, but neither required pericardiocentesis. Not obviously related to technique or sclerosant used.

31. BROWN DL, LUCHI RJ: **Cardiac Tamponade and Constrictive Pericarditis Complicating Endoscopic Sclerotherapy.** *Arch Intern Med* 1987, 147:2169–2170.

32. KNAUER CM, FOGEL MR: **Pericarditis: Complication of Esophageal Sclerotherapy. Report of Three Cases.** *Gastroenterology* 1987, 93:287–290.

33. TABIBIAN N, SCHWARTZ JT, SMITH JL, GRAHAM DY: **Cardiac Tamponade as a Result of Endoscopic Sclerotherapy: Report of a Case.** *Surgery* 1987, 102:546–547.

34. • TERADA T, NAKANUMA Y, YONEJIMA M, YOKOYAMA H, KOIKE N: **Portal, Mesenteric and Splenic Venous Thrombosis after Endoscopic Injection Sclerotherapy.** *J Clin Gastroenterol* 1990, 12:238–239.
Extensive thrombosis of the portal system is a rare but lethal complication of sclerotherapy. To be considered in patients developing severe and persistent abdominal pain with rapid deterioration in liver function tests after variceal sclerosis.

35. • SINGAL A, SARIN SK, SOOD GK, BROOR SL: **Ulcers after Intravariceal Sclerotherapy: Correlation of Symptoms and Factors Affecting Healing.** *J Clin Gastroenterol* 1990, 12:250–254.
Superficial mucosal ulceration was present in all patients 1 day after intravariceal injections of absolute alcohol. Only two-thirds had short-lived dysphagia, pain or fever. The ulcer size was directly related to the volume of sclerosant and all the ulcers healed within a few weeks.

36. • MADONIA S, TRAINA M, MONTALBANO L, D'AMICO G: **Variceal Ulceration Following Sclerotherapy: Normal Consequence or Complication.** *Gastrointest Endosc* 1990, 36:76–77.
This report again incriminates large volumes of sclerosant (sodium tetradecyl sulphate) in the development of deep ulceration. Perhaps a little and often (? titrated against the development of blanching during injection) is the best policy.

37. SARIN SK, NANDA R, KUMAR N, *ET AL.*: **Repeated Endoscopic Sclerotherapy for Active Variceal Bleeding.** *Ann Surg* 1985, 202:708–711.

38. SARIN SK, SACHDEV GK, NANDA R, MISTA SP, BROOR SL : **Endoscopic Sclerotherapy in the Treatment of Gastric Varices.** *Br J Surg* 1988, **75**:747–750.

39. COHEN LB, SIMON C, KORSTEN MA, *ET AL.*: **Esophageal Motility and Symptoms after Endoscopic Injection Sclerotherapy.** *Dig Dis Sci* 1985, **30**:29–32.

40. SORENSEN T, BURCHARTH F, PEDERSEN ML, *ET AL.*: **Esophageal Stricture and Dysphagia after Endoscopic Sclerotherapy for Bleeding Varices.** *Gut* 1984, **25**:473–477.

41. KOKUDO N, SANJO K, UMEKITA N, HARIHARA Y, TADA Y, IDEZUKI
• Y: **Squamous Cell Carcinoma after Endoscopic Injection Sclerotherapy for Esophageal Varices.** *J Gastroenterol* 1990, **85**:861–864.

A report of two cases of carcinoma of the oesophagus occurring 2 years after variceal sclerosis. This rare association is likely to be fortuitous but must be excluded in patients developing late dysphagia.

42. HOSKING SW, JOHNSON AG: **Gastric Varices: a Proposed Classification Leading to Management.** *Br J Surg* 1988, **75**:195–196.

43. CLARK AW, WESTABY D, SILK DBA, *ET AL.*: **Prospective Controlled Trial of Injection Sclerotherapy in Patients with Cirrhosis and Recent Variceal Haemorrhage.** *Lancet* 1980, **ii**:552–554.

44. MATHUR SK, DALVI AN, SOMESHWAR V, SUPE AN, RAMAKANTAN R:
• **Endoscopic and Radiological Appraisal of Gastric Varices.** *Br J Surg* 1990, **77**:432–435.

Gastric varices demonstrated by endoscopy and splenoportography in almost 80% of patients with oesophageal varices. In one-third, these became apparent only after sclerosis of the oesophageal varices. Predominantly lesser curve in site with only 10% in the fundus.

45. HASHIZUME M, KITANO S, YAMAGA H, KOYANAGI I, SUGIMACHI
• K: **Endoscopic Classification of Gastric Varices.** *Gastrointest Endosc* 1990, **36**:276–280.

A classification of gastric varices based on form, location and colour. Half were tortuous with one-third on the posterior wall of the cardia; 20% with overlying spot. Varices with a red spot, nodular in form and both in an anterior and greater curve location were more likely to bleed.

46. HESELTINE D, BRAMBLE M, COLE A, CLARKE D, CASTLE W: **Weber-**
• **Christian Disease Producing Splenic Vein Occlusion and Bleeding Gastric Varices: Successful Treatment with Sclerotherapy.** *Postgrad Med J* 1990, **66**:321–325.

A rare cause of bleeding gastric varices and long-term control with endoscopic sclerotherapy.

47. CHAWLA YK, DILAWARI JB, RAMESH GN, KAUR U, MITRA SK,
•• WALIA BNS: **Sclerotherapy and Extrahepatic Portal Venous Obstruction.** *Gut* 1990, **31**:213–216.

A large series of 104 patients with varices secondary to extrahepatic portal obstruction treated by sclerotherapy. Varices were eradicated in 91% of cases with a significant reduction in the number of bleeds per month per patient over a 2-year period. Low complication rate (perforation occurred in three children) and death from rebleeding in only 5.7% of patients.

48. RAIA S, MIES S, MACEDO SL: **Surgical Treatment of Portal Hypertension in Schistosomiasis.** *World J Surg* 1984, **8**:738–739.

49. SAKAI P, BOAVENTRUA S, ISHIOKA S, MIES S, SETTE H, PINOTTI
• HW: **Sclerotherapy of Bleeding Esophageal Varices in Schistosomiasis.** *Endoscopy* 1990, **22**:5–7.

Value of sclerotherapy for rebleeding after surgery for portal hypertension in schistosomiasis was compared with the outcome after sclerotherapy alone. Rebleeding was significantly less common in the post-surgical (mainly splenectomy) group.

50. STIEGMANN GV, GOFF JS, SUN JH, HRUZA D, REVEILLE RM: **En-**
•• **doscopic Ligation of Esophageal Varices.** *Am J Surg* 1990, **159**:21–26.

In a large study of 100 patients, endoscopic variceal ligation seemed to be as effective as sclerotherapy in controlling active bleeding (86%) and eradicating varices (68%). Its major advantage was the low incidence of early and late side-effects. A randomized trial comparing the two techniques is promised.

51. TAKASE Y, SHIBUYA S, CHIKAMORI F, ORII K, IWASAKI Y: **Recur-**
• **rence Factors Studied by Percutaneous Transhepatic Portography Before and After Endoscopic Sclerotherapy for Esophageal Varices.** *Hepatology* 1990, **11**:348–352.

A sclerotherapy technique which ensures sclerosis of not only the varix but also the feeder vein is followed by a lower varix recurrence rate (6.3%) over 2 years. The technique is more cumbersome than conventional sclerotherapy and a trial of the two methods is indicated.

52. HENDERSON JM, KUTNER M, MILLIKAN WJ, GALAMBOS JT, RIEPE
•• SP, BROOKS WS, BRYAN FC, WARREN WD: **Endoscopic Variceal Sclerosis Compared with Distal Splenorenal Shunt to Prevent Recurrent Variceal Bleeding in Cirrhosis.** *Ann Intern Med* 1990, **112**:262–269.

Both good- and poor-risk patients survived significantly longer after sclerotherapy than after shunt surgery. Rebleeding, however, was significantly less in the surgical group and uncontrolled bleeding after sclerotherapy was treated with a distal splenorenal shunt. Surgical rescue after variceal sclerosis gave patients with alcoholic cirrhosis a distinct survival advantage, but this was not true for patients with non-alcoholic cirrhosis.

53. SPINA GP, SANTAMBROGIO R, OPOCHER E, COSENTINO F, ZAMBELLI
• A, PASSONI GR, CUCCHIARO G, MACRI M, MORANDI E, BRUNO S, PEZZUOLI G: **Distal Splenorenal Shunt Versus Endoscopic Sclerotherapy in the Prevention of Variceal Rebleeding.** *Ann Surg* 1990, **211**:178–186.

Again the risk of rebleeding was significantly less after shunt surgery but the 2-year survival rates for both groups were similar.

54. RIKKERS LF, BURNETT DA, VOLENTINE GD, BUCHI KN, CORMIER RA: **Shunt Surgery Versus Endoscopic Sclerotherapy for Long-Term Treatment of Variceal Bleeding. Early Results of a Randomized Trial.** *Ann Surg* 1987, **206**:261–271.

55. CELLO JP, GRENDELL JH, CRASS RA, WEBBER TE, TRUNKEY DD: **Endoscopic Sclerotherapy Versus Portocavel Shunt in Patients with Severe Cirrhosis and Acute Variceal Haemorrhage. Long-Term Follow-Up.** *N Engl J Med* 1987, **316**:11–15.

56. TERES J, BORDAS JM, BRAVO D, *ET AL.*: **Sclerotherapy vs Distal Splenorenal Shunt in the Elective Treatment of Variceal Hemorrhage: a Randomized Controlled Trial.** *Hepatology* 1987, **7**:430–436.

57. PAQUET KJ, MERCADO MA: **Surgical Procedures for Bleed-**
• **ing Oesophagogastric Varices when Sclerotherapy Fails: a Prospective Study.** *Am J Surg* 1990, **160**:43–47.

This study supports the value of surgical rescue by a selective or non-selective shunt operation in those patients with continued bleeding in spite of chronic sclerotherapy. The long-term mortality rate for patients managed by continued sclerotherapy was significantly higher than those managed surgically (36% compared with 17%).

58. GRACE ND: **Prevention of Recurrent Variceal Bleeding —**
• **Is Surgical Rescue the Answer?** *Ann Intern Med* 1990, **112**:242–244.

A review of studies comparing chronic sclerotherapy with shunt surgery. Considers that initial treatment by sclerotherapy or β blockade has the advantage of preserving patient for liver transplantation. Surgical rescue was indicated for rebleeding in alcoholic cirrhosis; liver transplantation may be more appropriate for recurrent bleeding in non-alcoholic cirrhosis.

59. KOVACS TO, JENSEN DM: **Electrothermal Modalities in the**
•• **Treatment of Non-variceal Upper Gastrointestinal Bleeding.** *Eur J Gastroenterol Hepatol* 1990, **2**:87–93.

A good review of the various electrothermal techniques for controlling ulcer bleeding; supports the use of the heater or the bipolar probe as being both safe and effective.

60. BRANICKI FJ, COLEMAN SY, FOK PJ, PRITCHETT CJ, FAN ST, LAI
•• ECS, MOK FPT, CHEUNG WL, LAU PWK, TUEN HH, LAM SK, HUI WM, NG MMT, LAM DKH, TSE MCK, TANG APK, WONG J: **Bleeding Peptic Ulcer: a Prospective Evaluation of Risk**

Factors for Rebleeding and Mortality. *World J Surg* 1990, 14:262–270.
In a large prospective study of 701 patients with bleeding ulcers, the 'high-risk patient' again shown to be elderly (>60 years), sick from another illness or in shock. The 'high-risk ulcers' were large (>1 cm) and with endoscopic signs of recent haemorrhage. In the elderly, surgery for rebleeding had a mortality rate of 28.9%.

61. • LIN HJ, LEE FY, TSAI YT, LEE SD, LEE CH: **What Kind of Non-Bleeding Visible Vessel in a Peptic Ulcer needs Aggressive Therapy?.** *Endoscopy* 1990, 22:8–11.
Patients over the age of 60 years, in shock or requiring more than 500 ml of blood had a two to threefold increase risk of rebleeding from visible vessels. The authors make a plea for aggressive therapy (surgical or endoscopic) in this group of patients.

62. PANES J, VIVER J, FORNE R, *ET AL*: **Controlled Trial of Endoscopic Sclerosis in Bleeding Peptic Ulcers.** *Lancet* 1987, ii:1292–1294.

63. • PANES J, FORNE M, BAGENA F, VIVER J: **Endoscopic Sclerosis in the Treatment of Bleeding Peptic Ulcers with a Visible Vessel.** *Am J Gastroenterol* 1990, **85**:252–254.
Adrenaline and polidocanol injections again shown to be effective in stopping ulcer bleeding. The need for repeat endoscopic therapy, after rebleeding is emphasized. Bleeding was permanently controlled in 62% after a single treatment session and in another 28% after two sessions.

64. • BALANZO J, VILLANUEVA C, SAINZ S, ESPINOS JC, MENDEZ C, GUARNER C, VILLARDELL F: **Injection Therapy of Bleeding Peptic Ulcer. A Prospective, Randomized Trial 'Using Epinephrine and Thrombin.** *Endoscopy* 1990, 22:157–159.
Both treatments equally effective with rebleeding rates of 15.6% and 18.6%. Three-quarters of the patients were re-examined within 5 days — seven still with a visible vessel underwent further therapy without rebleeding. Harder evidence is required before this approach can be recommended.

65. • LIN HJ, LEE FY, KANG WM, TSAI YT, LEE SD, LEE CH: **Heat Probe Thermocoagulation and Pure Alcohol Injection in Massive Peptic Ulcer Hemorrhage: a Prospective Randomized Controlled Trial.** *Gut* 1990, 31:753–757.
Both treatments significantly reduce the need for surgery and the mortality when compared with conventional management. The heat probe proved to be more effective than alcohol injections in both the initial and long-term control of bleeding; the study's design, however, may have advantaged the heat probe results.

66. ASAKI S: **Endoscopic Hemostasis by Local Absolute Ethanol Injection for Upper GI Tract Bleeding — a Multi-Centre Study.** In *Endoscopic Surgery* edited by Okabe H, Honda T, Oshiba S. Amsterdam: Elsevier Science Publishers BB, 1984, pp 105–116.

67. • FULLARTON GM, BIRNIE GG, MACDONALD A, MURRAY WR: **The Effect of Introducing Endoscopic Therapy on Surgery and Mortality Rates for Peptic Ulcer Hemorrhage. A Single Centre Analysis of 1125 Cases.** *Endoscopy* 1990, 22:110–113.
A retrospective evaluation of conventional management was compared with a prospective study of outcome after the introduction of the heater probe. There was a significant reduction in the need for surgery and mortality in bleeding from gastric ulceration; patients with visible vessels fared best of all from endoscopic therapy.

68. • LIN HJ, LEE FY, KANG WM, YANG TT, LEE SD, LEE CH: **A Controlled Study of Therapeutic Endoscopy for Peptic Ulcer with Non-Bleeding Visible Vessel.** *Gastrointest Endosc* 1990, 36:241–246.
In a study of 60 patients with non-bleeding visible vessels, endoscopic therapy (heater probe) again was shown to reduce significantly the need for surgery; in the elderly, high-risk patients, there was a significant increase in the long-term control of bleeding.

69. • WINKELTAU G, ARLT G, TREUTNER KH, SCHUBERT T, SCHUMPELICK V: **Endoscopic Therapy and Early Elective Operation as a Therapeutic Regimen in Ulcer Bleeding.** *Hepatogastroenterology* 1990, 37:121–123.
Sixty-three patients with endoscopic signs of recent haemorrhage were treated by injections of adrenaline and polidocanol with control of bleeding in 98%. Thirty high-risk patients then proceeded to early elective surgery. Although claims are made for this approach, they are not convincing in the absence of a randomized trial.

70. BECKLY DE, CASEBOW MP, PETTENGELL KE: **The Use of a Doppler Ultrasound Probe for Localizing Arterial Blood Flow During Upper Gastrointestinal Endoscopy.** *Endoscopy* 1982, 14:146–147.

71. BECKLY DE, CASEBOW MP: **Prediction of Rebleeding from Peptic Ulcer: Experience with an Endoscopic Doppler Device.** *Gut* 1986, 27:96–99.

72. • FULLARTON GM, MURRAY WR: **Prediction of Rebleeding in Peptic Ulcers by Visual Stigmata and Endoscopic Doppler Ultrasound Criteria.** *Endoscopy* 1990, 22:68–71.
Endoscopic continuous wave Doppler ultrasound prediction of rebleeding, based on the demonstration of a positive arterial signal from the ulcer had a similar sensitivity (87%) and specificity (86%) to the endoscopic demonstration of a visible vessel. A clinical role for this investigation is yet to be shown.

73. SARIN SK, NANDA R, SACHDEV G: **Relative Efficacy and Safety of Absolute Alcohol and 50% Alcohol as Variceal Sclerosants.** *Gastrointest Endosc* 1987, 33:362–367.

74. JAPANESE RESEARCH SOCIETY FOR PORTAL HYPERTENSION: **The General Rules for Recording Endoscopic Findings on Esophageal Varices.** *Jpn J Surg* 1980, 10:84–87.

75. TERBLANCHE J, BORMAN PC, KAHN D: **The Failure of Long-Term Injection Sclerotherapy After Variceal Bleeding to Improve Survival.** *Lancet* 1983, ii:1328–1332.

76. WESTABY D, MACDOUGALL BRD, WILLIAMS R: **Improved Survival Following Injection Sclerotherapy for Esophageal Varices: Final Analysis of Controlled Trial.** *Hepatology* 1985, 5:627–631.

77. KORULA J, BALART LA, RADVAN G, *ET AL*: **A Prospective Randomized Controlled Trial of Chronic Esophageal Variceal Sclerotherapy.** *Hepatology* 1984, 5:584–589.

78. THE COPENHAGEN ESOPHAGEAL VARICES SCLEROTHERAPY PROJECT: **Sclerotherapy After First Variceal Hemorrhage in Cirrhosis: a Randomized Multicenter Trial.** *N Engl J Med* 1984, 311:1594–1600.

79. SODERLUND C, IHRE T: **Endoscopic Sclerotherapy Versus Conservative Management of Bleeding Esophageal Varices: a 5 Year Prospective Controlled Trial of Emergency and Long-Term Treatment.** *Acta Chir Scand* 1985, 151:449–456.

Lasers and tumor probes

M.H. Mellow

Department of Gastroenterology, Baptist Medical Center
and Presbyterian Hospital, Oklahoma City, Oklahoma, USA

Introduction

After the introduction of any novel treatment modality, initial enthusiasm is normally followed by varying degrees of sober reassessment. Once applicable patient populations are strictly defined and complications are emphasized, a treatment modality may fall by the wayside. To date, this has not happened with endoscopic laser therapy of gastrointestinal neoplasms. Review of this year's literature reveals that the early reports continue to be substantiated. Success rates (both technical success and, when tabulated, functional success) are very similar in all reports. Thus, at least in 'expert' hands, data are very reproducible. It must be comforting to the relative novice to see that the ranks of the 'experts' are enlarging rapidly. Furthermore, no new technology has emerged that surpasses results of endoscopic laser therapy in the palliation of gastrointestinal neoplasms (Fig.1).

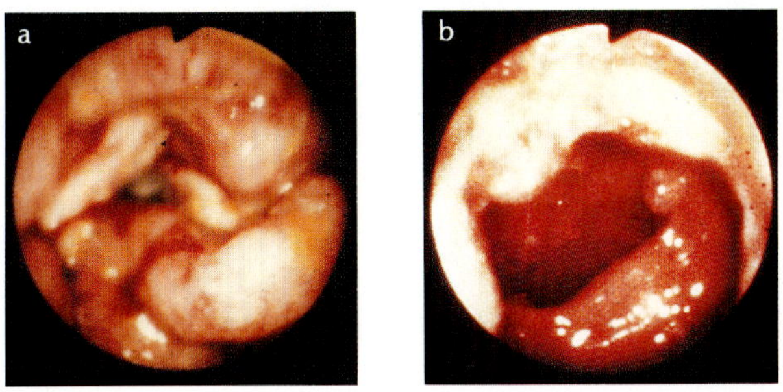

Fig. 1. Nearly obstructing rectosigmoid malignancy before (a) and after (b) laser therapy. Note bloodless coagulum in laser-treated area in (b).

	Neodymium-YAG (Present study)	Electrocoagulation (Madden and Kandalaft)
Mean patient age	76.6	66.5
Mean number of sessions	2.75	3.50
Cases with complications	12/100	22/77
Perforation	1	2
Rectovaginal fistula	1	2
Bleeding	3	17
Mortality	0	0
Setting	outpatient	inpatient
Anesthesia	IVS	spinal/general

Fig. 2 Comparative value of laser and electrocoagulation therapies. Published by permission [1].

Reviews of neodymium-YAG laser treatment in gastrointestinal neoplasms

Unger *et al.* [1•] report on results in 100 patients undergoing 275 procedures in the treatment of colorectal neoplasms. The number of treatments per patient varied greatly (between one and 22), but the majority had between two and six procedures. For the most part, treatments were carried out under intravenous sedation in an outpatient setting. Complications included one perforation, three hemorrhages, and one rectovaginal fistula. The authors compared their data with those reported previously for electrocoagulation of rectal cancer (Fig.2). Advantages of laser treatment included lower incidence of complications, ability to treat in an outpatient setting, with resultant lower cost. Performance status, evaluated by Karnofsky scale within 6 months of the first procedure, revealed that most patients were self-sufficient and many were able to work.

Loizou *et al.* [2•] treated 49 patients with rectosigmoid carcinoma who were considered unsuitable for surgery. The patients were divided into three groups, depending upon the degree of circumferential involvement on initial presentation. Three out of seven patients with small lesions had complete macroscopic and microscopic tumor eradication, at a mean of 20 months follow-up. In patients with more locally advanced lesions, initial success of laser treatment was significantly greater in those with non-circumferential involvement. However, initial tumor length and location did not have prognostic importance. Success rates tended to be greater in patients with rectal discharge than in those with obstructive symptoms. Overall, 91% of patients had symptomatic improvement, maintained by repeat laser sessions. Laser-induced perforation occurred in two patients (5%) with impassable circumferential lesions at the rectosigmoid junction, requiring defunctioning colostomy. The authors stressed the need for having patients return for procedures on a fixed schedule rather than retreat electively when symptoms reccurred. This is a very important point. By the time obstructive symptoms recur, it may be impossible to reattain luminal patency, especially in lesions that traverse the rectosigmoid angle. Labenz and Borsch [3•] treated 53 patients with a variety of rectal or rectosigmoid disease. The majority of these patients had rectal carcinoma. Three out of 22 patients with malignant obstruction were treatment failures (required colostomy, at an average of 7 months) because of recurrence not amenable to laser endoscopy. Bleeding was well con-

© Current Science Ltd ISBN 1-87045-32-7 ISSN 0952-6293

trolled. Out of 16 large, broad-based or flat colorectal adenomas, 14 were completely destroyed. Three patients experienced recurrence,1–36 months after initial treatment; recurrences were retreated, with two patients free of recurrence after 6 months. Gostout [4•] reviews the large Mayo Clinic experience with neodymium-YAG laser endoscopy, over 2000 procedures having been performed in the first 5 years. In photocoagulation of vascular malformations, Gostout emphasizes the real and theoretical advantages of neodymium-YAG laser. Being a non-contact device, laser therapy allows more efficient coagulation of multiple or large surface area lesions and avoids pretreatment mechanical disruption of such friable lesions. However, the author emphasizes that no prospective studies have compared long-term outcome of laser photocoagulation with other thermal endoscopic modalities. The Mayo Clinic data closely parallel other reported experience regarding technical and functional efficacy of treatment of esophageal and rectal malignancy.

Haruma *et al.* [5] report on the Japanese experience with neodymium-YAG laser therapy of early gastric cancer. Interestingly, they review a method for removing flat gastric lesions, developed by Tada. In order to excise a flat or depressed lesion endoscopically, a volume of 5–10 ml of saline is injected submucosally. This elevates the lesion so it can be resected by the usual endoscopic polypectomy technique.

Analysis of variables affecting outcome in treatment of gastrointestinal neoplasms

Several authors have attempted to define clinical and endoscopic tumor parameters that impact on immediate and long-term success in the palliative endoscopic management of malignancy. In an important study, Naveau *et al.* [6••] analyze, by unidimensional and multidimensional analysis, 11 variables' effect on symptomatic improvement 6 months after initial laser therapy in patients with esophageal carcinoma. One hundred and forty-four patients underwent neodymium-YAG therapy. Improvement of dysphagia was achieved in 83% after a median of 2.9 endoscopic sessions. For those with initial symptomatic improvement, the cumulative probability of remaining symptomatically improved at 3 and 6 months was 38 and 22%, respectively. Three variables were found to have independent prognostic value at 6 months. These included, not surprisingly, improvement after initial laser treatment. Adenocarcinoma was a positive predictor. Initial tumor length was negatively correlated with duration of symptomatic improvement (Fig.3). Among 82 patients who died during the time of observation, 50 had maintenance of their initial swallowing improvement until time of death.

Matthus-Vliegen and Tytgat [7•] retrospectively reviewed their experience with endoscopic neodymium-YAG photocoagulation of gastrointestinal neoplasms. The main points from their study were as follows: the difficulty of eradicating extensive benign colorectal adenomas — lesions encompassing greater than two-thirds of the circumference or growing in a flat tapestry-like pattern over more than 4 cm — were eradicated in only 43%. In colorectal cancer, hemostasis was obtained in 90% of 60 patients and successful palliation in 86% of 43 patients with obstructing cancer. Strange *et al.* [8•] analyzed determinants of survival in patients with esophageal carcinoma treated by neodymium-YAG laser therapy. Initial technical success was realized in 93% of 59 patients; treatment was functionally successful in 75%. In this series, survival did not relate to cell type, but related inversely to age. As expected, it related directly to the presence of distant metastases. The diameter of stenosis, both before and after initial treatment, related significantly to survival, as did severity of post-treatment dysphagia. It is noteworthy that patients receiving a percutaneous gastrostomy, because of inadequate caloric intake, had survival curves similar to those with good functional results of laser treatment. Therefore, if a patient cannot eat well following initial therapy, caloric access should be obtained rapidly (prosthesis or gastrostomy tube).

Review of neodymium-YAG laser treatment in gastrointestinal hemorrhage

Marcon [9•] reviews the literature, concentrating primarily on controlled trials involving both argon and neodymium-YAG lasers, on the photocoagulation of acute gastrointestinal hemorrhage. Salient points include the following: injection therapy alone produced results equivalent to injection plus laser therapy; repeat endoscopic therapeutic intervention is often of value in patients with recurrent bleeding. Despite theoretical concern, laser treatment in acute upper gastrointestinal hemorrhage appeared quite safe, with one out of 256 patients experiencing a perforation related to laser therapy. Wenk *et al.* [10•] report on 10 patients with radiation proctitis treated with neodymium-YAG laser therapy. One to five (mean 2.4) treatment sessions were required. Following laser treatment, no further blood transfusion was required in any patient. No complications were observed.

Naveau *et al.* [11•] report on long-term results of treatment of vascular malformations by neodymium-YAG laser photocoagulation in 60 patients (13 with hereditary hemorrhagic telangiectasia and 47 with angiodysplasias). Results were disappointing in those with hereditary hemorrhagic telangiectasia. No statistically significant decrease in transfusion requirements following treatment was observed. In patients with angiodysplasia, the cumulative probability of remaining free of blood loss recurrence at 24 months was 61%. Overall, three parameters had an independent prognostic value: the initial number of angiodysplasias, the presence of coagulation disorders and advanced age all impacted negatively on outcome. Van Cutsem reported a randomized crossover placebo controlled trial of combined estrogen and progesterone therapy in 10 patients with bleeding vascular malformations. Active therapy in these 10 patients (five of whom had hereditary hemorrhagic telangiectasia) resulted in a sig-

Variables	Patients (n)	Cumulative probablity of remaining symtomatically improved at 6 months	p
Age			
<67 years	54	18 ± 6	NS
≥67 years	51	26 ± 6	
Sex			
Female	85	23 ± 5	NS
Male	19	21 ± 9	
Location of upper end of tumor			
<27 cm	40	23 ± 5	0.07
≥27 cm	65	31 ± 7	
Initial tumor length			
<6 cm	49	33 ± 7	0.01
≥6 cm	56	12.5 ± 5	
Luminal patency in 5 grades			
≤3	65	30 ± 5	NS
>3	40	11 ± 5	
Endoscopic appearance			
Infiltrating	19	23 ± 10	NS
Exophytic	86	22 ± 5	
Histology			
Adenocarcinoma	41	41 ± 8	0.05
Squamous cell carcinoma	64	11 ± 4	
Kind of surgical contraindication			
Related in cancer	52	17 ± 5	NS
Not related with cancer	53	26 ± 6	
Previous radiotherapy			
Yes	22	5 ± 5	NS
No	83	25 ± 5	
Symptomatic result achieved by initial laser treatment			
Good	82	28 ± 5	0.0005
Fair	23	0	
Duration			
<2 weeks	57	26 ± 5	NS
≥2 weeks	48	18 ± 5	

Fig. 3 Cumulative probabilityof remanining symptomatically improved at 6 months according to 11 variables–unidimensional analysis. Published by permission [6].

nificant and impressive diminution in bleeding. Given the side effects of estrogen and progesterone, especially in the elderly, it might be worth reserving hormonal therapy for those who fail initial attempts at endoscopic coagulative therapy.

Comparison of techniques and use of laser in conjunction with other treatment modalities

Radford *et al.* [12] report on a prospective randomized evaluation of contact versus non-contact neodymium-

YAG laser therapy in palliation of esophageal carcinoma. Of the 20 patients evaluated, the authors found no significant difference in number of initial treatment sessions, length of treatment times, 1-month post-treatment dysphagia scores, or duration of palliation. There were two treatment failures using the contact method, one from inability to control tumor bleeding. The treatment area with the contact probe is limited to the small diameter of the contact tip itself, certainly a disadvantage for large, friable tumors. A laser-resistant guide probe could be helpful as an adjunct for contact laser therapy of very tight tumor stenoses. There is, of course, no reason why the two techniques should not simply be complementary.

Barr *et al.* [13••] report from their very active treatment unit on a randomized prospective evaluation of 46 patients referred for endoscopic palliative therapy of esophageal carcinoma. Patients were randomized to receive laser therapy only or initial laser therapy followed by endoscopic intubation. Twenty patients were treated in each group, with six exclusions. Data evaluated included pre and post-treatment dysphagia, quality of life index as assessed by both physician and patient, monthly post-treatment dysphagia grade, and complication rates. It should be noted that five of the six patients excluded from analysis could not have undergone initial prosthesis placement, because of either the proximity of the tumor to the upper esophageal sphincter or other technical problems preventing prosthesis passage. If patients required more than once-a-month laser treatment sessions, they were considered treatment failures and endoscopic intubation was performed. In those patients randomized to receive laser therapy followed by intubation, the major effort was simply to 'clear the esophagus' and allow proper anchoring and orientation of the tube. Intubation was performed 10–14 days after laser therapy to ensure that necrotic tissue treated by laser had separated, thus avoiding early slippage of the prosthesis. The authors found a significant improvement in post-treatment dysphagia grades with both methods. There was no significant difference in improvements between the two treatment groups; quality of life was similar in both groups. There was a significantly greater complication rate in the group treated with intubation following laser treatment. Four patients developed food bolus obstruction, requiring repeat endoscopy. One patient had tube dislodgement. In four patients, tumor overgrowth occurred, causing recurrent dysphagia. These were successfully treated by laser vaporization. Three patients had small pharyngeal perforations on routine contrast examination after intubation, but recovered on intravenous fluids and antibiotics. It is clear that both laser therapy and intubation are effective in relieving malignant dysphagia. Although intubation is theoretically a 'one time' treatment, it is associated with higher complication rates, often requiring repeated endoscopies. In fact, the authors did not find a significant difference in number of endoscopic sessions between the two groups. I believe, given equivalent technical expertise with both methods, that endoscopic laser therapy should initially be employed in patients undergoing palliative treatment for malignant dysphagia. On the other hand, as Naveau's article points out, it should become relatively clear that a subgroup of patients (not always easily identifiable by pretreatment characteristics) will not have functionally successful outcome following laser therapy. At that point, therapeutic alternatives (intubation and, in some instances, gastrostomy) must be considered. Semler [14•] combined palliative endoscopic laser therapy with afterloading irradiation in 22 patients with colorectal carcinoma. No significant complications occurred. Patients were not directly compared with those receiving laser therapy only or radiation therapy only. There may well be therapeutic advantage to this combined approach that needs to be further explored.

New uses of currently available laser technology

Radford *et al.* [15•] attempted endoscopic gastric vagotomy using neodymium-YAG laser in dogs. They found that although major vagal branches are identifiable for a distance of at least a centimeter as they course between longitudinal and circular muscle layers and that these branches are located within a predictable zone relative to the gastric emptying junction and midline of the lesser curvature, it was necessary, however, to produce a nearly full-thickness turn to interrupt the deep intramural vagal branches. Despite their efforts to control dosimetry, delayed perforations occurred in three out of the four dogs. The idea of focally ablating areas in the wall of the gut is an appealing one. Certainly the use of newer, near-infrared lasers, such as holmium or erbium-YAG, could produce a more precise tissue injury.

Neuhaus [16•] performed endoscopic laser therapy on malignant bile duct tumors using percutaneous cholangioscopy in three patients. No side effects were observed and stents were placed after successful recanalization of the malignant strictures. In a similar effort, Flowers *et al.* [17•] used a pulsed dye laser for purposes of fragmenting a large impacted intrahepatic stone in a patient who had already undergone cholecystectomy, choledochoduodenostomy, and choledochojejunostomy, the laser procedure being performed through the percutaneous transhepatic route. Following stone fragmentation of the large stone, a stone basket was used to remove fragments.

Photodynamic therapy

McCaughan *et al.* [18•] evaluated the use of photodynamic therapy for esophageal tumors. Forty patients were treated over a 5-year period. Luminal diameter, as judged by biopsy forceps measurement, increased from 6 mm to 9 mm 1 month after treatment. Thirty-five patients ingested at least a soft diet. Survival was in the range of 7 months. Complications included five sunburns, six pleural effusions, three tracheo-esophageal fistulas, a chylothorax and an endoscopic perforation. Thus, results were similar to those generally obtained with neodymium-YAG laser therapy, although complication rates appeared to be somewhat higher. Patrice *et al.* [19••] report their experience in 54 patients with inoperable gastrointestinal neoplasms. Both squamous cell and adenocarcinoma of the esophagus were treated, as were patients with rectosigmoid adenocarcinoma. Patients were considered inoperable because of associated medical conditions or recurrent disease after previous radiation therapy or surgery. Lesions, however, were small, all being less than 4 cm in their largest diameter. None showed detectable metastases at the time of diagnosis. Photodynamic therapy was delivered either by surface illumination or direct interstitial probe placement. Treatment was considered successful when there was complete local destruction of tumor and negative biopsy specimens were observed on two consecutive assessments. The vast majority of patients underwent photodynamic therapy just once. Six out of 54 patients received two courses. Complications included severe sunburn in three, esophageal stricture in five (four of whom responded to a single dilatation). One patient with late post-treatment colonic stenoses died after a bowel perforation following dilatation 33 months after initial photodynamic therapy. One patient exhibited spontaneous perforation a week after laser treatment. The points of interest in this study included the fact that no death occurred in patients with successful local response to photodynamic therapy that could be attributed to metastatic spread of tumor. Even in patients who relapsed, 11 of the 24 patients with squamous carcinoma of the esophagus had complete responses with a mean recurrence-free period of 11 months. Five out of 14 patients with adenocarcinoma had complete response with a recurrence free period of 15–1/2 months. Eight out of 16 patients with colorectal cancer had complete responses with a recurrence free period of 17 months. There was, as might be expected, a clear-cut relationship between complete local response and survival, with 50% survival rate at 2 years in the complete local responders. Several patients were given external radiation following their course of photodynamic therapy. One patient, an initial partial responder, became classified as a complete response. Perhaps the concurrent use of radiation therapy would be of value. The technique of photodynamic therapy certainly holds promise. Furthermore, the development of tissue photosensitizers that have more neoplastic tissue specificity, lack the current cutaneous toxicities, and allow deeper penetration into malignant tissue is required. Several photosensitizers in the range of 650–800 nM are undergoing preliminary testing.

Case report

No major advance was reported in this area. Laser lysis of an esophageal web was described by Krevsky and Pusateri [20•]. The patient in this study had required numerous endoscopic dilatations for recurrent dysphagia associated with a proximal esophageal web. Follow-up 4 months after laser therapy revealed no recurrence of dysphagia. Three patients with blue rubber bleb nevus syndrome who presented with recurrent gastrointestinal bleeding underwent neodymium-YAG laser treatment [21•]. As in the case with other diffuse vascular lesions of the gut, successful photocoagulation of 'reachable' vascular lesions does not ensure a long-term success. One of the three patients required laparotomy for treatment of bleeding small-bowel lesions.

Sander *et al.* [22•] emphasized the importance of polypectomy prior to laser therapy in broad-based villous adenomas. This is important for two reasons: first, endoscopic snare polypectomy is a more rapid way to remove tissue than laser therapy; second, it allows removal of a vast majority of the tumor, making histopathologic diagnosis somewhat more secure.

New applications of laser technology

Gana *et al.* [23•] report on the use of endoscopic laser-Doppler flowmetry in the measurement of resting focal gastric mucosal blood flow. Patients included healthy volunteers as well as those with dyspepsia and peptic ulcer. Blood flow was measured for 1 min at various endoscopic sites, including the first portion of the duodenum, prepyloric antrum, mid-antrum, and several areas of the gastric body, fundus and distal esophagus. Blood flow was highest in the fundus, followed by the body, and lowest in the antrum. The angularis had a high blood flow. Gana *et al.* found no correlation between age and blood flow, although no patients older than 66 were evaluated. For reasons that are unclear, the patients had modestly lower mucosal blood flows than the volunteers, whether or not gross disease was seen. Clearly more work needs to be done in this area. The basic principle of laser-Doppler flowmetry involves illumination of tissue by a helium neon laser light conducted through an optical fiber. The laser light is scattered by both moving red blood cells and static tissue. However, only the back-scattered light by red cells undergoes a shift in frequency according to the Doppler effect. This back-scattered light is collected by optical fibers and analyzed to give a stable signal linearly related to the flux of red blood cells over a radius of 1 mm of tissue. Flowmetry was performed by passing an endoscopic probe through the biopsy channel of the endoscope. This technique may be of value in documenting occlusion of treated vessels in bleeding ulcers and large vascular malformations. Extension of this technology to the elderly will also be very important. Good measurement of gastric or, perhaps more relevantly, the proximal jejunal blood flow may allow rapid diagnosis of ischemic bowel disease in the acutely ill patient with abdominal pain.

Cothren *et al.* [24••] have developed an endoscope-compatible optical fiber system used to obtain laser-induced fluorescent spectra of mucosal abnormalities during real time endoscopy. They have previously shown that laser-induced fluorescent tissue spectra *in vitro* are sufficiently unique to allow accurate diagnosis. Fluorescent spectra were obtained during colonoscopy in 20 patients. Thirty-one adenomas, four hyperplastic polyps, and 32 areas of normal mucosa were examined. The spectra could be used to correctly differentiate adenomas from normal colonic tissue and hyperplastic polyps in 97% of specimens studied, with an extremely high sensitivity, specificity, and positive predictive value. The spectroscopy probe, delivering monochromatic light at 370 nm pro-

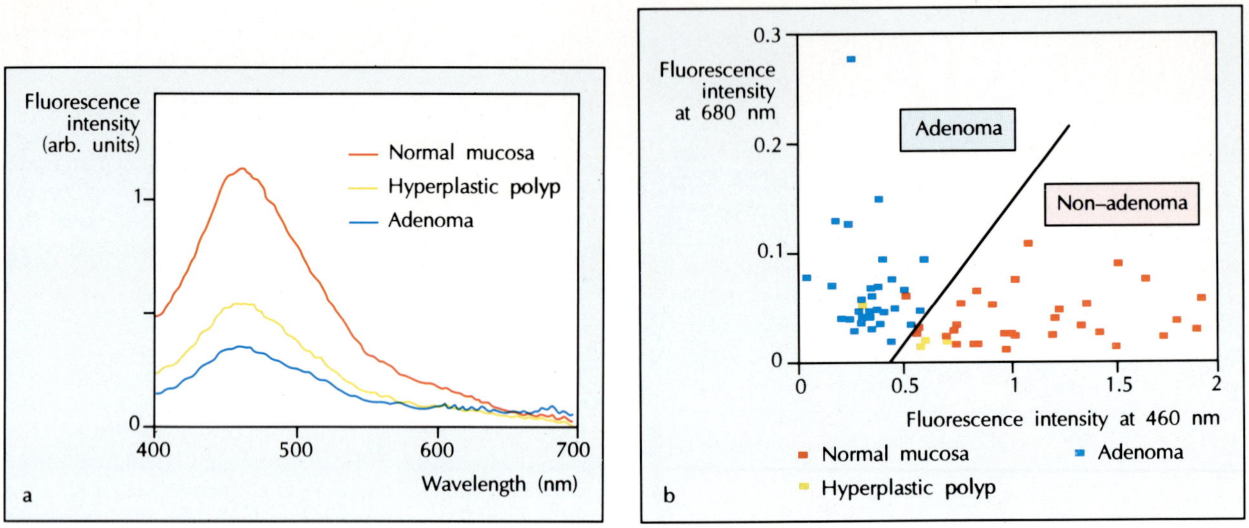

Fig. 4. (a) The hyperplastic polyp fluorescence intensity at 460 nm lies intermediate between the fluorescence intensities of adenoma and normal. At wave lengths greater than 650 nm, the fluorescence intensity of hyperplastic polyps closely approximates that of normal. (b) Two-dimensional scatter plot of the fluorescence intensity at 460 nm versus that at 680 nm for all 67 samples. The straight line represents the decision surface which minimizes the number of samples misclassified. One hyperplastic polyp and one normal mucosal specimen were misclassified as adenoma with a sensitivity, specificity, and predictive value of 100, 97,and 94%, respectively. After Cothren *et al.* [24••].

duced by a nitrogen pump dye laser, is passed through the biopsy channel of the endoscope and placed in direct contact with the surface of tissue to be evaluated. Fluorescence emission spectra were then collected from 350–700 nm, several probe placements were obtained on the same tissue site to evaluate reproducibility, and biopsies were then performed. Although the spectra of normal colon adenomas and hyperplastic polyps had similar line shapes, there were major differences in fluorescence intensity (Fig. 4). Fluorescence intensity of normal tissue was much greater at 460 nm, whereas at 650 nM adenoma fluorescence was greater than normals. There was excellent reproducibility of fluorescent spectra in all samples when the same site was retested on multiple occasions. The authors point out that real time spectral testing of diminutive polyps saves some time and certainly modest expense if one could accurately separate diminutive hyperplastic polyps from adenomas. Additionally, as premalignant changes associated with Barrett's esophagus and ulcerative colitis are histologically very similar to adenomas, it may be that similar fluorescent spectral patterns could be discerned in these situations. We await future developments in this area with great interest. Hopefully, the drawback of need for direct tissue contact (thus limiting 'area of interest' to a millimeter in size) can be eliminated.

Mang [25] investigates the effect of combination of photodynamic therapy with interstitial hyperthermia. Treatments were given sequentially and simultaneously in a mammary mouse tumor. Hyperthermia alone (44.5°C for 30 min) resulted in complete destruction of tumor with no subsequent regrowth in 7% of the mice treated; photodynamic therapy alone resulted in a cure rate of approximately 10%, but the simultaneous treatment with both modalities resulted in a 33% cure rate at 90 days, indicating a synergistic interaction. Endoscopic application of neodymium-YAG hyperthermia is somewhat cumbersome (although one can envisage use of multiple fibers through a rigid sigmoidoscope for distal rectal lesions), but one could certainly combine interstitial neodymium-YAG-induced hyperthermia with photodynamic therapy for intra-abdominal and/or cutaneous lesions. Moreover, the possibility exists that reduction in the concentration of hematoporphyrin derivative with concomitant increase in 630 nM light dose might result in a reduction of the cutaneous photosensitivity experienced by photodynamic therapy patients.

Hahl *et al.* [26•] report on the treatment of neodymium-YAG laser-induced hyperthermia in the destruction of malignant hepatic tumors. Laserthermia was performed during laparotomy using neodymium-YAG laser with contact sapphire probes at power settings of 6 watts. The probe was placed in the middle of the tumor with the temperature raised to between 41 and 45°C for 10 min, over a 1.5–2 cm area. In computed tomography scans obtained 4 weeks postoperatively, treated areas became more sharply bordered and hypodense as a sign of tumor necrosis. Necrosis was proved by fine-needle biopsies, but suspicion of viable cancer cells was still found in two of the patients. Important points include the need to strictly avoid coaxial air in interstitial work. One patient experienced a fatal air embolism. This has been reported earlier in interstitial treatment of uterine carcinoma as well. Thus, fluid cooling rather than air cooling is necessary. For this technique to be of greater practical importance, multifiber delivery systems must be developed so that one can greatly expand the field of injury.

Panjehpour *et al.* [27•] have developed a long, frosted contact probe in order to deliver interstitial neodymium-YAG laser-induced thermal injury in dogs. Their 13 mm

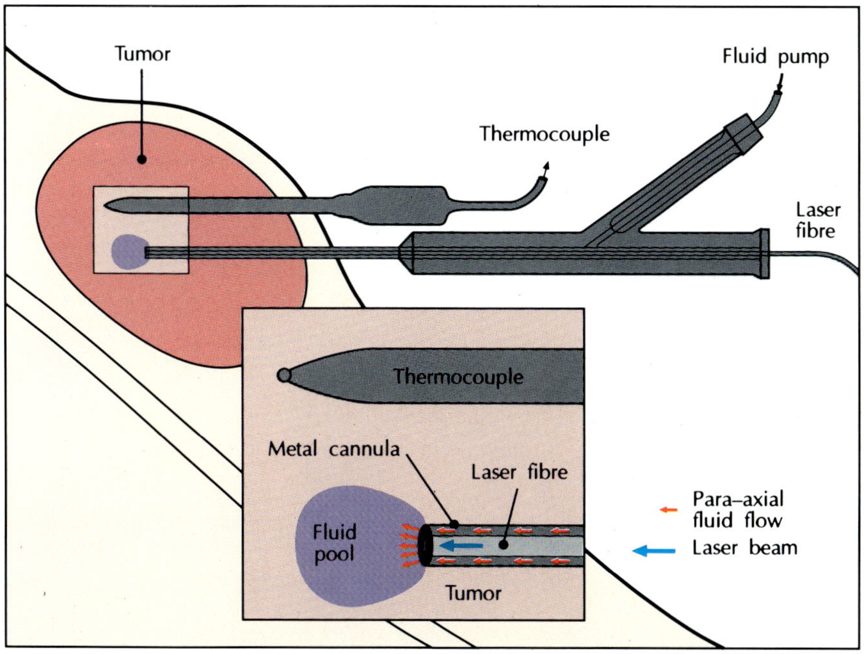

Fig. 5. Schematic drawing of the laser fiber placed inside a needle-cannula and 'Y'-shaped connector. Thermocouple is glued to the cannula and their tips are 3 mm apart. After Dowlatshahi *et al.* [28].

long probe produced hyperthermic temperatures in a 20 mm diameter around the probe, using 4–5 watts power. Given the probe's dimensions, the heating potential is a cylindrical volume of 20 mm diameter, having a 10 mm height and with its centeroid located at the tip of the contact probe. As discussed earlier, this type of probe might greatly enhance 'tumor kill' in photodynamic therapy.

Dowlatshahi *et al.* [28] have developed a system for protecting fiber function in interstitial laser therapy of malignant tumors. They have used neodymium-YAG laser and a 600 μm quartz fiber, stripping the terminal 5 cm of plastic coating, which is then inserted into a 5 cm long extra thin gauge 19 needle through a Y-shaped connector. The internal diameter of this needle cannula is large enough to allow for easy fiber placement as well as to permit para-axial flow of cooling fluid (Fig. 5). Using their system, 2 cm mammary tumors were treated in Sprague–Dawley rats. The authors found the optimal rate of saline flow to minimize probe tip damage and prevent excessive edema of the tumor was 1 ml per minute, at the 5 watt laser power setting. The fiber-needle complex was slowly withdrawn continuously throughout the treatment. Coaxial fluid cooling prevents the tissue from com-

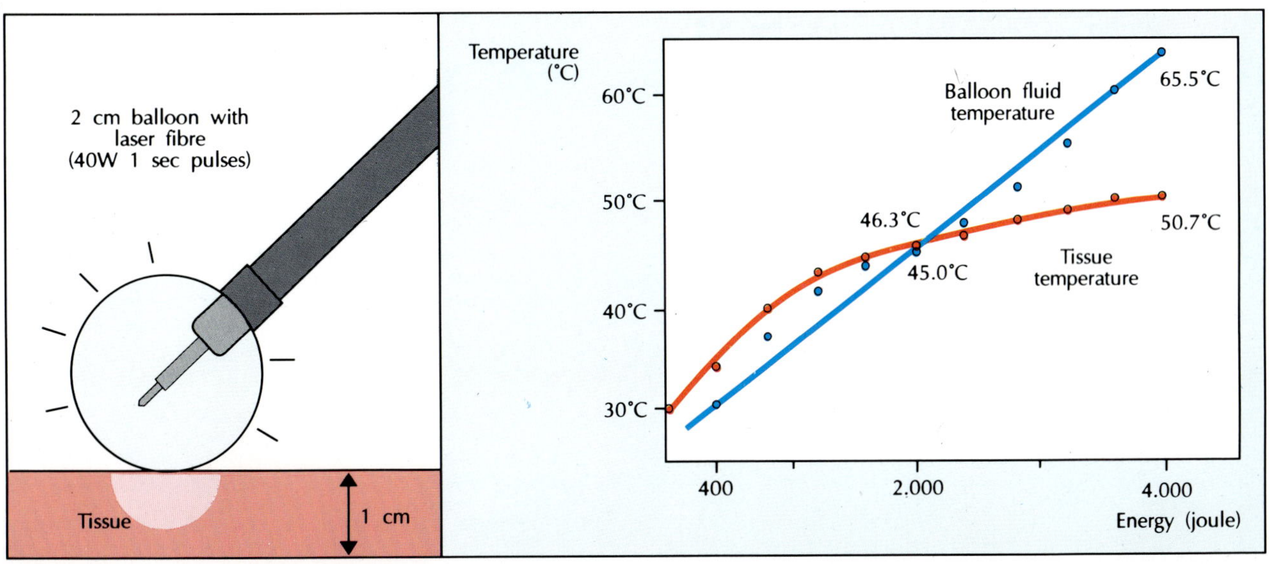

Fig. 6. Temperature (ordinate) of the balloon fluid and of rabbit liver parenchyma at 1cm depth during delivery of increasing pulses at 1 s intervals.

ing into direct contact with the fiber tip, thus allowing transmission of laser energy into the target tissue without causing a 'frying pan' effect. Continuous very slow needle withdrawal during laser delivery was advantageous both because a cooler zone of tumor was constantly entered and a smaller volume of fluid needed to cool the fiber. In addition, successive regions of tumor were lased, producing a coagulated column of necrotic tissue instead of a sphere of coagulation. Their ability to use power settings of up to 10 watts enabled the operator to coagulate significant volumes of tumor tissue over a much shorter period of time than would be possible at 1–3 watts output. An area of coagulation necrosis occurred in less than 2 minutes. This time conservation is a real advantage in the treatment of large tumors.

Shimamura *et al.* [29•] developed an endoscope equipped with a saline-filled latex rubber balloon at its tip, its purpose being to displace contaminating blood, bile or gastric contents during operative portoscopy, biliary endoscopy, or upper gastrointestinal endoscopy. A fiber with a tip inside the balloon transmitted energy from an neodymium-YAG laser for coagulation purposes (Fig. 6). We discussed the development of such a device by Fleischer in the 1990 *Annual of Gastrointestinal Endoscopy*. In addition to circumferential destruction of tumor tissue, one might be able to use this device for coagulation of gastrointestinal bleeding lesions, using the balloon for coaptation of vessels, a major disadvantage of non-contact YAG laser photocoagulation when compared with the commonly used contact devices.

References and recommended reading

Papers of special interest, published within the annual period of review, have been highlighted as:

- • Of interest
- •• Of outstanding interest

1. • UNGER SW, STERN JD, ARROYO PJ, RUSSIN DJ: **Endoscopic Nd:YAG Laser Treatment of Colorectal Neoplasms: A Four-year Longitudinal Study.** *Am Surg* 1990, **56**:153–157.
Retrospective evaluation of results, complications, and performance status in patients undergoing palliative neodymium-YAG laser treatment of colorectal neoplasms, with comparisons to historical data using electrocoagulation.

2. • LOIZOU LA, GRIGG D, BOULOS PB, BOWN SG: **Endoscopic Nd:YAG Laser Treatment of Rectosigmoid Cancer.** *Gut* 1990, **31**:812–816.
Review of a busy unit's experience with neodymium-YAG laser treatment of rectosigmoid cancer. The discussion is well worth reading.

3. • LABENZ J, BORSCH G: **Endoscopic Laser Therapy of Coloproctological Diseases.** *Coloproctology* 1989, **12**:132–136.
Review of experience with neodymium-YAG laser treatment of colorectal disorders.

4. • GOSTOUT CJ: **Gastrointestinal Laser Endoscopy: Future Horizons.** *Mayo Clin Proc* 1990, **65**:509–517.
Good review of the Mayo Clinic experience with gastrointestinal laser endoscopy, with speculation on future directions of laser development and uses.

5. • HARUMA K, SUMII K, INOUE K, TASHIMA H, KAJIYAMA G: **Endoscopic Therapy in Patients with Inoperable Early Gastric Cancer.** *Am J Gastroenterol* 1990, **85**:522–526.
Various endoscopic therapies including laser photoablation, drug injection, intralesional drug injection, and strip biopsy in the management of patients with inoperable early gastric cancer.

6. •• NAVEAU S, CHIESA A, POYNARD T, CHAPUT JC: **Endoscopic Nd:YAG Laser Therapy as Palliative Treatments for Esophageal and Cardial Cancer: Parameters Affecting Long-term Outcome.** *Dig Dis Sci* 1990, **35**:294–301.
Important article analyzing numerous variables that might affect long-term outcome of neodymium-YAG laser treatment of esophageal malignancies. Improvement after initial laser treatment and the presence of an adenocarcinoma were favorable parameters; initial tumor length was a predictor of treatment failure.

7. • MATHUS-VLIEGEN EMH, TYTGAT GNJ: **Analysis of Failures and Complications of Neodymium-YAG Laser Photocoagulation in Gastrointestinal Tract Tumors: A Retrospective Survey of 8 Years.** *Endoscopy* 1990, **22**:17–23.
Retrospective analysis of very large experience in the use of neodymium-YAG laser treatment of gastrointestinal tumors. Good discussion on when to suspect a malignancy in lesions initially considered to be benign.

8. • STRANGE EF, DYLLA J, FLEIG WE: **Laser Treatment of Upper Gastrointestinal Carcinoma: Determinants of Survival.** *Endoscopy* 1989, **21**:254–257.
Prospective study defining parameters of survival during laser treatment. Poor prognostic indicators included the presence of metastases; young patient; and both pre- and post-treatment degrees of stenosis.

9. • MARCON NE: **Lasers in Gastrointestinal Haemorrhage.** *Eur J Gastroenterol Hepatol* 1990, **2**:94–98.
Comprehensive review concentrating on controlled trials involving the use of argon and neodymium-YAG laser in photocoagulation of gastrointestinal bleeding.

10. • WENK H, LANGE V, HOHLBACH G, SCHILDBERG FW: **Endoscopic Laser Treatment of Bleeding Actinic Proctitis.** *Colorproctology* 1989, **12**:173–176.
The authors regard endoscopic neodymium-YAG laser therapy as the treatment of choice in troublesome symptomatic bleeding from radiation proctitis.

11. • NAVEAU S, AUBERT A, POYNARD T, CHAPUT JC: **Long-term Results of Treatment of Vascular Malformations of the Gastrointestinal tract by Neodymium-YAG Laser Photocoagulation.** *Dig Dis Sci* 1990, **35**:821–826.
Parameters having prognostic value in the long-term control of gastrointestinal bleeding from vascular malformations included (all negative) initial number of vascular malformations, presence of a coagulation disorder, and advanced age.

12. • RADFORD CM, AHLQUIST DA, GOSTOUT CJ, VIGGIANO TR, BALM RK, ZINSMEISTER AR: **Prospective Comparisons of Contact with Non-contact Nd:YAG Laser Therapy for Palliation of Esophageal Carcinoma.** *Gastrointest Endosc* 1989, **35**:394–397.
Little difference was observed between the two therapeutic modalities. Contact therapy can be very cumbersome with large, friable tumors.

13. •• BARR H, KRASNER N, RAOUF A, WALKER RJ: **Prospective Randomized Trial of Laser Therapy Only and Laser Therapy Followed by Endoscopic Intubation for the Palliation of Malignant Dysphagia.** *Gut* 1990, **31**:252–258.
A well-written article from an experienced endoscopic unit. Both groups fared similarly; there were more complications in the patients undergoing endoscopic intubation.

14. • SEMLER P: **Palliative Treatment of Cancer of the Colon with Laser Ablation and Afterloading Radiotherapy.** *Deutsch Med Wochenschr (DMW)* 1990, **115**:328–331.
Non-randomized observations regarding the use of endoscopic neodymium-YAG laser therapy with interstitial irradiation of colorectal malignancies.

15. • RADFORD CM, AHLQUIST DA, SARR MG, WOLD LE, ZINSMEISTER AR, GOSTOUT CJ: **Endoscopic Gastric Vagotomy: A Feasibility Study Using Laser in Dogs.** *Gastrointest Endosc* 1989, **35**:419–424.

Innovative but, unfortunately, unsuccessful attempt to focally destroy portions of gastric wall (vagus nerve elements). More precise lasers (e.g. holmium-YAG) might be applicable here.

16. NEUHAUS H: **Endoscopic Tumor Therapy.** *Endoscopy* 1989,
• 21:357–360.
Percutaneous cholangioscopy to vaporize bile duct tumor and allow subsequent stent placement.

17. FLOWERS BF, SASLAWSKY MJ, MATHES GL, TONKIN AK: **Use of the**
• **Pulsed Dye Laser and Ultrasonic Lithotriptor for Removal of Multiple Intrahepatic Gallstones.** *Surg Gynecol Obstet* 1990, 170:443–444.
Case report using percutaneous transhepatic endoscopy and pulse dye laser for fragmentation and removal of large intrahepatic gallstones.

18. MCCAUGHAN JS, NIMS TA, GUY GT, *ET AL*: **Photodynamic**
• **Therapy for Esophageal Tumors.** *Gastrointest Endosc* 1990, 36:85–86.
Review of the authors' extensive experience in the use of endoscopic photodynamic therapy for palliation of esophageal malignancies of various cell types. Results were comparable to those reported with neodymium-YAG laser.

19. PATRICE T, FOULTIER MT, YACTAYO S, ADAM F, GALMICHE JP,
•• DOUET MC, LEBODIC L: **Endoscopic Photodynamic Therapy with Hematoporphyrin Derivative for Primary Treatment of Gastrointestinal Neoplasms in Inoperable Patients.** *Dig Dis Sci* 1990, 35:545–552.
Encouraging results on the total ablation of relatively small gastrointestinal malignancies with endoscopic photodynamic therapy.

20. KREVSKY B, PUSATERI JP: **Laser Lysis of an Esophageal Web.**
• *Gastrointest Endosc* 1989, 35:451–453.
Case report of successful YAG laser photoablation of a previously recalcitrant esophageal web.

21. MAUNOURY V, TURCK D, BRUNETAUD JM, MARTI R, CORTOT A,
• FARRIAUX JP, PARIS JC: **Blue Rubber Bleb Nevus Syndrome.** *Gastroenterol Clin Biol* 1990, 14:593–595.
Successful coagulation of vascular lesions in this rare disorder.

22. SANDER R, POESL H, SPUHLER A, BRAIDA M: **The Importance of**
• **Polypectomy Prior to Laser Therapy in Broad-based Villous Adenomas.** *Gastrointest Endosc* 1990, 36:318.
Polypectomy specimens in large villous adenomas can allow more secure histologic diagnosis.

23. GANA TJ, SOENEN GM, KOO J: **A Controlled Study of Human**
• **Resting Gastric Mucosal Blood Flow by Endoscopic Laser-Doppler Flowmetry.** *Gastrointest Endosc* 1990, 36:264–267.
Mucosal blood flow may be measured via endoscopic laser-Doppler devices.

24. COTHREN RM, RICHARDS-KORTUM R, SIVAK MV, *ET AL*: **Gas-**
•• **trointestinal Tissue Diagnosis by Laser-induced Fluorescence Spectroscopy at Endoscopy.** *Gastrointest Endosc* 1990, 36:105–111.
Very important preliminary work from the Cleveland Clinic and Massachusetts Institute of Technology using laser light for induction of fluorescent spectra to be used in the differential diagnosis of mucosal abnormalities endoscopically.

25. MANG TS: **Combination Studies of Hyperthermia Induced**
• **by the Neodymium-Yttrium-Aluminium-Garnet (Nd:YAG) Laser as an Adjuvant to Photodynamic Therapy.** *Lasers Surg Med* 1990, 10:173–179.
Animal tumor model, showing a synergistic interaction between photodynamic therapy and neodymium-YAG-induced interstitial hyperthermia.

26. HAHL J, HAPPIAINEN R, OVASKA J, PUOLAKKAINEN P, SCHRODER
• T: **Laser-induced Hyperthermia in the Treatment of Liver Tumors.** *Lasers Surg Med* 1990, 10:319–321.
Intraoperative neodymium-YAG hyperthermia in humans with hepatocellular carcinoma.

27. PANJEHPOUR M, OVERHOLT BF, MILLIGAN AJ, SWAGGERTY MW,
• WILKINSON JE, KLEBANOW ER: **Nd:YAG Laser-induced Interstitial Hyperthermia Using a Long Frosted Contact Probe.** *Lasers Surg Med* 1990, 10:16–24.
A 13 mm probe developed for neodymium-YAG laser-induced tissue hyperthermia. Discussion is worth reading.

28. DOWLATSHAHI K, BANGERT JD, HAKLIN MF, RHODES CK,
•• WEINSTEIN RS, ECONOMOU SG: **Protection of Fiber Function by Para-axial Fluid Flow in Interstitial Laser Therapy of Malignant Tumors.** *Lasers Surg Med* 1990, 10:322–327.
Nice study using rat mammary tumor model for dosimetry of low power interstitial laser therapy.

29. SHIMAMURA Y, GUNVEN P, ISHII M, *ET AL*: **Endoscopic Laser**
• **Coagulation Through an Optical Laser Balloon.** *Lasers Surg Med* 1990, 10:25–27.
Preliminary work using a laser balloon for endoscopic purposes. Potential value includes circumferential irradiation of tumors and coaptive photocoagulation in gastrointestinal hemorrhage.

Endosonography

G.C. Caletti and L. Barbara

Academic Department of Medicine and Gastroenterology, University of Bologna, Bologna, Italy

New instruments such as thin echoprobes and the echocolonoscope have been described. It emerges that endosonography is an accurate and safe technique for evaluating upper and lower gastrointestinal pathology, particularly for staging neoplasms. Interesting new applications such as the assessment of portal hypertension are in progress.

Introduction

Endosonography is now 10 years old. Since the first reports in 1980 [1,2], experience has continued to broaden, and it is used in ever larger numbers of centers and patients.

During this time endosonography has shown itself to be a useful, accurate and safe technique for evaluating upper gastrointestinal pathology, and particularly for staging tumors [3•].

Instrumentation

Ultrasound endoscopes use mechanical sector scanners or linear arrays; the greatest experience is with the former. The Olympus GF-UM3/EU-M3, with a biopsy channel for endosonography-guided puncture and a switchable frequency from 7.5 to 12 MHz, is the most reliable instrument and the most suitable for clinical practice. No other systems are so widely used.

Despite excellent imaging quality, however, ultrasound endoscopes have a number of disadvantages, such as the cost and the fact that the ultrasound scanner is actually part of the endoscope. The consequence of this combination is that if a lesion is seen at endoscopy, the conventional endoscope must be removed and replaced with the ultrasound endoscope. A further disadvantage is that endosonography is inconvenient for the patient because of the larger diameter and the rigid tip of the instrument, which is more difficult to swallow than routine endoscopes.

For all these reasons, prototype echoprobes, which can be introduced down the working channel of conventional endoscopes, have been developed. Rösch and Classen [4•] have tested a miniature ultrasonic probe (Olympus Optical, Aloka, Japan), which has a diameter of 3.7 mm and a tiny rotating ultrasonic transducer that operates at a frequency of 7.5 MHz, generating a 360° view. The focal distance is stated to be 10 mm. This probe can be passed through a gastroscope with a large working channel (Fig. 1).

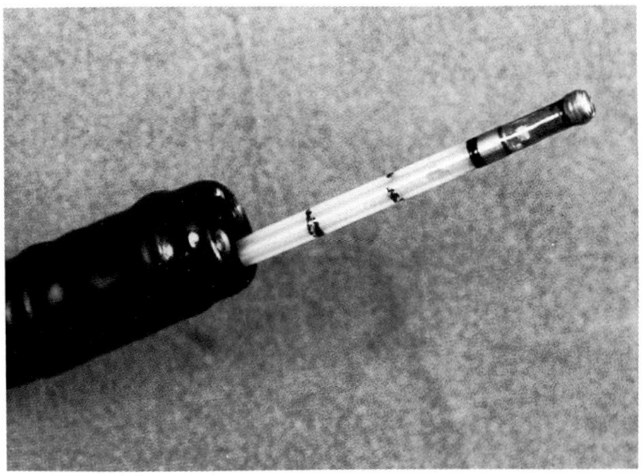

Fig. 1. Olympus catheter echoprobe passing through a forward-viewing large-channel gastroscope (Olympus GIF 1T10).

The authors reported that image resolution was slightly inferior to conventional endosonography, and extraluminal structures such as vessels or lymph nodes were seen only when they were located close to the gut wall. Compared with this probe, conventional endosonography has a greater depth of penetration and usually permits more complete delineation of the gastric wall circumference. Adequate contact with the wall is difficult to achieve in the esophagus because of the lack of a balloon. This probe therefore does not adequately visualize esophageal and gastric neoplasms of large diameter, their possible spread into neighboring organs, and perimural lymph nodes at some distance from the wall. The most important advantage of the probe is that it can be used in stenosed or narrowed hollow organs, where conventional endosonography fails (Fig. 2).

Kimmey *et al.* [5•] have developed a 20 MHz mechanical linear probe with an axial resolution of 0.2 mm, a lateral resolution of 0.5 mm, and a theoretical penetration of 1.5 cm. All five layers of the normal gastrointestinal wall are excellently imaged in the esophagus, stomach, duodenum, colon and rectum. Submucosal and subserosal vessels as small as 1.0 mm in diameter are also routinely seen. The probe obtains optimal images of rel-

© Current Science Ltd ISBN 1-870485-327 ISSN 0952-6293

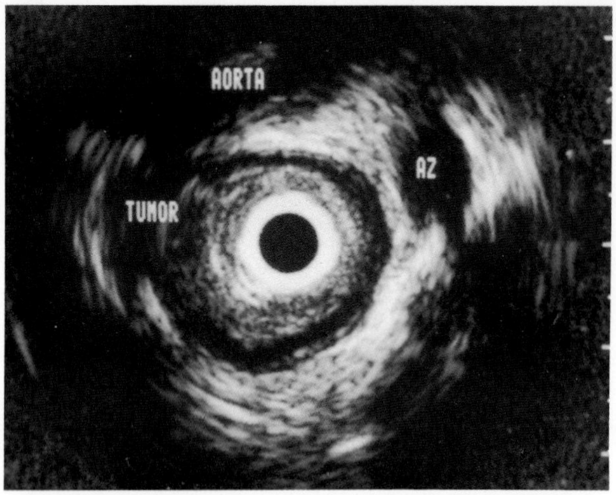

Fig. 2. Esophageal carcinoma. The patient presented with a stenosis which could not be passed with the echoendoscope; the probe was readily passed and showed semicircular thickening with irregular borders (TUMOR). The probe clearly demonstrated that the aorta (AORTA) and the azygos (AZ) were free of tumor.

atively small and flat endoscopically visible lesions such as early mucosal neoplasms and small intramural lesions.

Conversely, large intramural and extramural lesions such as leiomyomas and leiomyosarcomas may not be adequately imaged because of inadequate penetration of the ultrasound beam. Accordingly, the authors conclude that their probe would not be useful for screening large areas of tissue and would not achieve deep penetration into adjacent organs. It is therefore likely, they conclude, that a miniature ultrasound probe would have different indications and inherent advantages compared with dedicated ultrasound endoscopes; thus these instruments are complementary rather than competitive.

Miniature endoscopic ultrasound probes are at a very preliminary stage; they have limited penetration and very small acoustic field, and they need large-channel endoscopes which are not used in routine examination. However, the future of endosonography will no doubt rely on the development of a system which can couple all the advantages of both thin routine diagnostic endoscopes and reliable dedicated ultrasound endoscopes.

In the large bowel, endosonography has been performed to date only in the rectum, mainly with rigid instruments. Recently, a flexible ultrasound colonoscope has been developed (Olympus XCF-UM3, Olympus, Tokyo). It is a forward-viewing endoscope with a biopsy channel and a mechanical sector scanner at its tip which works with an ultrasound frequency of 7.5 or 12 MHz (rotation 10/s). The sonographic image approximates 320°. The focal distance is stated to be 30 mm, the lateral resolution 0.8 mm, and the axial resolution 0.4 mm. The rigid tip of the instrument is 40 mm long and has an outer diameter of 15 mm. A balloon attachment is also provided (Fig. 3). This new technique of colonoscopic ultrasonography is currently under evaluation, so that the results of clinical studies are still preliminary. They will be reported later in this chapter.

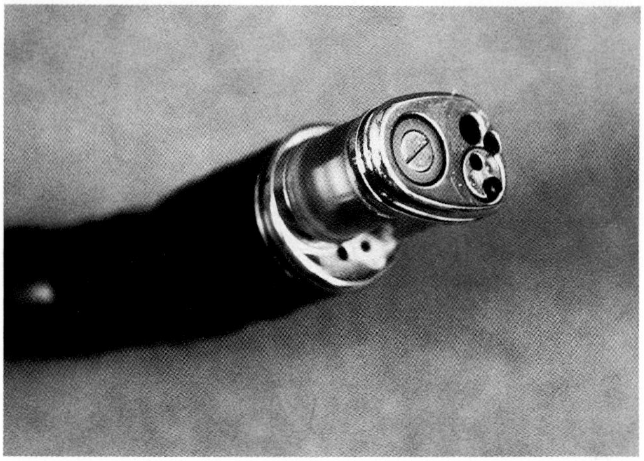

Fig. 3. Olympus forward-viewing colonoscope. The optical components and accessory channel are placed next to the ultrasound transducer. This reduces the sector scan from 360° to 320°.

New methods

Tanaka *et al.* [6•] report that in their series, endosonography of the upper gastrointestinal tract was unsuccessful in 15% of cases because of inaccurate guidance of the probe to small, shallow lesions, or because of difficulty in clearly demonstrating the surrounding layer structure and boundary of the lesion. In order to avoid these failures they injected saline solution into the submucosal layer of the esophagogastric wall. The ultrasonographic image of adjacent saline accurately guided the probe to the lesion. Moreover, injected saline enabled the mucosal layer to be distinguished from the muscularis propria surrounding the lesion and provided clear ultrasonographic imaging of the boundary between the lesion and the surrounding layer structure. In esophagogastric neoplasms, saline diffused and separated the tumor from the muscularis propria when the tumor in the submucosal layer merely touched the muscularis propria. On the other hand, saline did not separate the tumor from the muscularis propria when the tumor in the submucosa invaded the muscularis propria.

The failure rate of Tanaka *et al.* in upper gastrointestinal endosonography is markedly higher than that of most other authors. This is probably because they used front-viewing linear array equipment. In fact, using rotating radial scanners, orientation in the gut lumen is much easier to achieve. Moreover, the balloon or the water-filling techniques allow a good display of the esophagogastric wall layering in normal or disease situations. It seems that this new method can be used only in very limited cases, such as early cancers in which it is fundamental to know whether the muscularis propria is invaded.

The gut wall

It is widely accepted that a major advantage of endosonography is the ability to investigate the intestinal wall, which is made up of five ultrasonographic layers of different echogenicities. These layers are parallel to the mucosal surface in the image and are distinguished by their different echo texture and intensity. It has been definitively stated [7,8] (Fig. 4), that the correct interpretation of the ultrasonic image of the gastrointestinal wall is as follows:

- The first (innermost), hyperechoic, layer corresponds to the superficial mucosa;
- the second, hypoechoic, layer corresponds to the deep mucosa;
- the third, hyperechoic, layer corresponds to the submucosa plus the acoustic interface between the submucosa and the muscularis propria;
- the fourth, hypoechoic, layer corresponds to the muscularis propria minus the acoustic interface between the submucosa and the muscularis propria;
- the fifth hypoechoic, layer corresponds to the serosa and subserosal fat.

The endosonographic diagnosis of gastrointestinal diseases is made on the basis of changes in the layer structure of the gastrointestinal wall visualized by this technique. Neoplasms are detected as a disruption in the continuity of an ultrasound layer or by diffuse layer thickening. Infiltrating gastric neoplasms produce diffuse thickening of all ultrasound layers without causing layer disruption. A change in the echogenicity of the ultrasound layers is another sign of tissue pathology. Neoplasms are usually of intermediate echogenicity: less echogenic than the central layer, but more echogenic than the second and the fourth layers.

According to clinical endosonographic staging, tumor infiltration (T) of the first three layers is called 'T1' (cancer involving mucosa and submucosa), invasion of the fourth layer, T2 (cancer involving muscularis propria), invasion through the fifth layer, T3 (cancer penetrating the adventitia), and direct invasion of adjacent organs or structures, T4.

Esophageal carcinoma

The choice of treatment of esophageal carcinoma depends mainly on preoperative staging and grading of the tumor. Curative resection is possible in only a minority of patients, whereas several types of palliative treatment are available for patients with extensive tumor invasion. Survival after surgical resection is closely related to the stage or anatomical extent of this disease [9].

Most esophageal carcinomas in patients with subjective symptoms are advanced, and carcinomatous invasion to the surrounding tissues or lymph node metastasis is usually found at the time of surgery. Spread by way of the lymphatics is frequent, 30–45% even in early-stage carcinoma, and the prognosis in patients with lymph-node metastasis is poor. Moreover, the site of the metastatic lymph nodes is unpredictable because lymph drainage from the esophagus is extensive [10,11].

Conventional endoscopy allows direct visualization of the lesion, but this method is very inaccurate in assessing the tumor depth and extent. Computed tomography scanning has been accurate for local extension to mediastinal structures such as the trachea, aorta, and pericardium, and for distant metastasis to liver, lung, and adrenals. However, computed tomography has been disappointingly inaccurate in determining depth of wall penetration in early stages of disease and in assessing regional lymph node metastases [12,13]. Magnetic resonance imaging is

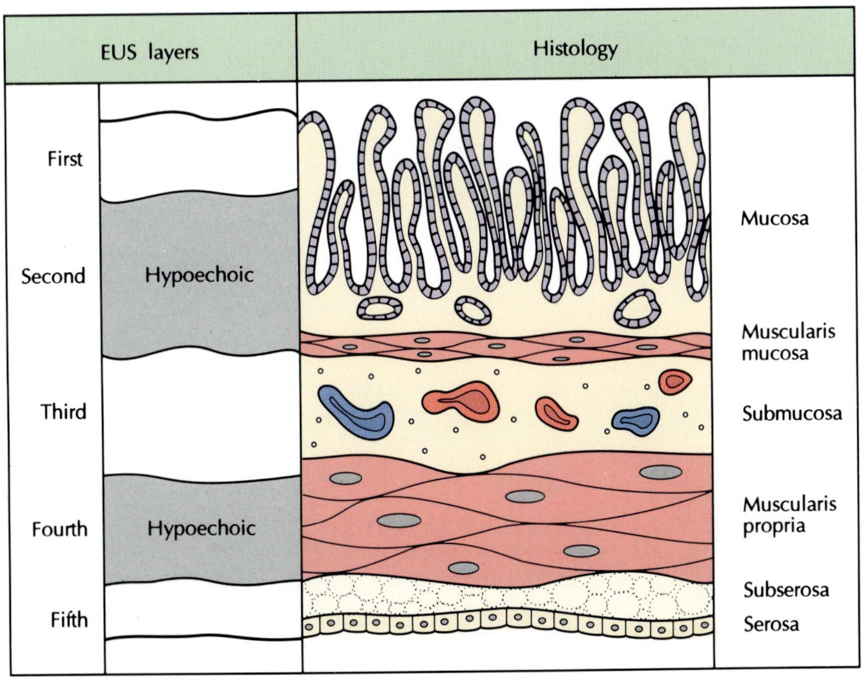

Fig. 4. A cross-section through the normal gastric wall showing the echographic layers corresponding to the structure of the gut wall.

in an early phase of evaluation, but seems to add little to computed tomography for staging esophageal cancer.

In an early report [14] endosonography was demonstrated to be superior to computed tomography in the evaluation of depth of tumor infiltration and in the assessment of regional lymph-node metastasis.

Four interesting papers appeared in 1990 on endosonography in the clinical staging of esophageal cancer [15•,16•,17••,18••]. In these studies the overall accuracy in assessing the depth of tumor infiltration was 89% [16•,17••], 90% [15•], and 92% [18••]. In the detection of regional lymph-node metastasis Tio reports an overall accuracy of 81% (sensitivity 95%, specificity 50%, positive and negative predictability 81 and 94%, respectively). Lightdale reported an accuracy of 88%, whereas Sugimachi found an accuracy of 93, 53 and 1% only, when the nodes were greater than 10, 5–9, and less than 5 mm in diameter, respectively. In staging distant metastases Tio reports an accuracy of 71% (sensitivity 60%, specificity 75%, positive and negative predictability 90 and 100%, respectively), and Lightdale's accuracy was 78%.

All these authors agree that endosonography represents a major advance in the clinical stage of esophageal cancer, whereas computed tomography is more accurate in staging distant metastasis. In fact in cases of severe stenosis, the instrument is unable to pass the tumor, and endosonographic staging of celiac axis lymph node metastases may be limited.

Another important indication for endosonography is the diagnosis of cancer recurrence at the surgical anastomosis. In fact, locally recurrent upper gastrointestinal cancer is a common and frustrating diagnostic challenge. Symptoms are indistinguishable from those due to postoperative sequences; endoscopy with biopsy can lead to a diagnosis only if recurrent cancer involves the mucosa or superficial submucosa. Lightdale and Botet [18••] have recently published their interesting experience with 40 patients whose esophageal or gastric cancer was resected and who were examined by means of endosonography. Twenty-four patients had recurrent cancer in the area of the surgical anastomosis (revealed by endoscopic biopsy in 16, repeat endoscopy in two, and surgery after negative endoscopy in six), and 16 patients had no anastomotic recurrence. With endosonography, locally recurrent cancer was correctly identified by nodular hypoechoic thickening at the anastomosis in 23 out of 24 patients, with one false-negative result; absence of anastomotic recurrence was correctly diagnosed in 13 out of 16, with three false-positive results. Sensitivity was 95%, specificity 80%, positive predictive accuracy 88% and negative predictive accuracy 92%. Furthermore, in six of their 23 patients with recurrent cancer diagnosed by endosonography, endoscopy with biopsy and brush cytology were negative.

Benign esophageal lesions

In a preliminary report [19] endosonography was proposed as a useful procedure in the diagnosis of achalasia. The authors affirmed that in five out of six patients with true achalasia a clear regular thickening of the muscular coat was found at the gastroesophageal junction (sensitivity 84%). It seems clear that their results were weighted by serious biases. First, a five-layer structure (as they saw) is very seldom seen in the esophagus, especially at the cardiac junction; on the contrary, because of focusing problems with the commercially available probes, only three layers are usually seen. The first, hyperechoic layer corresponds to the balloon-mucosa–submucosa and submucosa–muscularis propria interface together; the second, hypoechoic layer corresponds to the muscularis propria, and the third, hyperechoic layer to the outer border echo. Moreover, thickening of the layers, and particularly of the muscularis propria, is not steady but is strictly related to balloon inflation. In fact endosonography studies *in vivo* and *in vitro* [20] of normal esophagi have shown a sharp thickening of the muscularis propria at the cardiac level. Subsequent reports contradicted the results of Devière *et al.* [19], and stated that achalasia does not have a peculiar echopattern at endosonography [21,22•]. Recently Devière himself rectified his statement and reported a sensitivity of endosonography in achalasia of only 64% [23]. It therefore seems extremely difficult to diagnose achalasia by endosonography; however, it is generally agreed that it can be useful in distinguishing achalasia from pseudoachalasia in which there is tumor infiltration. In the early stage, tumors of the gastroesophageal junction may grow within the esophageal wall in such a way that mucosal integrity is maintained and biopsy forceps cannot reach them. From this type of tumor growth, a high-pressure zone in the gastroesophageal junction may result, and pathological patterns of esophageal motility that could imitate achalasia may develop [24] (Fig. 5).

Gastric disorders

Gastric carcinoma

The prognosis of patients with gastric carcinoma depends mainly on two variables: depth of tumor invasion and lymph node metastasis [25]. A strong correlation is also recognized between tumor size, depth of invasion, the stage of the disease, and the prognosis [26]. Prognosis after surgery in these diseases depends on the radicalness of the surgery. A sufficient distance from the tumor to the margins of resection is a prerequisite for radical surgery, as residual tumor at surgical margins reduces survival time [27,28].

Conventional endoscopy permits examination only of the stomach surface, and important data such as infiltration of the wall, local spread, and lymph-node involvement are not available with this technique.

Endosonography appears to be a useful tool for the preoperative staging of gastric cancer and lymphoma. It reveals not only tumor depth and local spread, but also the passage from a pathological to a normal wall. Moreover, endosonography is able to display the relationship

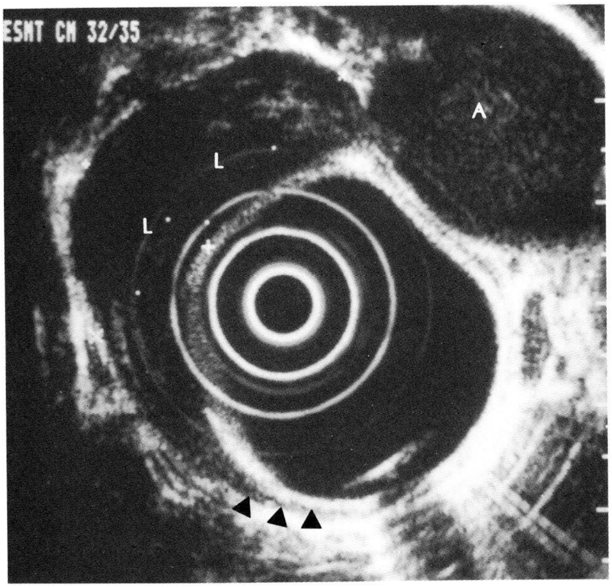

Fig. 5. Esophageal leiomyoma (L). Endoscopy showed bulging of the wall covered with normal mucosa. Endosonography shows a sharply delineated hypoechoic lesion originating from the muscular coat (arrows). A, aorta.

of the tumor to neighboring organs and early lymph-node metastasis [29].

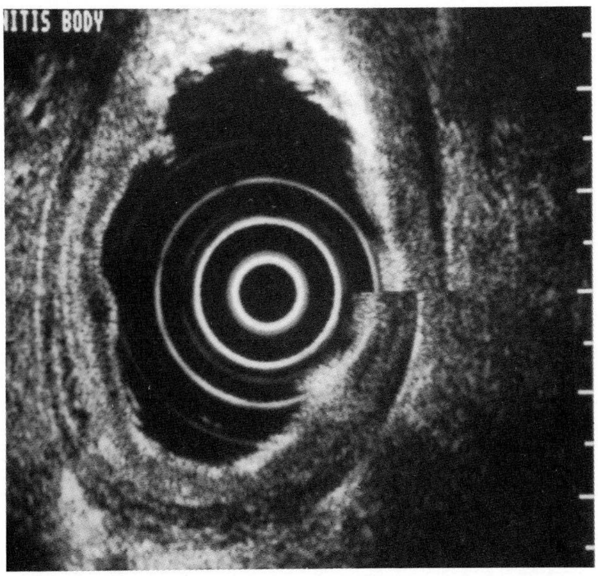

Fig. 6. Linitis plastica. Endosongraphy shows a diffuse gastric thickening of the second and third layers, while the fourth is intact. Histology of resected specimen showed a diffuse submucosal carcinoma.

Recent endosonography studies of this disease (cancer) demonstrated specific ultrasonographic features that allow correct diagnosis and staging in most patients [17] (Fig. 6). Tio *et al.* [17••] report that in staging tumor infiltration endosonography has an overall accuracy of 83% (79% for T1, 89% for T2, 84% for T3 and 78% for T4). Overstaging and understaging occurred in 9 and 8% of cases, respectively. In the detection of regional lymph-node metastasis, the authors report an overall diagnostic accuracy of 73%, with a sensitivity of 87%, a specificity of 48%, and a positive and negative predictive value of 74 and 68%, respectively. In detecting distant metastasis endosonography had an overall accuracy of 95% with a sensitivity of 43%, a specificity of 100%, and a positive and negative predictive value of 100 and 95%, respectively. This study shows that endosonography is accurate in the evaluation of the depth of tumor infiltration. The early stages of disease can be distinguished from advanced carcinomas according to images of intact or disrupted muscularis propria. Difficulties may arise in cases of inflammation around an early-stage carcinoma. Endosonography does not diagnose distant metastases accurately, particularly liver metastases or peritoneal dissemination, because of the limited penetration of ultrasound used with endosonography. Thus additional transcutaneous abdominal ultrasound or computed tomography are generally recommended for a complete staging of gastric cancer.

The endosonographic evaluation of regional lymph node in esophageal or gastric tumors is a problem far from being resolved. The sensitivity and negative predictive value of endosonography in metastatic lymph-node detection were low in our series and those of other authors [15•,18••,30], whereas Tio *et al.* [17••,31] reported better results in this field. This is probably because they used different criteria for detecting and assessing lymph-node involvement. In fact Tio *et al.* obtained a high sensitivity but a low specificity, which is the opposite of our results [32]. Moreover Tio *et al.* affirm that endosonography can discriminate between benign (inflammatory) and malignant nodes. Their conviction is not shared by other experts [33]. They state that irregularities of the outer margin or of the internal echo pattern of a lymph node are not reliable indicators of metastatic spread. Therefore, they recommend that endosonography should be used only to describe the size and location of the lymph nodes, and that the temptation of making histological diagnoses should be resisted.

Gastric ulcer

The ability to predict the healing or relapse of an ulcer has been a recurrent dream of gastroenterologists. With the development of endosonography, some Japanese authors believed that the endosonographic information on gastric ulcers might prove useful in differentiating between intractable ulcers and those that can be expected to heal [34].

Niwa *et al.* [35], in a complex and eccentric study, tried to assess this point again. They used endosonography to examine 16 patients with active, mainly recurrent gastric ulcers, before and after treatment, measuring the length and cross-sectional area of the ulcer on endosonographic photographs. From measurements of the contraction rate of the cross-sectional ulcer area during healing, they observed that the healed ulcers healed relatively rapidly and the non-healed cases had a poor contraction rate. They concluded that endosonography is useful for the quantitative estimation of histological changes associated with gastric ulcer healing. It seems clear that a healed ulcer has a more rapid contraction rate than a non-healed ulcer, and this fact has been known since the time of barium studies. Moreover, after a careful reading of this article it is difficult to understand the authors' message, and no clinical usefulness of endosonography in gastric ulcer management emerges from these results.

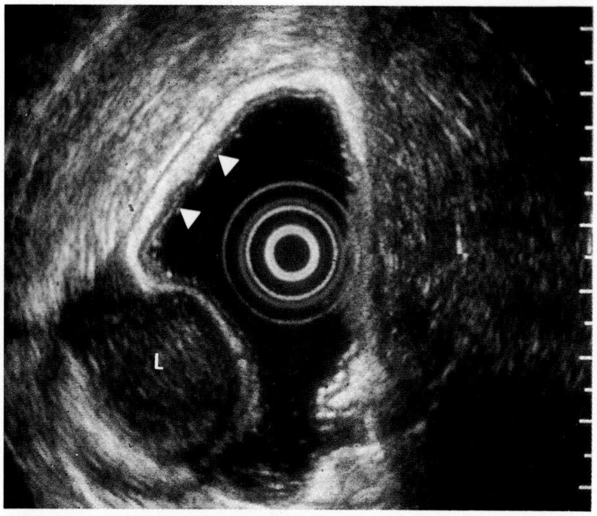

Fig. 7. Gastric leiomyoma (L). Endosonography shows a solid hypoechoic mass originating from the fourth layer, behind the first three layers which are normal (arrows).

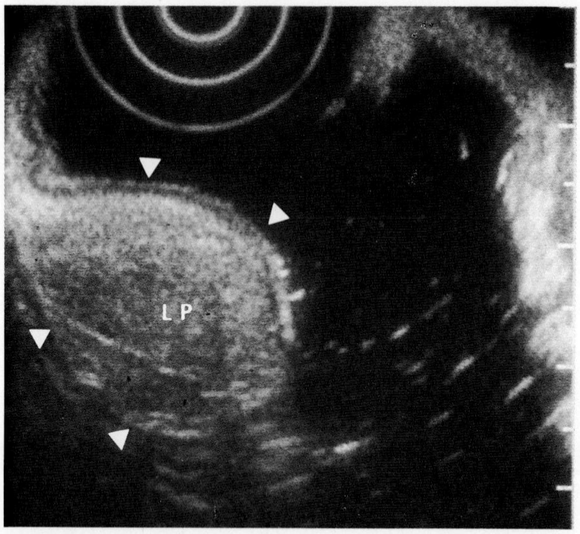

Fig. 8. Gastric lipoma (LP). Endosonography shows a solid hyperechoic mass originating from the third layer, behind the first two layers which, are normal (arrows). The fourth layer is clearly depicted and is normal (arrows).

Submucosal lesions

The diagnosis of a gastric submucosal tumor has always been difficult. An apparent tumor on the internal face of the gastric wall could be a benign or malignant pathological growth within the wall itself, or compression by a normal or diseased organ. Endoscopic examination is useful only in evaluating the luminal appearance of a non-epithelial neoplasm.

Multiple biopsy specimens are often inadequate for a histological diagnosis because of insufficient tissue depth and small sample size. Aggressive biopsy techniques may not be safe and are of no value in cases of extrinsic compression [36].

Endosonography can differentiate a submucosal tumor from extrinsic compression of the upper digestive tract and provides precise information about its site, size and nature (solid or liquid). The margins of the lesion can be defined more clearly than with other imaging modalities and, because of acoustic differences and identification of the wall layer of origin, the histological diagnosis is also suggested [37,38] (Figs 7 and 8).

The endosonographic appearance of a leiomyoma or a sarcoma of the stomach is that of a hypoechoic mass arising in the fourth, hypoechoic layer, interpreted as the muscularis propria coat [37,38]. Attempts to differentiate leiomyosarcoma from leiomyoma on the basis of size, shape and sonographic appearance have led to disappointing results.

Yasuda *et al.* [37,39•] report that a well-demarcated lesion located within the fourth, hypoechoic layer and with the same echodensity is likely to be a leiomyoma or a leiomyosarcoma. Unfortunately, the endosonographic appearance of these two lesions is the same, and the absence of distinguishing features makes differential diagnosis impossible. Aibe [40] reports that in malignant gastric submucosal tumor the wall layering is destroyed, although in benign gastric submucosal tumor the layers remain intact. Nakazawa *et al.* [41] state that irregularly shaped sonolucent areas within the tumor correspond to liquefaction necrosis; thus sonolucent areas may be indicative of leiomyosarcoma. Tio *et al.* [42•] point out that leiomyosarcoma or leiomyoblastoma are visualized at endosonography as a non-homogeneous hypoechoic large mass with sharply demarcated boundaries or irregular margins, occasionally associated with a central ulcer or fistulous tract. Although tumor size and the occurrence of gross necrosis or fistulization are suggestive of malignancy, only the biological behavior of the process (frank local infiltration or remote metastasis) defines true malignancy in those submucosal tumors. However, all these authors, in the absence of a histologic diagnosis, recommend a careful follow-up or, occasionally, surgical resection.

Recently, a new device for submucosal biopsy has been proposed with encouraging results: the Flexi-Temno guillotine needle biopsy [43] (Bauer, Italy). In cases of solid submucosal tumors discovered at endosonography, it allows a definitive diagnosis. Early malignancies can thus be detected when endosonography findings are not conclusive. In this way patients with asymptomatic solid gastric submucosal tumors can be regularly followed up and operated on only if necessary.

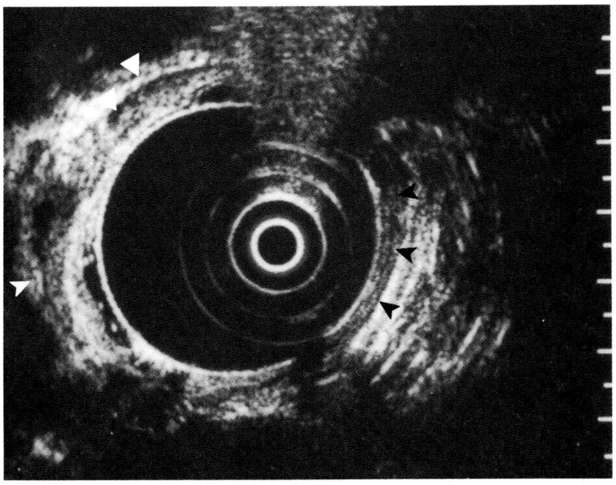

Fig. 9. Colonic cancer. The tumor mass invades the muscularis propria (white arrows). The black arrows indicate the normal wall.

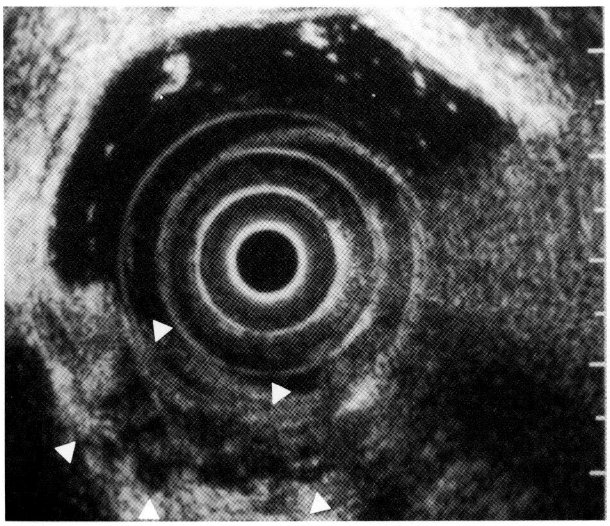

Fig. 10. Colonic angiodysplasia. Rounded echo-free venous-like structures are displayed in the colonic wall (arrows).

The lower gastrointestinal tract

In the large bowel, endosonography has been performed only in the rectum, mainly with rigid instruments, and a number of studies of cancer staging have been reported [44•].

Sophisticated treatments for rectal carcinoma, such as sphincter-preserving operations, preoperative irradiation or preoperative chemotherapy, require an exact pretherapy assessment of the tumor and its lymph node involvement. The possibility of performing a complete preoperative staging with assessment of the depth of tumor infiltration (90% of cases) and of lymph-node involvement (80% of cases) has an important clinical relevance. In advanced tumors the relationship of the tumor to adjacent organs can be assessed (97% of cases) and resectability can be estimated. In T4 and large T3 tumors preoperative irradiation can lead to a reduction of tumor mass and the success of irradiation can be assessed by endorectal ultrasonography. Patients with sonographically positive lymph-node involvement may enter adjuvant therapy studies. Moreover, endosonography may allow safer planning of local excision for villous adenomas and small rectal carcinomas.

Endorectal sonography opens up new perspectives for detecting and evaluating local recurrences after continence-saving rectal resections and local excisions for carcinomas [45]. The new flexible ultrasound colonoscope allows for the first time combined endoscopic and endosonographic evaluation of the entire large bowel. The normal colonic wall can be depicted in full detail in all regions of the large bowel including the ileocecal valve. Neighboring organs, including parts of the liver, pancreas, splenic vein, both kidneys, and urinary bladder, can be visualized endosonographically [46•] (Figs 9 and 10).

The major indication for colonic endosonography is the staging of large-bowel malignancy, even if it is uncertain whether local tumor staging by this technique will influence therapeutic decisions [47]. The depth of infiltration of a carcinoma was correctly predicted by this method by Rösch *et al.* [46]. In 21 out of 22 patients it was possible to differentiate benign from malignant growth.

Other potential applications of colonic ultrasonography that may be of clinical importance are the study of large sessile adenomas and follow-up examination of anastomoses after tumor resection. Rösch *et al.* [48••], in a series of seven large sessile colonic adenomas without evidence of carcinoma by biopsy, correctly identified with endosonography three lesions that proved to be malignant. Moreover, in 25 patients who had undergone resection of a colonic malignancy, endosonography was able to detect tumor recurrence at the anastomosis more often than endoscopy and computed tomography with only one false-positive result. As tumor recurrence often originates outside the bowel lumen, colonic endosonography may improve early detection of malignant disease in the follow-up of these patients.

Tio *et al.* [49•] reported that perianal fistulas and abscesses can be diagnosed sonographically. Trans-colorectal endosonography was carried out in 36 patients with Crohn's disease suspected clinically to have a fistula or abscesses. A hypoechoic or anechoic duct-like lesion immediately adjacent to the anorectal lumen compatible with a fistula was found in 32 patients. An anechoic cavity adjacent to or communicating with the fistula was visualized in 29 of the 36 patients. Endosonography appeared to be more accurate than fistulography because of the detailed visualization of the extent of the lesion, the ability to detect damage to the pelvic floor muscles or sphincters, and the accurate topographic mapping of the disease.

Whether endoscopic ultrasound of the colon will play a role in the diagnosis of chronic inflammatory bowel disease (for example, in differentiating between Crohn's disease and ulcerative colitis) remains to be seen. However, the ability of high-frequency endosonography to visualize mucosal lesions as well as alterations of various colonic wall layers seems to be promising (Fig. 9).

Pancreaticobiliary disease

Ultrasonography has contributed greatly to the diagnosis of pancreatic disease. Unfortunately, transabdominal scans of the pancreas are often limited by subcutaneous fat or digestive tract gas; moreover, tumors smaller than 2.0 cm are rarely detected, and carcinomas in the body and tail of the pancreas are difficult to recognize. Placement of a high-frequency ultrasound transducer close to the pancreas can provide images of the pancreatic parenchyma and adjacent retroperitoneal structures with a degree of resolution that is superior to conventional imaging methods. In theory it is possible to define lesions of 1.0 cm or less in diameter by endosonography.

Tio *et al.* [50] used endosonography for the preoperative TNM (1987) staging of tumors in 43 patients with pancreatic cancer and 24 patients with ampullary carcinomas. These results were correlated with the histologic findings of resected specimens. Early-stage tumors could be distinguished from advanced stages of cancer using endosonography. Detailed images of ductular and parenchymal abnormalities allowed distinction between pancreatic and ampullary carcinomas. The overall accuracy of endosonography in the assessment of tumor classification was 92 and 88% in pancreatic and ampullary carcinoma, respectively. The overall accuracy rate of endosonography in assessing regional lymph nodes of pancreatic carcinoma was 74% and the sensitivity was 91%, whereas the specificity was 42%. Positive and negative predictability were 75 and 71%, respectively. The overall accuracy rate of endosonography in assessing regional lymph nodes in ampullary carcinoma was 54%, the sensitivity was 80%, but the specificity was only 36%. The positive and negative predictability were 47 and 71%, respectively. Distant metastases were not revealed by this technique because of the limited depth of penetration of endosonography. Yasuda *et al.* [51] compared the ability of endosonography to detect pancreatic cancer with that of ultrasonography, computed tomography, endoscopic retrograde cholangiopancreatography (ERCP) and angiography in 50 patients. Endosonography detected all pancreatic tumors; the corresponding rates of positive diagnosis for the other imaging methods were as follows: ultrasonography 72%, ERCP 88%, computed tomography 78%, and angiography 75%. It must be emphasized that there were seven patients with cancer measuring less than 20 mm in diameter.

Bolondi *et al.* [52] described detection of neuroendocrine pancreatic tumors as small as 10 mm in diameter by endosonography. However, differentiation between neuroendocrine tumors and small pancreatic carcinomas by endosonography alone does not appear to be possible. Therefore, as concluded by Boyce and Sivak [53••], it can be confirmed that endosonography has a limited role in pancreatic disease. The technique may provide useful information when other imaging methods are inconclusive concerning the presence of a pancreatic lesion, especially when the suspected tumor is likely to be small. Although endosonography can be of assistance in differentiating focal areas of chronic pancreatitis from small pancreatic tumors, the accuracy of the procedure in these circumstances is uncertain. As current instruments and techniques make endosonography a relatively difficult procedure, it is not suitable for pancreatic cancer screening.

Endosonography has been put forward as a promising method for the diagnosis of extrahepatic cholestasis [54]. Amouyal *et al.* show, however, that the strategy for examination of patients in whom ultrasonography has not demonstrated the cause of the obstruction is still not defined. They state that transhepatic cholangiography and ERCP allow diagnosis of the cause, but can be dangerous. For these reasons endosonography, ultrasonography, and computed tomography were prospectively carried out in 52 patients with extrahepatic cholestasis. Endosonography was significantly more sensitive than ultrasonography or computed tomography (100% compared with 80 and 83%, respectively) in making a positive diagnosis of the obstruction. Endosonography was also significantly more accurate than ultrasonography or computed tomography (97% compared with 49 and 66%) in diagnosing the cause of the obstruction and more effective in the assessment of the locoregional spread of tumorous obstruction (75% compared with 38 and 62%). The authors conclude that endosonography is better than ultrasonography or computed tomography in the exploration of extrahepatic cholestasis. However, they suggest that ultrasonography should remain the initial screening procedure in cholestasis, and endosonography should immediately follow as the second choice in cases of negative ultrasound examination.

It is extremely difficult to accept this suggestion. Amouyal *et al.* [54] have compared apples with oranges, and thus their study has very little clinical relevance. In fact, ultrasonography was already the first choice in cholestasis, because it is a simple, safe and cheap method with a high success rate. Moreover, it is far from true that transhepatic and endoscopic cholangiography are associated with substantial morbidity and mortality, as stated by Amouyal *et al.* it would have been more useful to compare endosonography with ERCP, since they are both endoscopic procedures. At present, ERCP in good hands is a safe technique in the diagnosis of cholestasis. It is much quicker and cheaper than endosonography, and if necessary it can also be a therapeutic procedure. Endosonography should be performed only in cases where cholangiography has failed or when a precise assessment of the locoregional spread of tumors is needed.

Portal hypertension

A new and interesting application of endosonography is in the assessment of portal hypertension. We

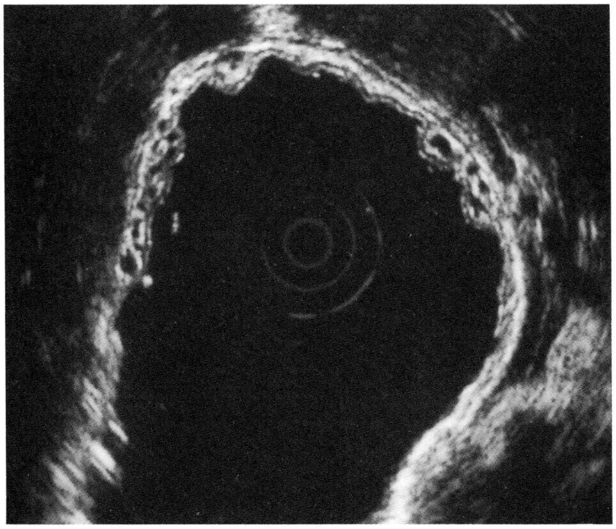

Fig. 11. Portal hypertensive gastropathy. Dilated veins within the gastric wall are displayed. Endoscopic findings of portal hypertensive gastropathy were present.

have demonstrated that endosonography can display esophageal and gastric varices and also periesophageal collateral veins [55]. More recently, Caletti *et al.* [56] have shown that endosonography can demonstrate small dilated vessels within the gastric wall in patients with portal hypertensive gastropathy (Fig. 11). As other vascular structures of the portal venous system are also displayed by endosonography, the authors undertook a prospective study [57••] to determine which structures of the portal venous system are visualized by this technique in patients with portal hypertension and in normal subjects. This study also attempted to correlate endoscopic and endosonographic findings in order to determine whether endosonography contributes to the assessment of portal hypertension.Endosonography was carried out in 40 patients with portal hypertension and in 48 control subjects. The azygos, splenic, mesenteric and portal veins were displayed in both groups. However, esophageal and gastric varices, periesophageal and perigastric collateral veins and submucosal gastric venules were displayed only in patients with portal hypertension. Endosonography was inferior to endoscopy in detecting and grading esophageal varices ($P < 0.0005$), but endosonography was superior in the detection of varices in the fundus of the stomach ($P < 0.0005$). Detection of periesophageal veins by endosonography increased with increasing diameter of esophageal varices at endoscopy (57% in grade 1, 89% in grade 2, 100% in grade 3) and there was a direct correlation between endoscopic grade and the diameter of the periesophageal collateral veins at endosonography. The diameter of the azygos vein by endosonography at its distal and proximal margins was significantly greater in patients with portal hypertension ($P < 0.001$); the endosonography diameter of the azygos vein was significantly larger with variceal grade 2 compared with grade 1 ($P < 0.02$ and $P < 0.01$, respectively). In portal hypertensive gastropathy, endoscopic and endosonography detection were coincident. No correlation was found between the presence of portal hypertensive gastropathy, endoscopic grade of esophageal varices, and detection of gastric varices at endosonography.

From this study it can be assumed that endosonography visualizes a large part of the portal venous system and is a safe, well-tolerated, relatively non-invasive technique that may be repeated several times. The azygos, splenic, mesenteric and portal veins are displayed in normal subjects and in patients with portal hypertension. However, esophageal and gastric varices, periesophageal and perigastric collateral veins and submucosal gastric venules are seen only with portal hypertension, as these structures are normally very small and undetectable by endosonography in normal subjects. The authors believe that endosonography will not supplant transabdominal ultrasonography in the study of the splenic, mesenteric and portal veins, because the latter technique is less time-consuming and provides better resolution. In fact, it is not possible to scan the entire course of the portal system by endosonography. The technique detected fundal varices with greater frequency than endoscopy. There was a direct correlation between variceal grade at endoscopy and the detection by endosonography of gastric varices. Endoscopy remains the most important technique for the assessment of esophageal varices. It is superior to endosonography for detection of varices and in grading of these vessels according to diameter and length. This may be in part attributable to problems with focusing the ultrasound display and to compression of the varices by the water-filled balloon at the ultrasound fiberscope. Furthermore, endosonography does not demonstrate the so-called red color signs that indicate an increased risk of bleeding. In our experience, endosonography has some value in confirming the eradication of esophageal varices and in assessing the patency and diameter of periesophageal collateral veins after a course of sclerotherapy.

In a retrospective study [58] endosonography was used to investigate the change in collateral circulation during non-shunting operations to clarify the inflow and outflow of esophageal varices. Devascularization procedures in the transabdominal approach can be more effectively carried out by using endosonography. Moreover, real-time observations of the intraoperative endosonography can confirm perfect devascularization.

It is clear from the literature that endosonography is a useful diagnostic technique with a wide range of present and potential applications. Further study is required to prove the overall value of the technique but it is predictable that endosonography will assume an important place in the future development of gastrointestinal endoscopy.

References and recommended reading

Papers of special interest, published within the annual period of review, have been highlighted as:

- • Of interest
- •• Of outstanding interest

1. DI MAGNO EP, BUXTON GL, REGAN PT, HATTERY RR, WILSON DA, SUAREZ JR, GREEN PS: **Ultrasonic Endoscopy.** *Lancet* 1980, 4:629–631.

2. STROHM WD, PHILLIP J, HAGENMÜLLER F, CLASSEN M: **Ultrasonic Tomography by Means of an Ultrasonic Fiberendoscope.** *Endoscopy* 1980, 12:241–244.

3. • NICKL NJ, COTTON PB: **Clinical Application of Endoscopic Ultrasonography.** *Am J Gastroenterol* 1990, **85**:675–682.
A complete review of the recent literature on endoscopic ultrasonography in approximately 2000 patients.

4. • RÖSCH T, CLASSEN M: **A New Ultrasonic Probe for Endosonographic Imaging of the Upper GI Tract.** *Endoscopy* 1990, 22:41–46.

5. • KIMMEY MB, MARTIN RW, SILVERSTEIN FE: **Endoscopic Ultrasound Probes.** *Gastrointest Endosc* 1990, **36**:S40–S46.
Two preliminary reports on prototype miniature (3.7 mm) endosonographic probes that can be used during conventional endoscopy, but only with endoscopes provided with large working channels.

6. • TANAKA M, BANDOU T, WATANABE A, SASAKI H: **A New Technique in Endoscopic Ultrasonography of the Upper Gastrointestinal Tract.** *Endoscopy* 1990, 22:221–225.
Injection of saline in the submucosa prior to performing endosonography for a better localization of the lesion and sonographic definition of the gastrointestinal wall structure.

7. BOLONDI L, CASANOVA P, SANTI V, CALETTI GC, BARBARA L, LABO G: **The Sonographic Appearance of the Normal Gastric Wall: an *In Vitro* Study.** *Ultrasound Med Biol* 1986, 12:991–998.

8. KIMMEY MB, MARTIN RW, HAGITT RC, WANG KY, FRANKLIN DW, SILVERSTEIN FE: **Histologic Correlates of Gastrointestinal Ultrasound Images.** *Gastroenterology* 1989 **96**:433–441.

9. SKINNER DB, FERGUSON MK, SORIANO A, LITTLE AG, STASZAK VM: **Selection of Operation for Esophageal Cancer Based on Staging.** *Ann Surg* 1986, **204**:391–401.

10. SUGIMACHI K, MATSUOKA H, OHNO S, MORI M: **Multifactorial Approach for Assessing the Prognosis of Clinical Oesophageal Carcinoma.** *Br J Surg* 1988, **75**:1115–1118.

11. SUGIMACHI K, OHNO S, MATSUDA H, MORI M, MATSUOKA H, KUWANO H: **Clinicopathological Study of Early-stage Esophageal Carcinoma.** *Surgery* 1989, **105**:706–710.

12. MOSS AA, SCHNYDER P, THOENI RF, MARGULIS AR: **Esophageal Carcinoma: Pretherapy Staging by Computed Tomography.** *AJR* 1981, **136**:1051–1056.

13. HALVORSEN RA, MAGRUDER-HABIB K, FOSTER WL JR, ROBERTS L JR, POSTLETHWAIT RW, THOMPSON W: **Esophageal Cancer Staging by CT: Long-term Follow-up Study.** *Radiology* 1986, **161**:147–151.

14. TIO COHEN P, COENE PP, UDDING J, DEN HARTOG JAGER FCA, TYTGAT GN: **Endosonography and Computed Tomography of Esophageal Carcinoma.** *Gastroenterology* 1989, **96**:1478–1486.

15. • SUGIMACHI K, OHNO S, FUJISHIMA H, KUWANO H, MORI M, MISAWA T: **Endoscopic Ultrasonographic Detection of Carcinomatous Invasion and of Lymph Nodes in the Thoracic Esophagus.** *Surgery* 1990, **107**:366–371.
A useful prospective correlation of endoscopic ultrasonography findings with intraoperative macroscopic and histopathologic findings of the resected specimens.

16. • TIO PL, COENE PPLO, DEN HARTOG JAGER FCA, TYTGAT GNJ: **Preoperative Classification of Esophageal Carcinoma by Endosonography.** *Hepatogastroenterology* 1990, **37**:376–381.

17. •• TIO TL, COENE PPLO, LUIKEN GJHM, TYTGAT GNJ: **Endosonography in the Clinical Staging of Esophagogastric Carcinoma.** *Gastrointest Endosc* 1990, **36**:S2–S10.
Two interesting and complete articles on the possibility of a preoperative TNM staging of esophagogastric malignancies by means of endoscopic ultrasonography.

18. •• LIGHTDALE CJ, BOTET JF: **Esophageal Carcinoma: Pre-operative Staging and Evaluation of Anastomotic Recurrence.** *Gastrointest Endosc* 1980, **36**:S11–S16.
A complete review of different techniques for staging esophageal cancer.

19. DEVIÉRE J, DUNHAM F, RICKAERT F, BOURGEOIS N, CREMER M: **Endoscopic Ultrasonography in Achalasia.** *Gastroenterology* 1989, **96**:1210–1213.

20. CALETTI GC, BOLONDI L, BARBARA L: **Instrumentation and Scanning Techniques.** In *Endoscopic Ultrasonography in Gastroenterology* edited by Kawai K. Tokyo-New York: Igaku-Shoin, 1988, pp 1–17.

21. PONSOT P, CHAUSSADE S, PALAZZO L, AMOUYAL P, GAUDRIC M, COUTURIER D, PAOLAGGI JA: **Endoscopic Ultrasonography in Achalasia.** *Gastroenterology* 1990, **98**:253.

22. • ZIEGLER K, SANFT C, FRIEDRICH M, GREGOR M, RIECKEN O: **Endosonographic Appearance of the Esophagus in Achalasia.** *Endoscopy* 1990, **22**:1–4.
A prospective study which clearly demonstrates that endosonography is not useful in the diagnosis of achalasia.

23. DEVIÉRE J, DUNHAM F, CREMER M: **Endoscopic Ultrasonography in Achalasia.** *Gastroenterology* 1990, **98**:253(Letter).

24. LORTAT-JAKOB JL, RICHARD CA, FEKETE F, TESTART J: **Cardiospasm and Esophageal Carcinoma: Report of 24 Cases.** *Surgery* 1969, **66**:969–975.

25. MARUYAMA K: **The Most Important Prognostic Factors for Gastric Cancer Patients. A Study Using Univariate and Multivariate Analyses.** *Scand J Gastroenterol* 1987, **22** (suppl 133):63–68.

26. SATO T, SAKAI Y, ISHIGURO S, FURUKAWA H: **Radiologic Manifestations of Early Gastric Lymphoma.** *AJR* 1986, **146**:513–517.

27. HORNIG D, HERMANEK P, GALL FP: **The Significance of the Extent of Proximal Margins of Clearance in Gastric Cancer Surgery.** *Scand J Gastroenterol* 1987, **22** (suppl 133):69–71.

28. KIRCHNER R, HENKE W, WITTEKIND C, FARTHMANN EH: **The Surgeon's Estimation of Radicality and Results of Pathologic Examination at Margins of Resection in Gastric Cancer Surgery.** *Scand J Gastroenterol* 1987, **22** (suppl 133):72–75.

29. ZIEGLER K, SANFT C, ZEITZ M, RIECKEN EO: **Preoperative Staging of Gastrointestinal Tumors by Endosonography.** *Surg Endosc* 1990, 4:154–160.

30. AIBE T, ITO T, IOSCIDA T, NOGUCHI T, OHTANI T, FUJI T, TAKEMOTO T: **Endoscopic Ultrasonography of Lymphnodes Surrounding the Upper GI Tract.** *Scand J Gastroenterol* 1986, **21** (suppl 123):164–169.

31. TIO TL, DEN HARTOG JAGER FCA, TYTGAT GNJ: **Endoscopic Ultrasonography of Non-Hodgkin Lymphoma of the Stomach.** *Gastroenterology* 1986, **91**:401–408.

32. CALETTI GC, BROCCHI E, GIBILARO M, FERRARI A, CARFAGNA L, BARBARA L: **Sensitivity Specificity and Predictive Value of Endoscopic Ultrasonography (EUS) in the Diagnosis and**

Assessment of Gastric Cancer. *Gastrointest Endosc* 1990, 36:194–195.

33. Dancyger H, Classen M: **Endoscopic Ultrasonography in Esophageal Diseases.** *Gastrointest Endosc* 1989, 35:220–225.

34. Nakazawa S, Segawa K, Yamanaka T: **Evaluation of Endoscopic Ultrasonography on the Histological Diagnosis of Gastric Ulcer.** *Curr Ther Res* 1986, 40:604–612.

35. Niwa Y, Nakazawa S, Yoshino J, Nakamura T, Ohashi S, Tsukamoto Y: **Quantification of Gastric Ulcer Healing by Endoscopic Ultrasonography.** *Gastrointest Endosc* 1990, 36:116–122.

36. Bjork JT: **Non Epithelial Neoplasms of the Stomach.** *Gastrointest Endosc* 1981, 23:162–163.

37. Yasuda K, Nakajima M, Yoshida S, Kiyota K, Kawai K: **The Diagnosis of Submucosal Tumors of the Stomach by Endoscopic Ultrasonography.** *Gastrointest Endosc* 1989, 35:10–15.

38. Caletti GC, Zani L, Bolondi L, Brocchi E, Rollo V, Barbara L: **Endoscopic Ultrasonography in the Diagnosis of Gastric Submucosal Tumor.** *Gastrointest Endosc* 1989, 35:413–418.

39. • Yasuda K, Cho E, Nakajima M, Kawai K: **Diagnosis of Submucosal Lesions of the Upper Gastrointestinal Tract by Endoscopic Ultrasonography.** *Gastrointest Endosc* 1990, 36:S17–S20.

A wide experience of miscellaneous submucosal lesions diagnosed by endosonography is described.

40. Aibe T, Takemoto T: **Benign Lesions of Gastrointestinal Tract.** In *Endoscopic Ultrasonography in Gastroenterology* edited by Kawai K. Tokyo, New York: Igaku-Shoin, 1988, pp 44–55.

41. Nakazawa S, Yoshino J, Nakamura T, Yamanaka T, Hase S, Kojima Y, Ohasi S, Niwa Y: **Endoscopic Ultrasonography of Gastric Myogenic Tumor. A Comparative Study Between Histology and Ultrasonography.** *J Ultrasound Med* 1989, 8:353–359.

42. • Tio TL, Tytgat GNJ, Den Hartog Jager FCA: **Endoscopic Ultrasonography for the Evaluation of Smooth Muscle Tumors in the Upper Gastrointestinal Tract: An Experience with 42 Cases.** *Gastrointest Endosc* 1990, 36:342–350.

Superiority of endosonography to other imaging techniques in the detection, staging, and follow-up of submucosal smooth muscle tumors is described.

43. Caletti GC, Guillini S, Brocchi E, Boccia S, Gibilaro M, Cantarini D, Ferrari A, Carfagna L, Barbara L: **Endoscopic Ultrasonography (EUS) with the Guillotine Needle Biopsy in the Diagnosis of Gastric Submucosal Tumors (GSMT).** *Gastrointest Endosc* 1990, 36:222.

44. • Glaser F, Schlag P, Herfarth Ch: **Endorectal Ultrasonography for the Assessment of Invasion of Rectal Tumours and Lymphnode Involvement.** *Br J Surg* 1990, 77:883–887.

A complete work on rectal cancer endosonographic staging by means of blind rigid, radial scanner.

45. Heintz A, Junginger Th, Böttger Th, Kreitner KF: **Endosonography for Diagnosis of Locoregional Recurrence After Anterior Rectal Dissection. Case Report.** *Coloproctology* 1990, 12:138–141.

46. • Rösch Th, Lorenz R, Suchy R, Dancygier H, Classen M: **Colonic Endoscopic Ultrasonography: First Results of a New Technique.** *Gastrointest Endosc* 1990, 36:382–386.

Detailed instructions on the technique of echocolonoscopy.

47. Shimizu S, Tada M, Kawai K: **Use of Endoscopic Ultrasonography for the Diagnosis of Colorectal Tumors.** *Endoscopy* 1990, 22:31–34.

48. •• Rösch Th, Lorenz R, Classen M: **Endoscopic Ultrasonography in the Evaluation of Colon and Rectal Disease.** *Gastrointest Endosc* 1990, 36:S33–S39.

A fundamental work on the indications and results of this technique in rectal and colonic disease.

49. • Tio TL, Mulder CJJ, Wijers OB, Sars PRA, Tytgat GNJ: **Endosonography of Peri-anal and Peri-colorectal Fistula and/or Abscess in Crohn's Disease.** *Gastrointest Endosc* 1990, 36:331–336.

An interesting new application of endosonography.

50. Tio TL, Tytgat GNJ, Cikot RJLM, Houthoff HJ, Sars PRA: **Ampullopancreatic Carcinoma: Preoperative TNM Classification with Endosonography.** *Radiology* 1990, 175:455–461.

51. Yasuda K, Mukai H, Fujimoto S, Nakajima M, Kawai K: **The Diagnosis of Pancreatic Cancer by Endoscopic Ultrasonography.** *Gastrointest Endosc* 1988, 34:1–8.

52. Bolondi L, Li Bassi S, Gaiani S, Campione O, Marrano D, Barbara L: **Diagnosis of Islet Cell Tumor by Means of Endoscopic Ultrasonography.** *J Clin Gastroenterol* 1990, 12:218–221.

53. •• Boyce GA, Sivak MV: **Endoscopic Ultrasonography in the Diagnosis of Pancreatic Tumors.** *Gastrointest Endosc* 1990, 36:S28–S32.

A complete review of the literature on the subject and a good guide to the technique of endosonographic scanning of the pancreas.

54. Amouyal P, Palazzo L, Amouyal G, Ponsot Ph, Mompoint D, Vilgrain V, Gayet B, Fléjou JF, Paolaggi JA: **Endosonography: Promising Method for Diagnosis of Extrahepatic Cholestasis.** *Lancet* 1989, 334:1195–1198.

55. Caletti GC, Bolondi L, Zani L, Brocchi E, Guizzardi G, Labo' G: **Detection of Portal Hypertension and Esophageal Varices by Means of Endoscopic Ultrasonography.** *Scand J Gastroenterol* 1986, 21 (suppl 123):74–77.

56. Caletti GC, Brocchi E, Zani L, Barbara L: **The Important Role of EUS in the Assessment of Patients with Portal Hypertension.** *Gastrointest Endosc* 1988, 34:154–155.

57. •• Caletti GC, Brocchi E, Baraldini M, Ferrari A, Gibilaro M, Barbara L: **Assessment of Portal Hypertension by Endoscopic Ultrasonography.** *Gastrointest Endosc* 1990, 36:S21–S27.

An important evaluation of the potential role of endosonography in the study of the portal venous system.

58. Nakamura H, Endo M, Shimojuu K, Goseki N, Inoue H: **Esophageal Varices Evaluated by Endoscopic Ultrasonography: Observation of Collateral Circulation During Non Shunting Operations.** *Surg Endosc* 1990, 4:69–75.

Endoscopy and pancreatic disease

G.A. Lehman and S. Sherman

Recent publications on prevention of post-endoscopic retrograde cholangiopancreatography (ERCP)-related pancreatitis, stenting for pancreatic disease, management of pancreatic calculi, and the relationship of gallstones to pancreatitis highlight this year's progress in reference to endoscopy and pancreatic disease.

Introduction

Recent reports and research continue to add building blocks to our overall knowledge of pancreatic physiology and pathophysiology. Although major gaps remain in our understanding and treatment of such diseases as pancreatic cancer, necrotizing pancreatitis, and chronic pancreatitis, progress is being made in these and other areas. Despite being still in their infancy, endoscopic therapies of pancreatic diseases are emerging. Pancreatoscopy, sphincter of Oddi manometry and new findings at pancreatography continue to stir great interest. Endoscopic pancreatic techniques can be expected to play increasing roles in patient care and research.

Pancreatography

There are many lessons to be learned from basic ductography. Morris *et al.* [1] reported a case of pseudo-double duct sign. This may be seen when the cystic duct take-off is very low (near the major papilla) and is involved with malignant obstruction near the take-off. The poorly filled cystic duct simulates an obstructed main pancreatic duct. Selective cannulation and contrast visualization of all ducts involved (including the pancreatic duct) will clarify the anatomy.

Gallstones are a well recognized cause of acute pancreatitis but are generally not thought to cause chronic pancreatitis. Misra *et al.* [2•] retrospectively evaluated the endoscopic retrograde cholangiopancreatography (ERCP) findings in 50 symptomatic patients with gallstone disease (current stones or history of cholecystectomy for stones) and compared them with 33 patients with jaundice from viral hepatitis. Patients with a history of alcohol consumption or other risk factors for pancreatitis were excluded. No patient had a clinical history of pancreatitis. Overall, gallstone patients had a 48% incidence of ductal abnormalities indicative of chronic pancreatitis (by Cambridge criteria). This contrasted with a 6% abnormality rate in the control group ($P < 0.001$). Pancreatitis severity was mild in all control patients. In gallstone patients, severity was mild in 32%, moderate in 10% and severe in 6% of cases. Overall, the data suggest that gallstone disease can indeed cause irreversible changes in the pancreatic ductal system. This study does not determine whether such ductal changes are clinically significant (i.e. cause pain) or are just scars from prior injury. These data need further confirmation in populations who do not live in Third World conditions.

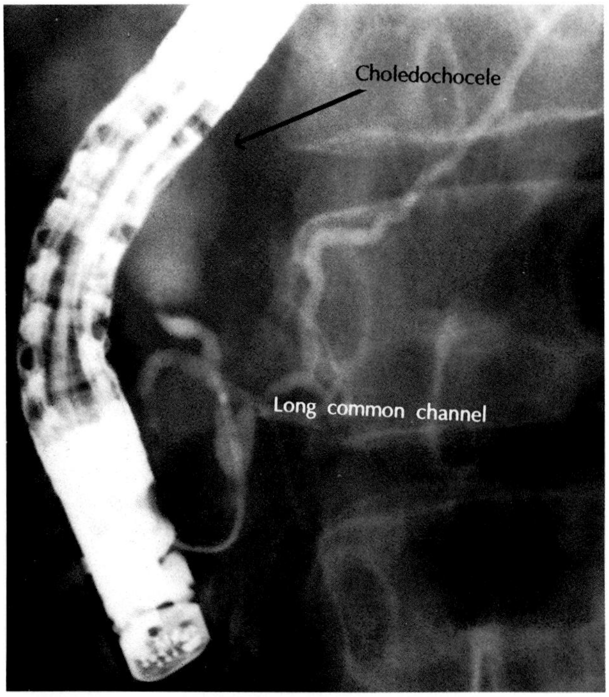

Fig. 1. Anomalous pancreatobiliary ductal union (long common channel) with choledochocele (type I).

Anomalous pancreatobiliary ductal union is a recognized congenital abnormality occurring in approximately 3% of patients. Misra and Dwivedi [3•] reviewed this entity and other variations of normal pancreatobiliary ductal anatomy. This excellent review reminds us that anomalous pancreatobiliary ductal union is associated with choledochoceles (Fig.1) and carcinomas of the gallbladder and bile duct. Such patients by definition have a common channel that is 15 mm or longer, with the pancreatobiliary ductal junction located outside the duodenal wall and not controlled by separate pancreatobiliary sphincters. This permits reflux of bile into the pancreatic duct and pancreatic juice reflux into the common bile duct. The latter is thought to be important in dissolving microcalculi at the expense of irritating bile duct mucosa. Separate main pancreatic duct and bile duct openings into the duodenum (i.e. no common channel) are

© Current Science Ltd ISBN 1-870485-32-7 ISSN 0952-6293

associated with a lower incidence of gallstone disease and lower incidence of gallstone pancreatitis but a higher incidence of chronic pancreatitis (especially alcoholic pancreatitis). It has been observed that a separate opening is more commonly associated with hyperplasia of pancreatic duct epithelium, which may help to cause obstruction to flow of juice.

A variety of other congenital anomalies of the pancreas are occasionally found at ERCP and reported because of their unusual nature. Many findings, such as ectopic pancreas [4], bifid dorsal duct [5], and partial agenesis [6] are generally of no clinical significance *per se*, but must be recognized to avoid confusion with malignancy or other serious disease (Fig. 2).

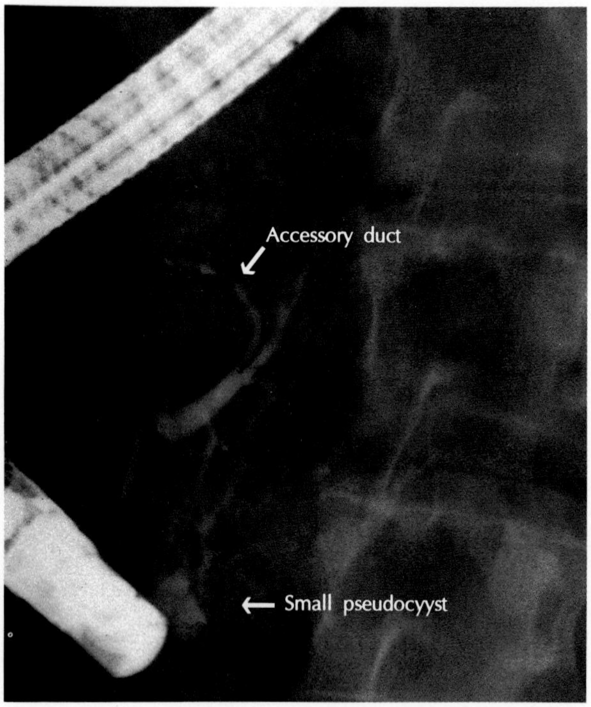

Fig. 2. This pancreatogram injected via the major papilla shows congenital absence of the body and tail of pancreas. Diffuse parenchymal calcifications are present (also evident prior to contrast injection). A small pseudocyst is seen in the uncinate process. A poorly developed accessory duct which fails to communicate with the duodenum is seen. The minor papilla was not patent by endoscopic probing and it emitted no juice after secretin stimulation. Computed tomography scan confirmed the above.

Pancreatic neoplasms

It is common clinical practice to manage patients with presumed pancreatic cancer (e.g. a pancreatic mass on computed tomography scan and/or ductal obstruction by ERCP) without histologic confirmation. In particular, in very elderly patients, tissue confirmation is generally considered unnecessary. In more surgically fit patients or in those in whom there is some confusion in the diagnosis, prompt histologic confirmation is essential or highly desirable. In pancreatic cancers causing biliary obstruction, Scudera *et al.* [7•] reported that brush cytology of the common bile duct was positive for malignant cells in five out of 10 cases. Foutch *et al.* [8•] similarly reported positive brushings in three out of five patients. Two larger abstracted series [9,10] with a total of 44 patients showed a bile duct brush cytology sensitivity in pancreatic cancer patients of only 36%. Gagnon *et al.* [9] added bile duct forceps biopsies to brush cytology in selected cases but found that diagnostic sensitivity rose from 36 to only 40%. It appears that many pancreatic neoplasms compress rather than invade the bile duct.

For pancreatic neoplasms, especially those not compressing the biliary tree, obtaining cytology and/or biopsy specimens directly from the pancreatic duct may be more appropriate. More than a decade ago Osnes *et al.* [11] obtained intrapancreatic duct cytology specimens in 29 pancreatic cancer patients in whom the pancreatic duct could be deeply cannulated. Positive cytology was found in 21 patients (63%). In approximately one-half of patients the brush could not be passed to the area of interest. Further studies are needed to determine whether the use of more modern cytology brush techniques (guidewire tipped or over the guidewire method) or the addition of intraductal forceps biopsy (with new malleable forceps which facilitate cannulation) in the pancreas will improve diagnostic yields. Although the safety of intrapancreatic brushings and biopsies needs to be established in larger series, early reports have not indicated complications.

Fine needle aspiration remains the best minimally invasive method to obtain pancreatic cytology. Sensitivities exceed 90% in many series. Fine needle aspiration is more difficult to perform in patients without an obvious pancreatic mass by computed tomography or ultrasound. Boustiere *et al.* [12] reported the use of simultaneous pancreatography to guide fine needle aspiration in patients with small pancreatic cancers. Nine out of 10 cancers were confirmed by this means.

Various malignant tumors, benign tumors, and inflammatory conditions of the pancreas may cause focal ERCP abnormalities that raise clinical concern about malignancy. Two recent reports [13,14] review the ERCP findings in islet cell tumors of the pancreas. These reports emphasize that benign or malignant islet cell tumors tend to cause low-grade, main or secondary pancreatic duct narrowing or displacement rather than the high-grade obstruction and gross ductal irregularities commonly seen with standard ductal origin adenocarcinomas. Such ductal distortion may mimic chronic pancreatitis. Ogawa *et al.* [13] report on an interesting technique of staging such tumors that involved placement of a balloon catheter in the distal main pancreatic duct and withdrawing the ERCP endoscope. Later, pancreatic ductography combined with portal venography was performed to evaluate tumor extension and resectability.

Lymphoma involvement of the pancreas was reviewed by Satake *et al.* [15], who described one new case and summarized 16 cases from the world literature. Moreira *et al.* [16] added an additional case. The pancreas may be primarily or secondarily involved with lymphoma. Computed tomography findings of large adjacent lymph nodes and a large pancreatic mass without vessel encasement serve to heighten suspicion toward lymphoma and away from carcinoma. The ERCP findings vary from an otherwise normal ductogram that only shows displacement to non-specific ductal irregularities, suggesting chronic pancreatitis, to frank ductal obstruction.

Cystic neoplasms of the pancreas constitute 5–15% of cystic lesions of the pancreas and 5% of pancreatic neoplasms. Pinson *et al.* [17] reported on 11 such cystic neoplasms, all of which caused variable degrees of focal narrowing of the main pancreatic duct at ERCP. None of these patients showed cyst communication with the duct however. Computed tomography scan features such as multiple honeycomb cysts, thick-walled cysts, central stellate calcification or associated mass suggested the correct neoplastic diagnosis. Mucinous cystadenomas or mucinous cystadenocarcinomas usually have a distinct ERCP appearance with a gaping papillary orifice emitting gelatinous mucus [18]. Dabezies *et al.* [19] reported on a typical case that communicated with the ductal system and showed focal saccular ductal dilatation at ERCP. Unfortunately, the ductograms do not differentiate the benign from the malignant cystic neoplasms [20]. Kohler *et al.* [21] used intraductal pancreatoscopy and forceps biopsy to diagnose a single case of cystadenoma. Nishida *et al.* [22] reported that percutaneous needle aspiration and CA 19-9 analysis of fluid clearly differentiated two cystadenocarcinoma patients from two cystadenoma patients, whereas cytology was non-diagnostic. Larger series evaluating the use of endoscopic intraductal cytology and biopsy for diagnosing such tumors are awaited.

Bastid *et al.* [23] recently summarized four cases of mucinous ductal ectasia of the pancreas. This condition with ductographic focal side-branch ectasia presented clinically as pancreatitis. Computed tomography scan showed clusters of tiny cystic structures that were consistent with small pseudocysts or dilatated ductules. The ERCP most typically showed a cluster of tiny cysts filling from side branches with or without intraductal mucus (filling defects). Two out of nine resected specimens showed focal adenocarcinoma. Benign lesions on resection showed a large number of mucus secreting cells in the cyst lining. Overall, this is thought to be a premalignant lesion, the cause of which is unknown.

Villous adenoma of the main pancreatic duct is another rare tumor that may present with abdominal pain or pancreatitis. Payan *et al.* [24] reviewed 10 cases from the world literature and added two more of their own. The ERCP diagnosis typically showed a filling defect in the distal duct with dilatation upstream. Ten out of 12 neoplasms were located in the head of the pancreas. Resection of the head of the pancreas is generally recommended, although 11 out of 12 neoplasms were benign.

ERCP findings in the above benign, premalignant, and malignant pathologic states are unfortunately often non-specific. Findings may be highly or only minimally suggestive of neoplasm. Studies are needed to determine whether ERCP associated techniques such as brush cytology, intraductal forceps biopsy, or intraductal juice aspiration for cytology, CEA, or CA 19-9 [25•] will be of value for identifying these less common neoplasms. In these difficult-to-diagnose cases, the ERCP may only be one small piece of the puzzle. The clinician should take full advantage of other diagnostic pancreatic tests. As many of the above neoplasms have a favorable course when appropriately treated by chemotherapy or resective surgery, the clinician must maintain a high index of suspicion so as not to overlook them.

Although debate continues about whether standard ductal adenocarcinoma of the pancreas represents a hopeless situation [26,27], Harrison and Hamilton [28] reported on the use of pancreatic duct stenting to relieve duct obstruction from carcinoma in the head of the pancreas. Placement of progressively larger stents (7, 8 and 10 French [F]) over a 5-month period appeared to relieve the patient's pain significantly. Such stents can probably be placed in only a small percentage of pancreatic cancers as gross disruption of the ductal system is often prohibitive to guidewire passage or stent placement. Also, intractable pain may occur from peripancreatic invasion without main duct obstruction. Nevertheless, when possible, this may offer the patient pain (and/or steatorrhea) palliation. Combining such techniques with intraductal radiation needs further evaluation.

Separation of pancreatic cancer patients from those with chronic pancreatitis can be problematic. Shemesh *et al.* [29] reviewed 10 patients with ductal adenocarcinomas coexisting with chronic pancreatitis and compared the ductography findings with 45 chronic pancreatitis patients observed during the same interval. Although not fully specific, the main feature that separated the cancer patients was high-grade localized irregularity and narrowing of the main duct and associated side branches out of portion to that diffusely found in other portions of the gland. Computed tomography scan or ultrasound detected a pancreatic mass in only 50% (50% false-negative rate) of cancer patients and demonstrated a mass in 13% of pancreatitis patients (13% false-positive rate for malignancy).

Flow cytometry has been used to characterize many neoplasms. Eskelinen *et al.* [30] reviewed paraffin block specimens from 46 patients with pancreatic cancer. In contrast to diploid tumors, aneuploid tumors showed a much poorer prognosis from multiple view points including more frequent (79 versus 36%) lymph-node involvement and poorer (0 versus 32%) 1 year survival. Whether flow cytometry evaluation of endoscopic specimens can give clinically helpful information remains to be evaluated.

Pancreatoscopy

Miniaturization of endoscopes continues to develop. The experience with daughterscope (generally 1–4 mm in diameter) evaluation of the pancreas has been limited. Foerster *et al.* [31] published their experience with the tiniest of pancreatoscopes. This instrument, measuring 0.5 mm in diameter, was passed through a standard 5 F catheter that had previously been passed up to the pancreatic tail. Passive viewing was performed as the catheter was withdrawn from the pancreatic tail. If areas of interest were observed, the pancreatoscope was withdrawn and tiny biopsy forceps, 1.5 mm in shaft diameter, were passed through the catheter and the duct biopsied. Specimens contained mostly ductal elements, but acinar cells were present in 14–23% of cases. Such miniscopes remain very fragile and costly for their current limited application. Whether or not intraductal viewing (with such tiny instruments that have limited resolution) will add significantly to current techniques of ductography and fluoroscopy-guided intraductal cytology or biopsy remains to be defined.

Pancreas divisum

Pancreas divisum occurs in approximately 7% of the general population. In such patients, the majority of the pancreatic juice must drain through a relatively small minor papilla. In a few such patients, the narrowing appears to be sufficiently small to cause relative pancreatic ductal obstruction.

The minor papilla has until recently served as an impediment to obtaining ductography at ERCP. Delhaye *et al.* [32] reported a large series with a minor papilla cannulation success rate of 80–90%. Benage *et al.* [33•] reported on a series of 120 dorsal ductograms in such patients. Overall, 30% of these patients had an abnormal dorsal ductogram generally consisting of variants of chronic pancreatitis. Of 43 patients presenting with clinical pancreatitis documented by an elevated pancreatic serum enzyme level, 53% had abnormal dorsal ductograms. When patients presented with pancreatobiliary pain only (with no enzyme abnormality), only 13% had abnormal dorsal ductograms. Similarly, 6% of biliary disease patients had dorsal duct abnormalities. Five out of six (83%) patients with mass lesions seen on computed tomography scan had abnormal dorsal ductograms; three out of five of which were cancers. With use of short, blunted, 23 or 25 gauge needle-tipped tapered catheters (with or without use of secretin stimulation to assist minor papilla orifice identification) cannulation rates of 90% should be readily achievable by experienced endoscopists.

Warshaw *et al.* [34••] updated their large series of 88 pancreas divisum patients treated by minor papilla sphincteroplasty. Overall, they reported a good, fair, or poor outcome in 74, 8, and 18% of patients, respectively, who presented with attacks of pain consistent with acute pancreatitis. Patients who presented with chronic pain did less well, having 38, 18, and 44% good, fair, and poor surgical outcomes, respectively. These authors used the technique of intraoperative lacrimal probe evaluation of minor papilla patency. The orifice was considered stenotic when it resisted passage of a 0.75 mm diameter probe. Only six out of 22 patients without minor papilla stenosis (27%) had a good or fair outcome from surgical sphincteroplasty. This contrasted ($P < 0.001$) with an 85% good or fair response in 66 patients who had documented stenosis. These authors continue to report that the secretin stimulated ultrasound test will predict surgical results. Ninety-two per cent of patients with a positive secretin ultrasound test had a good or fair response, whereas only 40% of those with a negative test had a beneficial outcome from surgery ($P < 0.001$). These data indicate that patient selection strongly influences outcome.

Initial series reporting use of endoscopic sphincterotomy for minor papilla stenosis in pancreas divisum are reviewed in Fig. 3. Improvement in frequency and/or severity of pancreatitis or pain occurred in approximately two-thirds of patients with relatively short follow-up. In our own series (IUMC), patients presenting with documented pancreatitis were more likely to benefit from sphincterotomy (75 versus 35%) than those presenting with chronic pain without abnormal serum enzymes.

Lans *et al.* [35••] recently abstracted their results of a randomized controlled trial of long-term (12 months) stenting of the minor papilla in patients with recurrent pancreatitis. Follow-up of stented patients continued for at least 12 months after stent removal. Stented patients had fewer hospitalizations and episodes of pancreatitis ($P < 0.05$) and were more frequently clinically judged to be improved (90 versus 10% for controls).

Year	Author	No of patients n	Patients improved	Follow-up (months)
1978	Cotton	1	100%	3
1984	Cotton	5	20%	7
1986	Soehendra	6	83%	6
1986	Liguory	11	63%	12–30
1990	IUMC	41	66%	6–60

IUMC, Indiana University Medical Center

Fig. 3. Endoscopic sphincterotomy of the minor papilla for symptomatic pancreas divisum.

Factors which increase risk for pancreatitis	Techniques to possibly avoid/limit pancreatitis
1. Sphincter of Oddi disease or variant anatomy as manifested by: a. abnormal manometry b. prolonged contrast drainage time c. dilated pancreatic duct d. difficult cannulation	1. Limit dye volume, rate of injection, number of injections and cannulation time. Limit intraductal manometry time in pancreas to less than 3 min. Aspirate water during manometry. Stent pancreatic duct before or after extensive manipulation
2. Endoscopic sphincterotomy performed in setting of non-dilated bile duct	2. Limit coagulation current near pancreatic orifice. Also see no. 1 above.
3. History of prior post-ERCP pancreatitis	3. Use low osmolarity and/or non-ionic contrast media, Also see no. 1 above
4. Recent or current pancreatitis of any cause	4. Wait 1–2 weeks after pancreatitis resolution if possible. Also see no. 1 and no. 3 above
5. Pseudocyst	5. Prophylactic antibioticst. Limit contrast media filling of pseudocys. Schedule pseudocyst decompression within 24 hours
6. Pancreatic duct stricture	6. See no. 5 above.
7. History of contrast media reaction	7. Premedicate with steroids (2 doses. Give) antihistamines. See no. 3 above.

Patient factors which increase the risk of post-procedure pancreatitis and techniques to avoid or limit this complication. Modified from Sherman S, Lehman GA. Complications of ERCP and endoscopic sphincterotomy-management and prevention. In: Barkin *Advanced Therapeutic Endoscopy* edited by Barkin JS, O'Pehlan CA. New York: Raven Press, 1990, pp 201–210.

Fig. 4. ERCP and sphincterotomy-related pancreatitis.

Siegel and colleagues [36] reported on their series of minor papilla endoscopic therapy for symptomatic pancreas divisum patients. Although this sizable series has potential to shed light on this difficult group of patients, the report is unclear about the type of patients studied (pancreatitis versus pain only), size of stents used, duration of stent therapy, and the simultaneous use (or not) of endoscopic sphincterotomy of the minor papilla. Clarification of the above data is awaited.

Gregg *et al.* [37] preliminarily reported follow-up results in 45 pancreas divisum patients who had endoscopic (sphincterotomy, seven; balloon dilatation, five) or surgical therapy (minor papilla sphincteroplasty) for minor papilla stenosis. Manometric evaluation revealed total sphincter ablation in 27 patients. Residual sphincter pressure of less than 35 mmHg was present in 13 patients, whereas nine patients had stenosis of their minor papilla (presumably with sphincter pressure greater than 35 mmHg). All patients with restenosis had recurrent pain or pancreatitis. Intraductal secretin-stimulated juice was collected and analyzed for flow rate, bicarbonate concentration, or γ glutamyl transpeptidase. Thirty-two out of 40 patients were considered to have an abnormal secretory study, but correlation with clinical outcome (pain relief) was poor.

Overall, the published surgical and endoscopic series have reported outcomes varying from excellent to poor. Patient selection criteria, the length of follow-up, and restenosis of the minor papilla are especially important factors. The two most important questions in this controversial area remain. First, are there non-operative tests which can select patients who will have a favorable response of minor papilla ablation? Second, what is the most effective method of opening the minor papilla?

ERCP, endoscopic sphincterotomy, and sphincter of Oddi manometry-induced pancreatitis

During ERCP and endoscopic sphincterotomy (ES), the pancreas is subjected to many types of potential injury: mechanical, chemical, hydrostatic, enzymatic, microbiologic, allergic and thermal. The potential role of each etiologic factor in the development of ERCP and ES-induced pancreatitis was recently detailed [38••]. A variety of clinical settings that may increase the risk for post-procedure pancreatitis and techniques attempting to minimize this complications are presented (Fig. 4).

There has been a long search for an agent that will prevent or resolve pancreatitis no matter what the cause. ERCP has the advantage of permitting treatment prior to, during, and after the intervention. Studies with antibiotics, aprotinin, calcitonin, and glucagon have generally failed to show any decrease in post-ERCP hyperamylasemia or pancreatitis. The initial enthusiasm for prophylactic somatostatin or its analog [39] has been dampened by two recent preliminary reports. In a multicenter randomized placebo-controlled trial assessing the efficacy of octreotide (Sandostatin, Sandoz Pharmaceuticals Corp., East Hanover, New Jersey, USA; 100 µg intravenously prior to ERCP and 100 µg subcutaneously 45 min later) in reducing the incidence of post-ERCP pancreatitis, 84 patients were evaluated [40•]. Overall, pancreatitis occurred in 11% of the control group and 35% of the treatment group ($P < 0.01$). In the treatment group, pancreatitis occurred in 15% after-ES (versus 16% in the placebo group) and 59% following diagnostic ERCP (versus 6% in the placebo group). The treatment and control groups were similar with respect to the duration of ERCP, number of cannulations of the pancreatic duct, and volume of contrast injected. Approximately 2% of patients evaluated had an elevated serum amylase and/or lipase level prior to the procedure, but no evidence of clinical pancreatitis. The frequency of pancreatitis following ERCP with or without endoscopic sphincterotomy was disturbingly high in this series and may in part reflect an inappropriately sensitive definition of post-procedure pancreatitis (any elevation of serum amylase or lipase with abdominal pain and tenderness as early as 2 h following the procedure). In another randomized, double-blind, placebo-controlled trial of 63 patients undergoing ERCP, octreotide (200 μg subcutaneously 25 min prior to and 8 and 16 h after ERCP) had no effect on the development of post-procedure chemical (23 versus 25%) and clinical pancreatitis (6 versus 0%) [41•]. Other potential prophylactic treatments, such as antioxidants, await further clinical evaluations.

Sphincter of Oddi manometry (SOM) is a useful adjunct in the evaluation of patients with unexplained pancreaticobiliary pain and idiopathic pancreatitis, and may predict which patients will respond to endoscopic sphincterotomy [42]. Unfortunately, pancreatitis may be provoked by SOM. Rolny *et al.* [43•] found a disturbingly high frequency of post-SOM pancreatitis. In this retrospective review of the complications following 207 attempted SOM studies in 146 patients, 11% of the pancreatic duct evaluations were complicated by pancreatitis in contrast to only 1% of the bile duct studies. Patients with chronic pancreatitis were at significant risk (26% incidence of pancreatitis following SOM). Based on the hypothesis that increased pancreatic duct hydrostatic pressure from prolonged perfusion is the major cause of the pancreatitis, a modified triple lumen aspirating SOM catheter was developed [44•]. This catheter allows for aspiration of the perfused fluid from end and side holes that simultaneously record pressures from the two remaining side ports. This catheter was evaluated in 26 patients who had pancreatic duct SOM performed by the standard perfusion technique and the aspirating technique in random sequence. The mean basal pancreatic sphincter pressure, phasic amplitude, phasic duration, and phasic frequency when measured by both techniques were similar. A prospective randomized study was performed to determine whether routine use of this catheter would reduce the frequency and severity of post-manometry pancreatitis and pancreatic enzyme elevation [45••]. Seventy-six patients with unexplained pancreaticobiliary pain or idiopathic pancreatitis were randomly assigned to undergo SOM with the standard perfusion catheter (infused group) or the aspiration catheter (aspiration group). Sphincter of Oddi manometry and ERCP were performed on separate days. After SOM, there were significantly more patients in the infused group with both amylase and lipase values elevated at least two times the upper limits of normal at 2 ($P < 0.001$), 6 ($P = 0.01$) and 18 hours ($P = 0.03$) after the procedure. The overall incidence of post-SOM pancreatitis was 14.5%. As compared with the standard perfusion system, the aspiration catheter was associated with a decreased frequency of clinical pancreatitis (23.5 versus 3%, $P = 0.01$). When manometry was performed only in the bile duct, no episodes of clinical pancreatitis occurred in either group. In contrast, when the pancreatic duct was evaluated (with or without a bile duct study) 30.8% of patients in the infused group developed post-SOM pancreatitis in contrast to only 3.8% in the aspiration group ($P = 0.01$). These results suggest that the aspiration catheter should be used for SOM particularly when the pancreatic duct sphincter is being evaluated.

Because of the significant risk of pancreatitis Rolny *et al.* [47•] state that pancreatic duct manometry should not be performed, especially in patients with chronic pancreatitis. However, this recommendation excludes the possibility that pancreatic sphincter manometry may be clinically helpful and necessary. In a small series on patients with abnormal sphincter of Oddi manometry and acute recurrent pancreatitis, seven out of nine patients had the abnormality confined to the pancreatic duct segment [46•]. Similarly, Rolny noted that 53% of patients with an abnormal basal sphincter pressure had differing pancreatic and biliary pressures. In a preliminary report [48], 67 patients with possible sphincter of Oddi dysfunction were evaluated by both pancreatic and biliary manometry. Correlation between basal biliary and pancreatic sphincter pressures occurred in 57 patients (85%); both basal sphincter pressures were normal in 32 (48%) and abnormal in 25 patients (37%). Ten (29%) of the 35 patients with an elevated basal sphincter pressure had the abnormality restricted to one of the segments. There were no clinical or laboratory features that could predict which sphincter segment would be abnormal. Thus, one sphincter may be dysfunctional while the other is normal.

As a result, in certain situations, pancreatic duct manometry may be critical. Moreover, use of the aspiration catheter in the pancreatic duct reduces the complication rate to a level similar to that associated with ERCP. The reduction of pancreatitis with use of this catheter and the very low incidence of pancreatitis following a bile duct study lends support to the notion that increased pancreatic duct hydrostatic pressure is probably the major cause of this complication.

Acute gallstone pancreatitis

The pathogenesis of acute gallstone pancreatitis remains controversial. In a short communication, Neuhaus and Classen [49] describe some of the lines of evidence favoring the gallstone migration theory. They coined the term 'acute obstructive pancreatitis' to emphasize the acute stage of the disease and the 'mechanical occlusion' as the decisive pathogenic mechanism. The authors describe the use of ERCP to confirm the 'obstructive' nature of the pancreatitis and the benefit of endoscopic sphincterotomy. Emphasis was placed on avoiding pancreatic duct visualization to minimize complications. However, cautious pancreatic duct filling may be relatively safe. In a recent randomized prospective controlled trial for acute biliary pancreatitis [50], unintentional pancreatic duct filling (often incomplete) occurred in 50% of severe cases and 90% of mild cases without undue complications. Moreover, additional pathologic findings of the pancreas may be discovered and useful information in cases possibly requiring surgery (e.g. fistulization) may be provided [51,52]. Further studies are necessary to confirm the safety and use of pancreatic duct visualization in the setting of acute gallstone pancreatitis.

As noted, papillary obstruction to pancreatic juice flow is believed to be the major pathogenic factor in acute gallstone pancreatitis. It follows that a patent accessory duct (of Santorini) and minor papilla may allow for pancreatic duct decompression and a lower incidence of pancreatitis in patients with choledocholithiasis. This theory was prospectively evaluated in 67 patients undergoing urgent ERCP (within 24 hours of admission) for acute gallstone pancreatitis [53••]. AT ERCP, the anatomy of the pancreatic duct was evaluated and special attention was paid to the patency of the accessory duct as a potential outflow for the pancreatic juice. The cholangiogram revealed choledocholithiasis in 32, choledocholithiasis and cholecystolithiasis in 24 and cholecystolithiasis alone in 11. A pancreatogram was obtained in 47 of these patients. The control groups comprised 100 consecutive patients in whom a pancreatogram was obtained during ERCP for suspected biliary pathology but no evidence of pancreatitis (46 had cholecystolithiasis and/or choledocholithiasis and 54 were post-cholecystectomy without evidence of common duct stones). Patency of the accessory duct and minor papilla were found in only 17% of patients with acute gallstone pancreatitis, in contrast to 69% of the control group (P <0.001, Fig. 5). The Santorini duct was absent in 72% of acute gallstone pancreatitis patients and 19% of controls ($P < 0.001$). The authors concluded that the lack of this additional draining channel for pancreatic juice may be an important pathogenic factor in acute gallstone pancreatitis. The complications of pancreatic duct injection were not reported. The importance of this outflow tract is also reflected by the lower incidence of post-ERCP pancreatitis in patients with a patent minor papilla and Santorini duct [54,55].

The management of acute gallstone pancreatitis remains controversial, as evidenced by the differing opinions of an expert biliary endoscopist and world-class biliary surgeon [56•]. Both agree that the natural history of acute gallstone pancreatitis is variable and urgent intervention may not be necessary, particularly for mild cases. Moreover, both felt that methodologic problems exist in the literature, as the differentiation of acute pancreatitis secondary to gallstones from acute biliary disease with an elevated amylase is not always corrected made. However, on the basis of the results of a recently published prospective randomized control trial for acute gallstone pancreatitis [50] the endoscopist advocated early ERCP diagnosis and therapy. Surgery should be reserved for delayed elective cholecystectomy when indicated. The surgeon, however, felt that the major drawback of ERCP and endoscopic sphincterotomy in the setting of acute gallstone pancreatitis were the risks of exacerbating the pancreatitis and the possibility of introducing infection into peripancreatic devitalized tissue. As a result, percutaneous transhepatic cholangiography was recommended in those who do not respond rapidly. If calculus obstruction of the ampulla is demonstrated, endoscopic sphincterotomy was felt to be a reasonable therapeutic option.

Chronic pancreatitis

Pancreatic stones

Two forms of chronic pancreatitis have been described [57]. Chronic calcifying pancreatitis is marked by the presence of intraductal plugs and calcified calculi in the lumen of acini and ducts. Conversely, in obstructive pancreatitis (i.e. the gland changes are noted upstream to the obstruction), pancreatic calculi are not observed and intraductal plugs are not characteristic. Lorente *et al.* [58] report a case of obstructive pancreatitis and pancreatic stone formation. A 20-year-old woman with recurrent bouts of acute pancreatitis was found at ERCP to have a main pancreatic duct stricture with upstream dilatation and a radiolucent stone. The cause for the pancreatitis and the stricture were not uncovered. A pancreatojejunostomy was performed with no further episodes of acute pancreatitis.

There is debate about whether pancreatic calculi aggravate the clinical course of chronic pancreatitis (mani-

Santorini duct	ABP No. of patients (%)	Control group No. of patients (%)	Significance
Patent	8 (17)	69 (69)	$P < 0.001$
Obliterated	5 (11)	13 (13)	NS
Absent	34 (72)	15 (15)	$P < 0.001$
Total	47	100	

ABP, acute biliary pancreatitis [53].

Fig.5 . Patency of the accessory duct (of Santorini) in patients with ABP and in the control group.

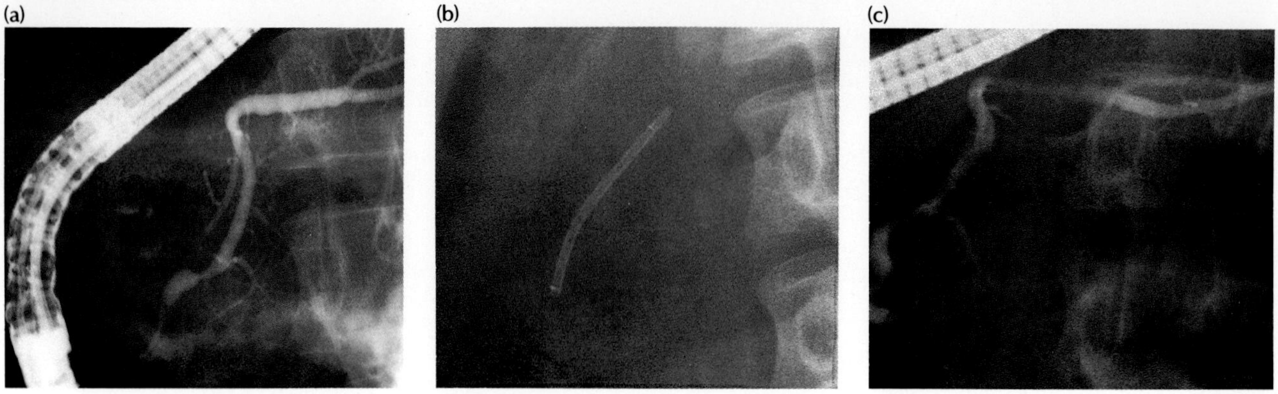

Fig. 6. (a) A 32-year-old man with idiopathic pancreatitis has main duct stricture of the head and small pseudocyst in the head. (b) A 7 F multiside hole straight 5 cm length stent has been placed. The patient's pain was moderately improved until stent occlusion occurred 2 months later. (c) Follow-up ductogram at the time of stent removal shows persistence of focal duct narrowing in the head (brush cytology negative for malignant cells) and edematous changes throughout the main duct of the head. Further follow-up is needed to determine whether such short-term stenting intervals are of any long-term benefit.

fested as increased abdominal pain and/or recurrent attacks of acute pancreatitis) or are just the inevitable sequelae of ongoing gland destruction. It has been postulated that increased intraductal pressure upstream from an obstructed focus within the pancreatic duct, as with a pancreatic duct stone, is one of the potential mechanisms responsible for attacks of acute pancreatitis or exacerbations of chronic abdominal pain in patients with chronic pancreatitis [59]. Reports [60,61] indicating that endoscopic removal of pancreatic calculi resulted in improvement in symptoms support this notion. Two recent preliminary reports confirm and expand the role of endoscopic therapy for the management of main pancreatic duct calculi. In the largest reported series [62•], 104 patients with chronic pancreatitis (80% due to alcohol) and obstructing main pancreatic duct stones with proximal dilatation were treated with extracorporeal shock wave lithotripsy (ESWL) and pancreatic duct endoscopic sphincterotomy and stone fragment extraction. Stones were successfully disintegrated in 99%, but complete clearance of the fragments from the main pancreatic duct occurred in onl· 54%. Duct dilatation decreased in 82% and continuous pain disappeared in all patients. Adverse effects occurred in 27% of patients (generally mild) and the mortality rate was 0%. Haber *et al.* [63•] attempted to identify those patients with predominantly main pancreatic duct stones most amenable to endoscopic removal and to determine the effect on the patient's clinical course with such removal. Twenty-six patients with ductographic evidence of chronic pancreatitis and pancreatic duct stones underwent attempted endoscopic removal (extraction, flushing and/or fragmentation) after sphincterotomy, minor or major (pancreatic and/or biliary). Eleven patients also had stents or nasopancreatic drains used. The stones were successfully removed in 18 (70%) with symptomatic improvement (moderate or complete pain relief) in 60% (mean follow-up, 2 years). Failure to remove the stones occurred in eight patients and was due to stricture (three) or inability to capture the stone (five), largely because of stone impaction. Three of these patients benefited from sphincterotomy alone with or without placement of a pancreatic stent. Factors favoring stone removal included the following: (a) three stones or less; (b) stones confined to the head and/or body of the pancreas; (c) absence of a downstream stricture; (d) stone diameter 10 mm or less; (e) absence of impacted stones. These results suggest that removal of pancreatic duct stones may result in symptomatic improvement. A long-term follow-up will be necessary to determine wetherf endoscopic success results in longstanding clinical improvement and/or permanent regression of the morphologic changes of chronic pancreatitis. Ultimately, controlled trials will be needed to compare the various therapies (medical, endoscopic, ESWL, surgical) for chronic pancreatitis when complicated by the presence of calculi.

Pancreatic stent induced changes of the pancreatic duct simulating chronic pancreatitis

Pancreatic stents and drains are now being applied to a variety of benign pancreatic disorders (e.g. dominant structures, pancreas divisum, pseudocyst drainage) [64–67] (Fig. 6). Complications related directly to stent therapy have focused primarily on stent occlusion or migration with one report documenting the development of dorsal duct changes compatible with chronic pancreatitis in a previously normal duct [65]. The anatomic alterations of the pancreatic duct induced by pancreatic stents was evaluated by Kozarek [68•]. Thirty-four patients had 38 ductal stents placed for: disrupted pancreatic ducts with pseudocysts (11), hypertensive pancreatic duct sphincter after biliary sphincter ablation (11), pancreatic duct stricture (seven), recurrent pancreatitis with pancreas divisum (five). The stents were polyethylene, 5–7 F, with additional side holes. Stents were removed or exchanged at a mean of 4 months (2 weeks–24 months). Nine patients were found to have occluded stents, six of whom had new ductal changes: diffuse ductal dilatation (four), new pseudocyst (one), enlargement and infection of an existing pseudocyst (one). With stent change or removal, five of the six ductal changes resolved, while one duct remained moderately dilatated (at 6 months after stent removal). Three patients developed changes characteristic of chronic pancreatitis (main duct stenosis with side branch ectasia) at anatomical sites contiguous with the stent. At follow-up (after stent removal) the pancreatic duct was normalized in one patient (at 3 months), improved in another (strictures and side branch changes persist at 6 months) and was mildly dilated in a third (at 3 months). The latter patient had an abnormal p-aminobenzoic acid (Chymex) test for pancreatic insufficiency whereas the first two were normal. As the results of pre-stent p-aminobenzoic acid pancreatic function testing are not detailed, it is not clear whether the abnormal result is new. A preliminary report [69] confirms these stent-induced changes in previously normal pancreatic ducts. In this series, 36 patients were treated with 5–7 F stents, 3–12 mm long, for 4–22 months (exchanges at 1–9 month intervals). Mild to marked pancreatic ductal changes were noted in 30 patients (83%) at the time of stent removal. Of the 14 patients having follow-up ERCP (6–12 months after-stent removal), 12 (86%) had normalization of their pancreatogram. Although therapeutic benefit has been reported for pancreatic stenting, these studies reveal that morphologic changes of the pancreatic duct directly related to this therapy occur in the majority. Despite the tendency of these ductal changes to improve with time following stent change and/or removal, it remains uncertain what the long-term consequences of these stent changes are. We believe that current experience is still too limited to recommend general use of pancreatic stents particularly in patients with normal pancreatic parenchyma, i.e. no chronic pancreatitis. Numerous questions need to be answered about correct stent diameter, length, composition, number of side holes, duration of therapy and patient selection.

Therapy of distal common bile duct structure secondary to chronic pancreatitis

Intrapancreatic common bile duct strictures have been reported to occur in 2.7–45.6% of patients with chronic pancreatitis [70]. In the past, operative biliary drainage was often recommended to prevent the possible development of acute cholangitis and secondary biliary cirrhosis. On the basis of the absence of increased morbidity associated with conservative management in these patients, Stahl *et al.* recommended operative biliary drainage only when acute cholangitis, biliary cirrhosis and/or persistent jaundice were present [70]. Devière *et al.* [71•] evaluated the use of biliary stenting in 25 patients with common bile duct obstruction and significant (alkaline phosphatase greater than two times normal) cholestasis secondary to chronic pancreatitis. Nineteen patients had jaundice and seven presented with cholangitis. The patients were treated by endoscopic sphincterotomy followed by insertion of one or two biliary stents of 10 F size placed across the stricture. The stents were changed when clinical or ultrasonographic (every 3 months) evidence of blockage was present. Cholestasis, hyperbilirubinemia, and cholangitis resolved in all patients following stent replacement. The late follow-up (mean 14 months, 4–72 months) on 22 patients was much less satisfactory. One patient died 1 month following treatment from acute cholecystitis and post-surgical complications while a second died 3 months after stenting from sepsis felt to be due to stent blockage or dislodgement. Stent migration occurred in 10 patients (mean time, 11 weeks) and stent blockade in eight (mean 6.5 months) resulting in cholestasis with or without jaundice (12), cholangitis (four), or no symptoms (two). These patients were treated by stent replacement and/or surgery (seven). Ten patients continued to have a stent in place (mean follow-up, 8 months) and remained asymptomatic although three required no further stents because of resolution of their biliary stricture. The salient point of this study was that biliary drainage is an effective therapy for resolving cholangitis or jaundice in patients with chronic pancreatitis and biliary stenosis, but the long-term efficacy of this treatment is much less satisfactory because stricture resolution rarely occurs. Although the Stahl and the Devière studies are retrospective, both appear to indicate that it is preferable to use operative intervention (rather than endoscopic) as a long-term solution in such patients.

In conclusion

Endoscopic aspects of pancreatic disease continue to evolve. Diagnostic aspects have expanded to include more routine use of manometry and intraductal sampling of juice and tissue. Endoscopic therapeutic aspects of pancreatic disease that include stenting of stenotic sphincters, strictures and pseudocysts as well as pancreatic stone fragmentation and extraction are exciting new areas. Endoscopists are reminded to exercise caution in application of newer pancreatic techniques as serious complications — especially pancreatitis — may occasionally occur.

References and recommended reading

Papers of special interest, published within the annual period of review, have been highlighted as:

- • Of interest
- •• Of outstanding interest

1. MORRIS JB, ZOLLINGER RM JR, STELLATO TA, YANG P: **The Pseudo-Double Duct Sign: an ERCP Finding in Pancreatic Carcinoma.** *Gastrointest Endosc* 1990, **36**:408–409.

2. MISRA SP, GULATI P, CHOUDHARY V, ANAND BS: **Pancreatic • Duct Abnormalities in Gall Stone Disease: an Endoscopic Retrograde Cholangiopancreatographic Study.** *Gut* 1990, **31**:1073–1075.

Ductographic changes of chronic pancreatitis were found in 48% of gallstone patients versus only 6% of control (viral hepatitis) patients.

3. MISRA SP, DWIVEDI M: **Pancreaticobiliary Ductal Union.** *Gut* • 1990, **31**:1144–1149.

Excellent review of this entity and its associated pathologic states such as choledochoceles.

4. GILMORE PR, AGARWAL VP: **Endoscopic Evaluation of Heterotopic Pancreas.** *Gastrointest Endosc* 1989, **35**:563–565.

5. HALPERT RD, SHABOT JM, HEARE BR, ROGERS RE: **The Bifid Pancreas: a Rare Anatomical Variation.** *Gastrointest Endosc* 1990, **36**:60–61.

6. NISHIMORI I, OKAZAKI K, MORITA M, MIYAO M, SAKAMOTO Y, KAGIYAMA S, YAMAMOTO Y, YAMAMOTO Y: **Congenital Hypoplasia of the Dorsal Pancreas: with Special Reference to Duodenal Papillary Dysfunction.** *Am J Gastroenterol* 1990, **85**:1029–1033.

7. SCUDERA PL, KOIZUMI J, JACOBSON IM: **Brush Cytology Eval- • uation of Lesions Encountered During ERCP.** *Gastrointest Endosc* 1990, **36**:281–294.

Sensitivity and specificity of brush cytology of the bile duct reported in 25 patients, of whom 10 had pancreatic cancer.

8. FOUTCH PG, KERR DM, HARLAN JR, MANNE RK, KUMMET TD, • SANOWSKI RA: **Endoscopic Retrograde Wire-guided Brush Cytology for Diagnosis of Patients with Malignant Obstruction of the Bile Duct.** *Am J Gastroenterol* 1990, **85**:791–795.

Over-the-wire brush cytology technique used to evaluate 39 bile duct strictures. Brush cytology sensitivity for cholangiocarcinoma, pancreatic cancer and metastatic obstruction was 100, 60 and 22%, respectively.

9. GAGNON P, PONCHON T, LABADIE M, BERGER F, CHAVAILLON A, BOUSTIERE C: **Value of Endobiliary Brushing Cytology and Biopsies of Bile Duct Stenosis.** *Gastrointest Endosc* 1990, **36**:200A.

10. RYAN ME: **Cytologic Brushings of Ductal Abnormalities Identified During ERCP.** *Gastrointest Endosc* 1989, **35**:168A.

11. OSNES M, SERCK-HANSSEN A, KRISTENSEN O, SWENSEN T, AUNE S, MYREN J: **Endoscopic Retrograde Brush Cytology in Patients with Primary and Secondary Malignancies of the Pancreas.** *Gut* 1979, **20**:279–284.

12. BOUSTIERE C, PONCHON T, VALETTE PJ, GENIN G, GAGNON P, LABADIE M: **Percutaneous Fine Needle Aspiration Cytology of Main Pancreatic Duct Stenosis Guided by Wirsungography.** *Gastrointest Endosc* 1990, **36**:200A.

13. OGAWA Y, TANAKA M, MATSUMOTO S, YAMAUCHI S, IKEDA S, YOSHIMOTO H: **Islet Cell Tumors of the Pancreas.** *Int J Pancreatol* 1990, **6**:49–60.

14. KAUFMAN AR, SIVAK MV, FERGUSON DR: **Endoscopic Retrograde Cholangiopancreatography in Pancreatic Islet Cell Tumors.** *Gastrointest Endosc* 1988, **34**:47–52.

15. SATAKE K, ARIMOTO Y, FUJIMOTO Y, NISHIWAKI H, NISHINO H, UMEYAMA K, INOUE T, MITSUHASHI T: **Malignant T-cell Lymphoma of the Pancreas.** *Pancreas* 1991, **6**:120–124.

16. MOREIRA VF, ROMAN AL-S, LEDO L, MERONO P, ERDOZAIN JC: **Retroperitoneal Lymphoma Causing Pancreatic Ductal Obstruction in Endoscopic Retrograde Cholangiopancreatography.** *Gastrointest Endosc* 1990, **36**:80–81.

17. PINSON CW, MUNSON JL, DEVENEY CW: **Endoscopic Retrograde Cholangiopancreatography in the Preoperative Diagnosis of Pancreatic Neoplasms Associated with Cysts.** *Am J Surg* 1990, **159**:510–513.

18. ISAACS PET: **Unique Appearance of the Duodenal Papilla in Pancreatic Cystadenocarcinoma.** *Endoscopy* 1989, **21**: 102–104.

19. DABEZIES MA, CAMPANA T, FRIEDMAN AC: **ERCP in the Diagnosis of Ductectatic Mucinous Cystadenocarcinoma of the Pancreas.** *Gastrointest Endosc* 1990, **36**:410–411.

20. KATOH H, ROSSI RL, BRAASCH JW, MUNSON JL, SHIMOZAWA E, TANABE T: **Cystadenoma and Cystadenocarcinoma of the Pancreas.** *Hepatogastroenterology* 1989, **36**:424–430.

21. KOHLER B, KOHLER G, RIEMANN J: **Pancreoscopic Diagnosis of Intraductal Cystadenoma of the Pancreas.** *Dig Dis Sci* 1990, **35**:382–284.

22. NISHIDA K, SHIGA K, KATO K, KUNIHIRO K, FUJII T, TOMII T, YAMAMOTO H, YAMANE E, NISHIOKA B, YOSHIKAWA T, KONDO M: **Two Cases of Pancreatic Cystadenocarcinoma with Elevated CA 19-9 Levels in the Cystic Fluid in Comparison with Two Cases of Pancreatic Cystadenoma.** *Hepatogastroenterology* 1989, **36**:442–445.

23. BASTID C, BERNARD JP, SARLES H, PAYAN MJ, SAHEL J: **Mucinous Ductal Ectasia of the Pancreas: a Premalignant Disease and a Cause of Obstructive Pancreatitis.** *Pancreas* 1991, **6**:15–22.

24. PAYAN MJ, XERRI L, MONCADA K, BASTID C, AGOSTINI S, SASTRE B, SAHEL J, CHOUX R: **Villous Adenoma of the Main Pancreatic Duct: a Potentially Malignant Tumor?** *Am J Gastroenterol* 1990, **85**:459–463.

25. STEINBERG W: **The Clinical Utility of CA 19-9 Tumor-asso- • ciated Antigen.** *Am J Gastroenterol* 1990, **85**:350–356.

Excellent review of the clinical utility of CA 19–9 for the detection of pancreatic cancer.

26. ZERA RT: **Is Pancreatic Cancer Hopeless?** *Gastrointest Endosc* 1990, **36**:161.

27. VENNES J: **Bile Duct Cancer is not Hopeless?** *Gastrointest Endosc* 1989, **35**:267–268.

28. HARRISON MA, HAMILTON JW: **Palliation of Pancreatic Cancer Pain by Endoscopic Stent Placement.** *Gastrointest Endosc* 1989, **35**:443–445.

29. SHEMESH E, CZERNIAK A, NASS S, KLEIN E: **Role of Endoscopic Retrograde Cholangiopancreatography in Differentiating Pancreatic Cancer Coexisting with Chronic Pancreatitis.** *Cancer* 1990, **65**:893–896.

30. ESKELINEN M, LIPPONEN P, COLLAN Y, MARIN S, ALHAVA E, NORDLING S: **Relationship Between DNA Ploidy and Survival in Patients with Exocrine Pancreatic Cancer.** *Pancrease* 1991, **6**:90–95.

31. FOERSTER EC, STOMMER P, SCHNEIDER MU, MATEK W, GERNER G, DOMSCHKE W: **Transpapillary Miniscopy and Mini-biopsy of the Pancreatic Duct.** *Endoscopy* 1990, **22**:78–80.

32. DELHAYE M, ENGELHOUN L, CREMER M: **Pancreas Divisum: Congential Anatomic Variant of Anomaly?** *Gastroenterology* 1985, **89**:951–956.

33. BENAGE D, MCHENRY R, HAWES RH, O'CONNOR KW, LEHMAN • GA: **Minor Papilla Cannulation and Dorsal Ductography in Pancreas Divisum.** *Gastrointest Endosc* 1990, **36**:553–557.

Authors report 90% success rate of minor papilla cannulation and correlate the frequency of ductography abnormalities with the presenting features of the patients.

34. WARSHAW AL, SIMEONE JF, SCHAPIRO RH, FLAVIN-WARSHAW B: •• **Evaluation and Treatment of the Dominant Dorsal Duct Syndrome (Pancreas Divisum Redefined).** *Am J Surg* 1990, **159**:59–66.

Summary of large surgical series of pancreas divisum patients treated by minor papilla sphincteroplasty. The secretin-stimulated ultrasound test predicted which patients were likely to respond to intervention.

35. •• LANS JI, GEENEN JE, JOHANSON JF, HOGAN WJ: **Endoscopic Therapy in Patients with Pancreas Divisum and Acute Pancreatitis: a Prospective, Randomized, Controlled Clinical Trial.** *Gastroenterology* 1991 (in press).
Important randomized controlled trial that evaluates stenting the minor papilla in pancreas divisum patients with recurrent pancreatitis. Stented patients had significantly fewer pancreatitis episodes.

36. SIEGEL JH, BEN-ZVI JS, PULLANO W, COPPERMAN A: **Effectiveness of Endoscopic Drainage for Pancreas Divisum: Endoscopic and Surgical Results in 31 Patients.** *Endoscopy* 1990, 22:129–133.

37. GREGG JA, STERN JS, GREGG L: **Correlation of Postoperative Dorsal Duct Pancreatic Sphincter Manometry and Intraductal Secretin tests with Relief of Pain in Pancreas Divisum.** *Am J Gastroenterol* 1990, **85**:1249A.

38. •• SHERMAN S, LEHMAN GA: **ERCP and Endoscopic Sphincterotomy Induced Pancreatitis.** *Pancreas* 1991 (in press).
Detailed review of the multiple pathogenic processes potentially involved in this procedure related complication. Proposed techniques to limit pancreatitis are given.

39. BORDAS JM, TOLEDO V, MONDELO F, RODES J: **Prevention of Pancreatic Reactions by Bolus Somatostatin Administration in Patients Undergoing Endoscopic Retrograde Cholangio-Pancreatography and Endoscopic Sphincterotomy.** *Horm Res* 1988, **29**:106–108.

40. • STERNLIEB J, ARONCHICK C, RETIG J, DABEZIES M, SAUNDERS F, GOOSENBERG R, INFANTOLINO A, IONNA S, MAISLIN G, WRIGHT S, LIPSHUTZ W: **A Multicenter, Randomized, Controlled Trial to Evaluate the Effect of Octreotide on Post-ERCP Pancreatitis.** *Am J Gastroenterol* 1990, **85**:1259A.
Preliminary report indicating no efficacy to octreotide therapy in preventing post-ERCP pancreatitis.

41. • TAYLOR DH, BRODMERKEL GJ: **Role of Octreotide in ERCP Associated Pancreatitis.** *Am J Gastroenterol* 1990, **85**:1260A.
Preliminary report indicating no efficacy of octreotide therapy in preventing post-ERCP pancreatitis.

42. GEENAN JE, HOGAN WJ, DODDS WJ, TOOULI J, VENU RP: **The Efficacy of Endoscopic Sphincterotomy After Cholecystectomy in Patients with Sphincter of Oddi Dysfunction.** *N Engl J Med* 1989, **320**:82–87.

43. • ROLNY P, ANDERBERG B, IHSE I, LINDSTROM E, OLAISON G, ARVILL A: **Pancreatitis After Sphincter of Oddi Manometry.** *Gut* 1990, **31**:821–824.
A retrospective review of the complications following 207 attempted sphincter of Oddi manometries in 147 patients. Acute pancreatitis was the only complication and occurred in 8% of the patients examined. The risk of a complication was considerable when the pancreatic duct was evaluated (11%) particularly in patients with chronic pancreatitis (32%).

44. • SHERMAN S, TROIANO FP, HAWES RH, LEHMAN GA: **Does Continuous Aspiration from an End and Side Port in a Sphincter of Oddi Manometry Catheter Alter Recorded Pressures?** *Gastrointest Endosc* 1990, **36**:500–502.
A modified triple lumen aspirating manometry catheter was developed. The mean basal pancreatic sphincter pressure, phasic amplitude, phasic duration, and phasic frequency were similar when measured by perfusion and aspiration techniques.

45. •• SHERMAN S, TROIANO FP, HAWES RH, LEHMAN GA: **Sphincter of Oddi Manometry: Decreased Risk of Clinical Pancreatitis with the Use of a Modified Aspirating Catheter.** *Gastrointest Endosc* 1990, **36**:462–466.
A prospective randomized study was conducted to determine whether routine use of the aspirating sphincter of Oddi manometry catheter would reduce the frequency and severity of post-manometry pancreatitis. The aspiration catheter was associated with the following: (1) decreased frequency of clinical pancreatitis (23.5% versus 3%, $P = 0.01$) and pancreatic enzyme elevation; (2) reduced hospital stay; (3) milder pancreatitis.

46. • RADDAWI HM, GEENEN JE, HOGAN WJ, DODDS WJ, VENU RP, JOHNSON GK: **Pressure Measurements from Biliary and Pancreatic Segments of Sphincter of Oddi — Comparison Between Patients with Functional Abdominal Pain, Biliary, or Pancreatic Disease.** *Dig Dis Sci* 1991, **36**:71–74.
Authors found that five out of eight patients with abnormal basal sphincter pressure had that abnormality confined to the biliary portion of the sphincter. Seven out of nine recurrent pancreatitis patients with abnormal basal sphincter pressure had that abnormality confined to the pancreatic portion of the sphincter.

47. • ROLNY P, ARLEBACK A, FUNCH-JENSEN P, KRUSE A, JARNEROT G: **Clinical Significance of Manometric Assessment of Both Pancreatic Duct and Bile Duct Sphincter in the Same Patient.** *Scand J Gastroenterol* 1989, **24**:751–754.
In one-half of patients with abnormal sphincter of Oddi manometry, the bile duct sphincter and the pancreatic duct sphincter in the same patient did not show the same abnormality. Measurement of pressure in both sphincters may be needed.

48. SILVERMAN WB, RUFFOLO TA, SHERMAN S, HAWES RH, LEHMAN GA: **Correlation of Basal Sphincter Pressure Measured from Both Bile Ducts and Pancreatic Duct in Patients with Suspected Sphincter of Oddi Dysfunction (SOD).** *Gastrointest Endosc* 1991 (in press).

49. NEUHAUS H, CLASSEN M: **Endoscopy in the Diagnosis and Therapy of Acute Obstructive Pancreatitis.** *Ital J Gastroenterol* 1989, **21**:273–275.

50. NEOPTOLEMOS JF, LONDON NJ, JAMES D, CARR-LOCKE DL, BAILEY IA, FOSSARD DP: **Controlled Trial of Urgent Endoscopic Retrograde Cholangiopancreatography and Endoscopic Sphincterotomy Versus Conservative Treatment for Acute Pancreatitis due to Gallstones.** *Lancet* 1988, ii:979–983.

51. SAFRANY L, SCHMEDING K, SCHOTT B: **Endoskopische Papillotomie bei Akuter Biliarer Pankreatitis.** *Med Welt* 1989, **40**:171–174.

52. TONAK J, LUX G, GEBHARDT CH: **A Surgical Approach to Hemorrhagic Necrotizing Pancreatitis Based on Endoscopic Retrograde Pancreatography.** *Gastrointest Endosc* 1986, **32**:104–106.

53. •• NOWAK A, NOWAKOWSKA-DUTAWA E, RYBICKA J: **Patency of the Santorini Duct and Acute Biliary Pancreatitis: a Prospective ERCP Study.** *Endoscopy* 1990, **22**:124–126.
The importance of a patent duct of Santorini and minor papilla in limiting the frequency of acute gallstone pancreatitis was assessed in 67 patients. The outflow tract was present in only 17% of the patients with acute gallstone pancreatitis in contrast to 59% of the control group.

54. ARAKAWA S, VENO F, IWAMURA K: **Evaluation of the Role of Santorini's Duct by Digital Subtraction Endoscopic Retrograde Pancreatography.** *Am J Gastroenterol* 1988, **83**:1072A.

55. MAIROSE UB, WURBS D, CLASSEN M: **Santorini's Duct — an Insignificant Variant from Normal or an Important Overflow Valve?** *Endoscopy* 1978, **10**;24–29.

56. • ZIMMON D, RANSON JHC: **What is the Role of Endoscopy in the Management of Biliary Pancreatitis and when Should it be Utilized?** *Am J Gastroenterol* 1990, **85**:9–11.
The management of acute gallstone pancreatitis is discussed by an expert biliary endoscopist and a world-class biliary surgeon. The biliary endoscopist advocates early ERCP diagnosis and therapy, while the surgeon is concerned about this approach because of the possibility of exacerbating the pancreatitis and introducing infection into devitalized tissue.

57. SARLES H: **Etiopathogenesis and Definition of Chronic Pancreatitis.** *Dis Sci* 1986, **31**:915–1075.

58. LORENTE JA, DEL ARBÓL LR, MORELRA VF, GARCIA-PLAZA A: **Recurrent Pancreatitis in a Young Patient Associated with a Solitary Nonopaque Concretion in the Main Pancreatic Duct.** *Gastrointest Endosc* 1990, 36:63–65.

59. SCHNEIDER MU, LUX G: **Floating Pancreatic Duct Concrements in Chronic Pancreatitis.** *Endoscopy* 1985, 17:8–10.

60. FUJI T, AMANO H, HARIMA K, AIBA T, ASAGAMI F, KINUKAWA K, ARIYAMA S, TAKAMOTO T: **Pancreatic sphincterotomy and pancreatic endoprosthesis.** *Endoscopy* 1985, 17:69–72.

61. PONSKY JL, DUPPLER DW: **Endoscopic Sphincterotomy and Removal of Pancreatic Duct Stones.** *Am Surg* 1987, 53:613–616.

62. DELHAYE M, VANDERMEAREN A, GABBRIELLI A, CREMER MP
• **Lithotripsy and Endoscopy for Pancreatic Calculi: the First 104 Patients.** *Gastroenterology* 1990, 98:A216.

Preliminary report of excellent clinical results from extracorporeal shock wave lithotripsy of pancreatic calculi followed by endoscopic extraction of stone fragments.

63. HABER G, SHERMAN S, MILLER L, HAWES R, PONICH T, KORTAN R,
• LEHMAN G: **Pancreatic Duct Stones: Frequency of Successful Removal and Improvement in Symptoms.** *Gastrointest Endosc* 1990, 36:202–203A.

Preliminary report of endoscopic removal of pancreatic calculi with symptom improvement in 60% of patients.

64. HUIBREGTSE K, SCHNEIDER B, VRIJ AA, TYTGAT GNJ: **Endoscopic Pancreatic Drainage in Chronic Pancreatitis.** *Gastrointest Endosc* 1988, 34:9–15.

65. MCCARTHY J, GEENE JE, HOGAN WJ: **Preliminary Experience with Endoscopic Stent Placement in Benign Pancreatic Diseases.** *Gastrointest Endosc* 1988, 34:16–18.

66. KOZAREK RA, PATTERSON DJ, BALL TJ, TRAVERSO LW: **Endoscopic Placement of Pancreatic Stents and Drains in the Management of Pancreatitis.** *Ann Surg* 1989, 209:261–266.

67. GRIMM H, MEYER WH, NAM VCH, SOEHENDRA N: **New Modalities for Treating Chronic Pancreatitis.** *Endoscopy* 1989, 21:70–74.

68. KOZAREK RA: **Pancreatic Stents Can Induce Ductal Changes**
• **Consistent with Chronic Pancreatitis.** *Gastrointest Endosc* 1990, 36:93–95.

Pancreatic stents induce ductal changes that simulate chronic pancreatitis. This is a worrisome consequence of pancreatic stenting.

69. DERFUS GA, GEENEN JE, HOGAN WJ: **Effect of Endoscopic Pancreatic Duct Stent Placement on Pancreatic Ductal Morphology.** *Gastrointest Endosc* 1990, 36:206A.

70. STAHL TJ, ALLEN MO, ANSEL HJ, VENNES JA: **Partial Biliary Obstruction Caused by Chronic Pancreatitis: An Appraisal of Indications for Surgical Biliary Drainage.** *Ann Surg* 1988, 207:26–32.

71. DEVIÈRE J, DEVAERE S, BAIZE M, CREMER M: **Endoscopic Biliary**
• **Drainage in Chronic Pancreatitis.** *Gastrointest Endosc* 1990, 36:96–100.

The value of biliary stenting for common bile duct obstruction secondary to chronic pancreatitis was evaluated in 25 patients. Cholestasis and cholangitis initially resolved in all patients but recurred with stent occlusion or migration. Only three patients required no further stents because of resolution of pancreatitis and biliary structure. This retrospective study indicates that operative intervention is preferable as a long-term solution in such patients.

Endoscopic management of gallstone disease

D.E.F. Tweedle and D.F. Martin

Departments of Surgery and Radiology, Gastroenterology Unit, Withington Hospital, University Hospital of South Manchester, Manchester, UK

Advances in the management of cholecystolithiasis and choledocholithiasis continued to enable an ever greater proportion of patients to be managed without conventional surgery. The role of laparoscopic cholecystectomy is gradually being established as is the range of adjunctive procedures. Successful endoscopic extraction of larger bile duct stones is increasing.

Introduction

Undoubtedly one of the major events of 1990 in the field of gastroenterology was the universal adoption of laparoscopic cholecystectomy. In biliary tract disease this procedure has already produced a revolutionary effect comparable to the introduction of endoscopic retrograde cholangiopancreatography (ERCP) in 1974. The technique of laparoscopic cholecystectomy and other more immediate details are dealt with in this issue by Boyce. However, it is already apparent that laparoscopic removal of the gallbladder will have significant consequences for the biliary endoscopist [1••] and these will be dealt with in more detail later in this chapter. The endoscopist is now able to remove more than 90% of gallstones from the biliary tract. During the past year, the major concerns have been how to deal with stones demonstrated in the biliary tree that cannot be removed by standard techniques; how to achieve success in the small numbers of patients in whom the whole or part of the biliary tree seems inaccessible and the subsequent function or the need to remove a retained gallbladder (regardless of whether it contains stones or not).

Retained stones

Other studies [2] have demonstrated that the complication rate following endoscopic sphincterotomy for choledocholithiasis is increased when clearance of the biliary tree is not achieved at the initial ERCP. This has recently been confirmed in 128 patients undergoing this procedure in whom the complication rate was 11.4% in the 70 patients whose ducts were cleared at the initial endoscopy, but was 32.8% in the 58 in whom clearance was not achieved [3]. It is rare to experience difficulty in removing stones up to 1 cm in size, unless there is a stricture below the stone. Many stones larger than 2 cm prove to be very difficult to remove. The standard technique for such stones usually involves mechanical lithotripsy and three different types of mechanical lithotriptors have been used in 93 patients over the last 8 years by Siegel *et al.* [4••], with 94% success in clearing the common duct. Mechanical lithotripsy is now more easily performed using the newly devised system in which a basket is initially introduced into the bile duct through a Teflon sheath over which the outer, larger diameter, coiled spring sheath is then advanced (Fig. 1). An alternative method in patients in whom it proves difficult to gain access to a stone after sphincterotomy is to use a basket that has a 3–4 cm distal soft tip (Fig. 2) and is inserted into the common duct. The tip may then be left in the common duct when the basket containing the stone is withdrawn into the duodenum. The stone can then be released without losing access to the common duct [5•]. This basket is manufactured in a form that allows it to be used with a so-called emergency lithotriptor. These modifications to existing equipment will enable fragmentation and extraction to be performed in some patients in whom previously this was not technically feasible. There are still patients in whom mechanical lithotripsy and extraction is impossible and a number of techniques have been devised to deal with these retained stones. An impacted distal stone is an emergency, as complete obstruction of the bile duct in a patient with stones is almost always followed by cholangitis. If the patient has a T-tube *in situ*, obstruction and cholangitis are less likely to occur. A three-stage interventional radiological technique has been devised to overcome this difficulty [6•].

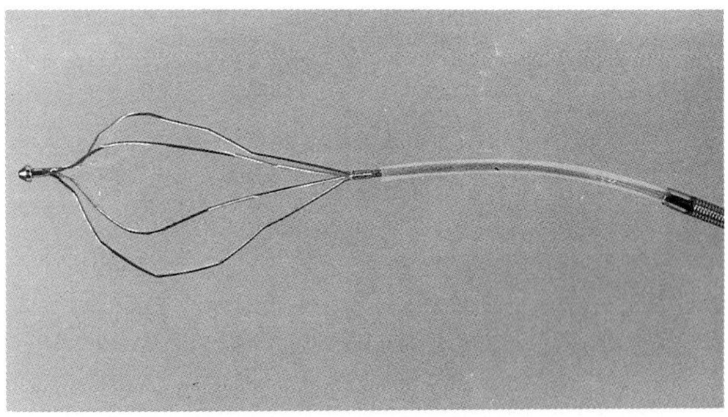

Fig. 1. Mechanical lithotriptor with a Teflon sheathed basket to facilitate duct cannulation and stone entrapment.

A further method to deal with large stones in either the bile duct or intrahepatic ducts is to use a pulsed dye laser to disintegrate the stones, as in the two case reports by Berci *et al.* and one by Flowers *et al.* [7•,8•,9•].

© Current Science Ltd ISBN 1-870485-32-7 ISSN 0952-6293

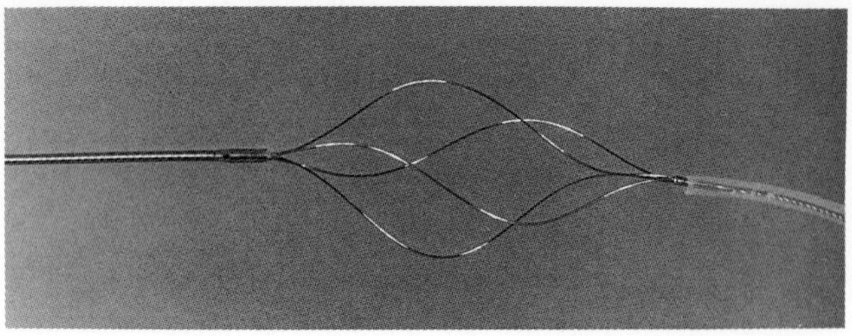

Fig. 2. Soft guide-wire tipped basket for maintaining bile duct cannulation during stone extraction.

These procedures may be performed along the T-tube track using a choledochoscope or a flexible ureteroscope and the stones can be disintegrated under direct vision within a few seconds. An alternative to using laser lithotripsy is electrohydraulic lithotripsy. Initially this technique was associated with significant mucosal damage, but in a series of 21 patients [10•] 18 of the patients underwent successful disintegration and extraction of fragments. One patient suffered a minor attack of acute pancreatitis but there was no other complication. If the patient does not have a T-tube in the common bile duct, an impacted stone may be dealt with by pre-cut papillotomy (see elsewhere in this chapter). In the future, contact lithotripsy will be performed more often under direct vision using 'mother and baby' endoscopes. This system allows direct visualization of lithotripsy and has the advantage of allowing the endoscopist to see other lesions in the biliary tree and to take brushings and biopsies from these. The major disadvantage is that it requires two endoscopists and can be very time-consuming [11•]. Many institutions do not have these sophisticated techniques available for distintegration of large stones. If the common bile duct cannot be cleared at ERCP we agree with Siegel *et al.* [3] that a biliary endoprosthesis should be inserted for temporary drainage. A pernasal catheter can also be left *in situ* and extracorporeal shock-wave lithotripsy (ESWL) undertaken. Our own experience with this mode of lithotripsy is encouraging, but indicates that ERCP is needed to clear fragments after ESWL, a sentiment echoed by Kohlberger *et al.* [12•], using a Wolf piezoelectric lithotriptor. The major concern in leaving a stone in the common duct is that it might impact and produce cholangitis. As indicated above, in order to prevent this possibility an endoprosthesis may be inserted into the bile duct. Long-term-follow-up [13•] (median 26 months) of 26 elderly patients (mean age 81) showed that 10 patients died 2–28 months after the insertion of the endoprosthesis from causes unrelated to biliary pathology, five patients required surgical treatment and the remaining 11 patients were alive and free of symptoms. If an endoscopist working in a hospital with limited facilities is unable to extract a large stone, perhaps the sensible approach is to insert an endoprosthesis to prevent impaction and refer the patient to a specialist centre where there are facilities for various forms of lithotripsy. Although Soomers *et al.* [13•] describe the use of 10 French (F) endoprostheses, we prefer to use 7 F double pigtail endoprostheses (Fig. 3). These can be inserted using a standard 3.2 mm channel endoscope after ERCP and this avoids the need to change to a larger channel endoscope during the procedure.

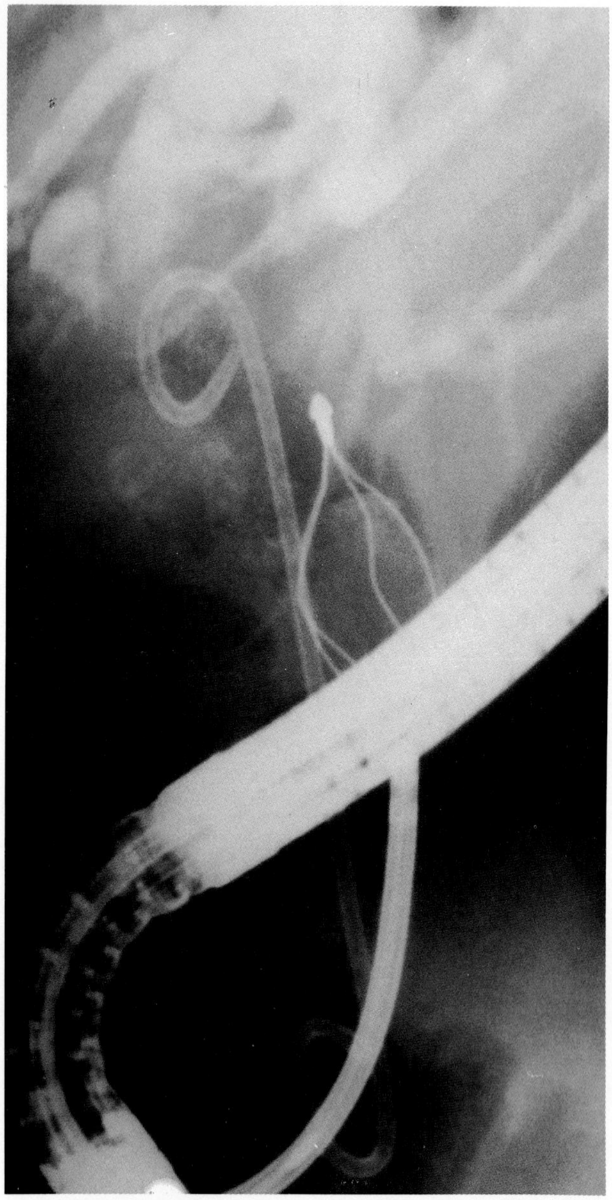

Fig. 3. Radiograph showing a 7 F double pigtail endoprosthesis previously inserted to prevent stone impaction. A mechanical lithotriptor is about to crush the stone.

Pre-cut papillotomy

Since a very cautionary editorial was published suggesting this was a risky technique to be used by experts only experts only [14], there has been another important publication concerning the use of this technique in patients with impacted common bile duct stones at the ampulla [15••].

Conventional papillotomy had failed because of an impacted ampullary stone in 20 out of 510 (4%) patients with common bile duct stones. Diagnostic cannulation had been successful in only seven of these patients. All patients were suffering from acute cholangitis. Following pre-cut papillotomy, immediate extraction of the stone was possible in 16 patients. In three patients a naso-biliary catheter was inserted for temporary drainage and extraction was ultimately successful. Extraction failed in only one patient who underwent surgery. No perforation, cholangitis or clinical pancreatitis resulted from pre-cut papillotomy. This paper emphasizes how this technique is being adopted successfully by experts to treat highly selected patients in whom endoscopic sphincterotomy has failed. Our belief [16] is that pre-cut papillotomy is excellent in assisting sphincterotomy when deep cannulation is difficult, although a wire guided sphincterotome (Fig. 4) may avoid this need. Pre-cut papillotomy for diagnostic cholangiography should only be undertaken when there is firm clinical and radiological evidence of duct obstruction which may be treatable endoscopically.

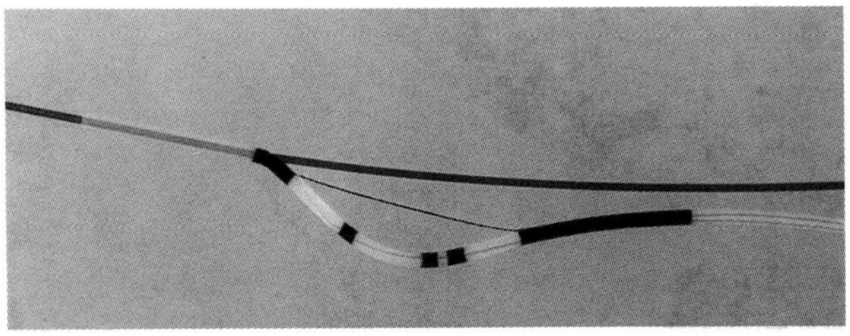

Fig. 4. A wire-guided sphincterotome (our preferred design).

Cholangitis and pancreatitis

Surgical decompression for acute cholangitis can be associated with a mortality of up to 50%. The excellent results obtained by pre-cut papillotomy in 20 patients from Hong Kong with cholangitis due to an impacted stone at the ampulla have been described already [15••]. In a further series of 30 patients from Denmark, 25 (83%) were successfully treated by endoscopic sphincterotomy and stone extraction [17•]. Four patients required surgical exploration and extraction. All these patients survived. One elderly patient who also had a cholangio-carcinoma died. In Australia, 13 (81%) out of 16 patients showed rapid resolution of cholangitis following successful endoscopic sphincterotomy [18•]. Of three other patients requiring surgical decompression, one died. Although there has not been a randomized controlled trial of endoscopic versus surgical decompression in patients with acute cholangitis, these and other studies show clearly that endoscopic decompression carried a much lower mortality and morbidity.

During the past year there was one published study [19] of a large consecutive series of patients undergoing endoscopic sphincterotomy for biliary pancreatitis. One hundred and forty-eight patients underwent this procedure within 24 hours of admission to hospital. The mortality rate was impressive, with only five deaths. However, only 17 of these patients had a Ranson score of four or more and could be considered to be suffering from severe pancreatitis. The role of endoscopic sphincterotomy in patients with acute biliary pancreatitis remains to be established by a controlled trial, but these results are very encouraging. In an interesting paper Baillie *et al.* [20•]described the use of sphincterotomy to clear the ducts of five patients with calculous biliary obstruction presenting during mid to late pregnancy. All patients were successfully treated and delivered normal children. The authors rightly stress the importance of limiting radiation dose to the fetus and describe how this can be very easily undertaken. Our own experience with three patients presenting with obstructive jaundice in early pregnancy is equally encouraging. In these three patients the monitored radiation dose to the fetus was less than that which would be anticipated from a maternal frontal chest radiograph.

Technique

Impaction of endoscopic basket

This complication is fortunately very infrequent and usually occurs during the attempted extraction of a large stone. Luckily most stones can be disimpacted by pushing the basket back up the bile duct with the tip of the duodenoscope angled firmly against the sphincterotomy. When the basket reaches the hepatic duct confluence, it is opened by an assistant, tends to fold over and distort and then releases the stone. If this manoeuvre does not work, the basket can be left *in situ*, the endoscope removed and the stone crushed using a spiral steel oversheath-type emergency lithotriptor. If this does not work and insertion of a drainage tube or endoprosthesis fails, then the patient is usually left with an obstructed duct with a very high risk of cholangitis and septicaemia. Urgent treatment is required. Many of these patients have undergone surgery when more conservative methods have failed. Successful treatment of this complication by disintegrating the stone using extracorporeal shock wave lithotripsy is another alternative that has recently been described [21•]. Patients should be referred urgently to a centre where this and other techniques and expertise are available before undergoing surgery. The sentiment expressed by Landreneau and McClelland [22•] on their experience of a single patient—that surgery should be considered as primary treatment of complex biliary stone problems because of the risk of basket impaction—is not one with which most biliary endoscopists or indeed biliary surgeons would have sympathy.

Foreign bodies

In our experience it is not uncommon to identify and remove at ERCP suture material in patients who have undergone surgical exploration of the bile ducts, surgical sphincteroplasty or choledochoduodenostomy. The removal of prolene sutures has been described in two patients who also underwent endoscopic sphincterotomy and extraction of a stone that may have formed around the suture [23•]. (In Britain, surgeons are trained never to use non-absorbable sutures in the bile duct.) A much more dramatic and clearly symptomatic foreign body, a piece of gauze left following exploration of the bile duct 6 years previously, has also been successfully removed [24•]. This latter foreign body had the radiological appearances of a large stone in the common bile duct on ERCP.

Outpatient endoscoic sphincterotomy

In most centres, endoscopic sphincterotomy is usually performed as an inpatient procedure, the patient remaining overnight because of concern for potential complications. In our own hospital (Withington Hospital, Manchester), we often perform endoscopic sphincterotomy on patients referred from other hospitals, who travel to and from our institution on the same day as sphincterotomy. Most complications of endoscopic sphincterotomy are apparent within the first few hours following the procedure. A study from Canada [25] of 137 selected patients undergoing outpatient sphincterotomy over a 4-year period showed a similar rate of complications to those occurring in inpatients. Complications were noted within 2–4 hours of endoscopic sphincterotomy in 6.6% of outpatients, compared with 7.3% of inpatients. Those patients in whom it was intended to perform the procedure on an outpatient basis, but who developed complications, were admitted. No delayed complications after 4 hours were noted and none of the patients died. Four patients developed pancreatitis, three bled, one developed cholangitis and perforation occurred in another. In addition, five other patients were admitted overnight with abdominal pain that settled spontaneously without any obvious cause. Thus 123 (90%) of the patients were able to be discharged within 4 hours of sphincerotomy. From this study it appears that the majority of patients requiring sphincterotomy can be discharged within 4 hours at procedure providing that they have appropriate escort and accommodation to which to return, they are fit and well and there is no other medical reason that might predispose to complications (e.g. coagulopathy or deficient immunocompetence). Clearly, outpatient sphincterotomy should only be performed by the experienced endoscopist and it is essential that the patient can return immediately for appropriate medical and surgical treatment should any serious complication arise.

The retained gallbladder

Although the management of the *in situ* gallbladder after endoscopic common duct clearance has been contentious, further evidence has emerged that cholecystectomy is not routinely indicated and is ultimately required in only a minority [26•]. Our own data on over 200 patients [27] followed for up to 100 months indicate that symptomatic cholecystectomy is needed in 5.2%, but that 25% die from non-biliary disease, reflecting the poor health of this elderly group in whom routine cholecystectomy would surely do little other than shorten their existence.

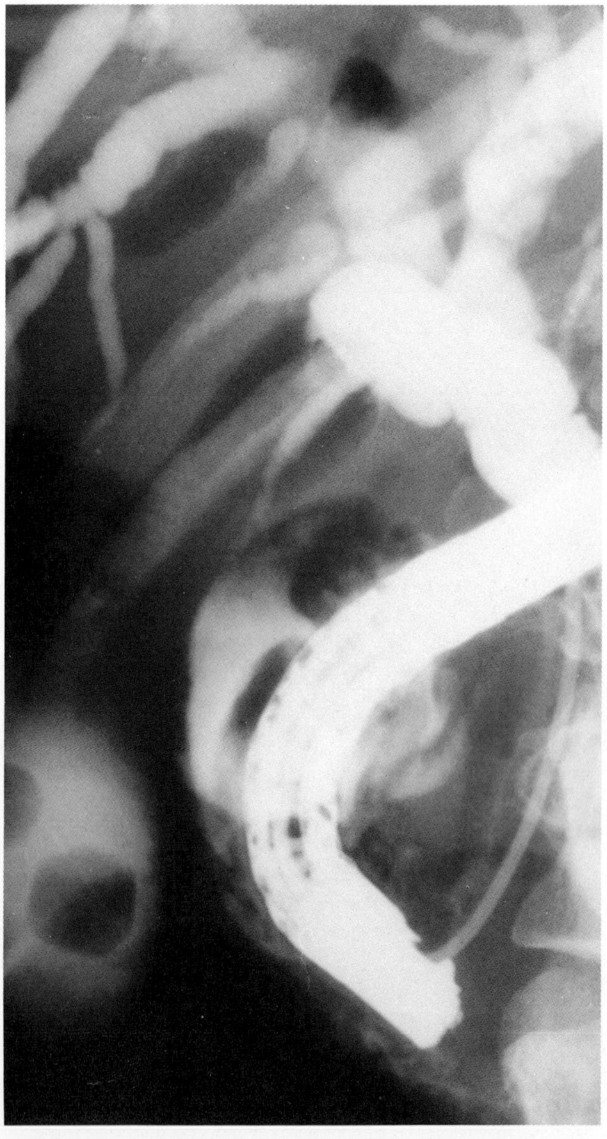

Fig. 5. Mirizzi's syndrome successfully treated endoscopically by pushing the large impacted stone back into the gallbladder with subsequent fragmentation by extracorporeal shock-wave lithotripsy ESWL followed by laparoscopic cholecystectomy.

It may be that stones in the gallbladder can be managed endoscopically. Soehendra *et al.* [28••] and McCarthy *et al.* [29•] have contributed to the literature describing endoscopic retrograde gallbladder cannulation, which can then allow direct contact dissolution with methy tert-butyl ether (MTBE) imaging for ESWL. What happens to gallbladder function after sphincterotomy and is it clinically relevant? The answer to the first question is still unclear, although data suggesting reduced function have been recorded by Desa *et al.* [30•] using Technetium HIDA. This study has been criticized on methodological and semantic grounds, but will no doubt stimulate further investigation. The question of clinical relevance will have to wait a while.

Laparoscopic cholecystectomy

The philosophical approach of many surgeons to the possibility of co-existent pathology in the bile ducts when performing open cholecystectomy for cholecystolithiasis differs radically. The majority of experts in the field favour peroperative cholangiography, arguing that any disease noted radiologically before surgery may have changed by the time of operation. Others will perform a cholecystectomy without any radiological assessment of the bile duct. Between these two extremes are surgeons who will accept radiological assessment performed a short while (up to 3 months) before operation. Perhaps it is not surprising that a similar philosophical approach is emerging in those surgeons who are performing laparoscopic cholecystectomy. In a series of 105 patients undergoing laparoscopic cholecystectomy, unsuspected stones were discovered in 8% [31••]. Peroperative cholangiography is technically feasible in more than 90% of patients undergoing laparoscopic cholecystectomy. This procedure also makes the laparoscopic dissection safer, demonstrating unsuspected anatomical variations such as the origin of the cystic duct from the right hepatic duct. The right hepatic duct may also be divided when mistaken for the cystic duct at open cholecystectomy. If unsuspected stones are found in the common duct during laparoscopic cholecystectomy, it is possible to remove these in some patients with or without disintegration using some form of lithotripsy. It is likely that sophisticated choledochoscopic techniques for dealing with this situation will be developed further in the future. At present, the majority of patients in whom unsuspected stones are found in the duct at laparoscopic cholecystectomy will be referred for postoperative endoscopic sphincterotomy. In an ideal world, patients otherwise suitable for laparoscopic cholecystectomy would undergo endoscopic cholangiography and, if necessary, endoscopic sphincterotomy and stone extraction (Fig. 5) immediately before laparoscopic cholecystectomy, possible in the operating theatre.

References and recomended reading

Papers of special interest, published within the annual period of review, have been highlighted as:

- • Of interest
- •• Of outstanding interest

1. •• REDDICK EJ, OLSEN D, ALEXANDER W, BAILEY A, BAIRD D, PRICE N, PRUITT R: **Laparoscopic Laser Cholecystectomy and Choledocholithiasis.** *Surg Endosc* 1990, **3**:133–135.
Common duct stones suspected before laparoscopic cholecystectomy and those demonstrated by intraoperative cholangiography are best managed by ERCP, although intraoperative choledochoscopy is useful in patients with sufficiently large cystic ducts.

2. MARTIN DF, MCGREGOR JC, LAMBERT ME, TWEEDLE DEF: **Stone Extraction after Endoscopic Sphincterotomy—an Active Policy is Best.** *Gut* 1987, **25**:85.

3. KULLMAN E, BORCH K, LIEDBERG G: **Long Term Follow Up after Endoscopic Management of Retained and Recurrent Common Duct Stones.** *Acta Chir Scand* 1989, **155**:395–399.

4. •• SIEGEL JH, BEN-ZVI JS, PULLANO WE: **Mechanical Lithotripsy of Common Duct Stones.** *Gastrointest Endosc* 1990, **36**:351–356.
Three different types of mechanical lithoptriptors were used endoscopically in 93 patients with 94% success in clearing the common duct. Good description of techniques.

5. • SCHWARTZ HM, BARKIN JS: **Wire Guided Basket Extraction of Common Bile Duct Stones.** *Gastrointest Endosc* 1990, **36**:296–298.
Triple case report of the use of a 4 cm guidewire tipped basket that allows access to the common duct to be maintained while the stone is withdrawn into the duodenum.

6. • MALONE DE, BURHENNE HJ: **Technical Problems: Impacted Retained Distal Common Duct Stone.** *Clin Radiol* 1990, **41**:130–133.
Case report of a three-stage procedure successfully allowing T-tube track extraction of impacted bile duct stones.

7. • BERCI G, HAMLIN JA, DAYKHOVSKY L, PAZ-PARTLOW M: **Common Bile Duct Laser Lithotripsy.** *Gastrointest Endosc* 1990, **36**:137–138.
Case report of pulsed dye laser lithotripsy of a bile duct stone via T tube track.

8. • BERCI G, HAMLIN JA, GRUNDFEST W, DAYHKHOVSKY L, PAZ-PARTLOW M: **Percutaneous Endoscopic Laser Lithotripsy of Retained Stone in the Left Hepatic Duct.** *Surg Endosc* 1990, **4**:36–38.
A flexible ureteroscope inserted through a T tube track allowed pulsed dye laser lithotripsy of intrahepatic stones.

9. • FLOWERS BF, SASLAWSKY MJ, MATHES GL, TONKIN AK: **Use of the Pulsed Dye Laser and Ultrasonic Lithotriptor for Removal of Multiple Intrahepatic Gallstones.** *Surg Gynecol Obstet* 1990, **170**:443–444.
Case report of a complex patient treated by transhepatic pulsed dye laser lithotripsy via a flexible nephroscope to fragment and clear intrahepatic duct stones.

10. • SIEGEL JH, BEN-ZVI JS, PULLANO WE: **Endoscopic Electrohydraulic Lithotripsy.** *Gastrointest Endosc* 1990, **36**:134–136.
Describes 86% success (21 patients) using balloon guided transduodenoscopic electrohydraulic lithotripsy on stones 1–1.5 cm in diameter.

11. • PONSKY JL, SCHEERES DE, SIMON I: **Endoscopic Retrograde Cholangioscopy.** *Am Surg* 1990, **56**:235–237.
Describes the use of the 'mother and baby' system in five patients with bile duct stones and speculates on the usefulness of the system.

12. KOHLBERGER EJ, RADECKE J, SALM R, WANINGER J: **Large-Bile-**
• **Duct Stones—Extracorporeal Piezoelectric Lithotripsy as Adjuvant Measure for Endoscopic Basket Extraction.** *Surg Endosc* 1990, 4:20–22.

Describes 75% (nine out of 12 patients) success in clearing previously unextractable stones from the common duct using a piezolith lithotriptor. Additional endoscopic procedures were usually required to assist ESWL.

13. SOOMERS AJ, NAGENGAST FM, YAP SH: **Endoscopic Placement**
• **of Biliary Endoprostheses in Patients with Endoscopically Unextractable Common Bile Duct Stones.** *Endoscopy* 1990, 22:24–26.

Thirty-four patients (eight lost to follow-up) with common duct stones treated by stent insertion. Five required surgery, 10 died of unrelated causes, the remainder required no other therapy.

14. COTTON PB: **Precut Papillotomy—A Risky Technique for Experts Only.** *Gastrointest Endosc* 1989, **35**:578–579.

15. LEUNG JWC, BANEZ VP, CHUNG SCF: **Precut (needle knife)**
•• **papillotomy for impacted common bile duct stone at the ampulla.** *Am J Gastroenterol* 1990, **85**:991–993.

Describes how the judicious use of pre-cut papillotomy for impacted stones can turn failure to success in experienced hands.

16. TWEEDLE DEF, MARTIN DF: **Pre-Cut Papillotomy for Endoscopic Sphincterotomy and Cholangiography.** *Gastrointest Endosc* (in press).

17. DITZEL H, DE MUCKADELL OBS: **Endoscopic Sphincterotomy**
• **in Acute Cholantitis Due to Choledocholithiasis.** *Hepatogastroenterology* 1990, **37**:204–207.

Thirty patients with acute cholangitis were managed endoscopically with success in 25 patients. One with a cholangio-carcinoma died, four others underwent surgery.

18. WORTHLEY CS, TOOULI J: **Endoscopic Decompression for**
• **Acute Cholangitis due to Stones.** *Aust NZ J Surg* 1990, 60:355–359.

Reports 81% success in the management of 16 patients with acute cholangitis (11 severe). Two endoscopic failures requiring surgery died.

19. SAFRANY L, SCHMEDING K, SCHOTT B: **Endoskopische Papillotomie bei Akuter Biliarer Pankreatitis.** *Med Welt* 1989, 40:171–174.

20. BAILLIE J, CAIRNS SR, COTTON PB: **Endoscopic Management of**
• **Choledocholithiasis During Pregnancy.** *Surg Gynecol Obstet* 1990, 171:1–4.

Five patients in mid to late pregnancy with biliary obstruction successfully managed endoscopically. Important and useful discussion of radiation dose limitation.

21. MERRETT M, DESMOND P: **Removal of Impacted Endoscopic**
• **Basket and Stone from the Common Bile Duct by Extra Corporeal Shock Waves.** *Endoscopy* 1990, 22:92.

Case report of ESWL successfully fragmenting a 2 cm stone trapped in a basket.

22. LANDRENEAU RJ, MCCLELLAND RN: **Impaction of the Endo-**
• **scopic Basket.** *Am Surg* 1990, **56**:388–393.

Single case report describing surgery to remove an impacted basket. Attempts to argue for primary surgical management in complex problems with stones in the common duct because of the risk of this complication, and largely ignores recent advances.

23. HEARNE SE, STUMP DL: **Endoscopic Removal of Proline Su-**
• **tures from the Common Bile Duct During Endoscopic Retrograde Cholangiography.** *Gastrointest Endosc* 1990, **36**:301.

Two case reports of suture material removed with stone fragments at ERCP.

24. SAKAI P, ISHIOKA S, ZAMBRANO M, MARONE P, ZITRON C: **Endo-**
• **scopic Removal of an Atypical Common Bile Duct Foreign Body.** *Endoscopy* 1990, **22**:93.

Report of a case in which a crumpled gauze swab left in the bile duct after cholecystectomy 6 years previously was removed endoscopically.

25. PODOLSKY I, KORTAN P, HABER GP: **Endoscopic Sphincterotomy in Outpatients.** *Gastrointest Endosc* 1989, **35**:372–376.

26. SHEMESH E, KLEIN E, CZERNIAK A, CORET A, BAT L: **Endoscopic**
• **Sphincterotomy in Patients with Gallbladder In Situ: The Influence of Periampullary Duodenal Diverticula.** *Surgery* 1990, **107**:163–166.

Fourty-four patients (mean age 77 years) with gallbladders in position followed up for 25 months (mean) after endoscopic duct clearance. Only two patients required cholecystectomy, which was performed without complication.

27. HILL J, MARTIN DF, TWEEDLE DEF: **What are the Risks of Leaving the Gallbladder *in situ* after Endoscopic Sphincterotomy for Bile Duct Stones.** *Br J Surg* (in press).

28. SOEHENDRA N, SCHULZ H, NAM VCH *ET AL*: **ESWL and Gall-**
•• **stone Dissolution with MTBE via a Naso-Vesicular Catheter.** *Endoscopy* 1990, **22**:176–179.

Ninety per cent success in cannulating and catheterizing the gallbladder via the duodenoscope. Describes the use of MTBE and ESWL to treat gallbladder stones with complete stone clearance in 60% (20 out of 34); there were five complications (three pancreatitis, one cystic duct perforation, one guidewire impaction).

29. MCCARTHY JH, MILLER GL, LAURENCE BH: **Cannulation of**
• **the Cystic Duct and Gallbladder [Letter].** *Endoscopy* 1990, 22:191.

Letter describing techniques of gallbladder catheterisation.

30. DESA LA, GRACE PA, HENDERSON B, THOMPSON JN, VIPOND MN:
• **Gallbladder Function after Endoscopic Sphincterotomy.** *Br Med J* 1990, **300**:1111.

Six patients studied shortly after sphincterotomy using technetium HIDA to assess gallbladder filling. All had gallbladder filling at the time of ERCP but none showed filling by technetium HIDA.

31. BERCI G: **Extra Corporeal Shock Wave Lithotripsy of Gall-**
•• **stones and the Importance of Operative Cholangiography During Laparoscopic Cholecystectomy.** *Surg Endosc* 1990, 4:131–132.

Reports an 8% rate of unsuspected duct stones and emphasizes the risk of anatomical variants.

Endoscopic management of biliary strictures

J.W.C. Leung

Department of Medicine, Prince of Wales Hospital, The Chinese University of Hong Kong, Shatin, New Territories, Hong Kong

Endoscopy has opened new avenues in the management of difficult biliary strictures and fistulae. Although endoscopic stenting is useful palliative therapy for malignant jaundice in elderly high-risk patients, there is growing evidence to support conventional surgery for young and fit patients. The problem of late stent clogging has prompted clinicians to design and develop new stents.

Introduction

Therapeutic endoscopy has made a significant impact in the management of patients with biliary strictures. Stenting has an established role in the palliation of malignant jaundice and is also useful in promoting healing of biliary fistulas. Balloon dilatation and stenting have achieved good short- and intermediate-term results in patients with benign biliary strictures. However, long-term follow-up studies are necessary to compare the results with surgical treatment. Clogging is a major complication affecting all kinds of plastic stents and limits its use for long-term stenting of benign strictures. Different methods, including surface modification and new stent designs, are being tested in an attempt to prevent or delay clogging. Although results of randomized controlled studies will help to define the relative benefits of individual therapy in treating biliary strictures, we must remember that these results only apply to a certain patient population in a special centre under a particular setting.

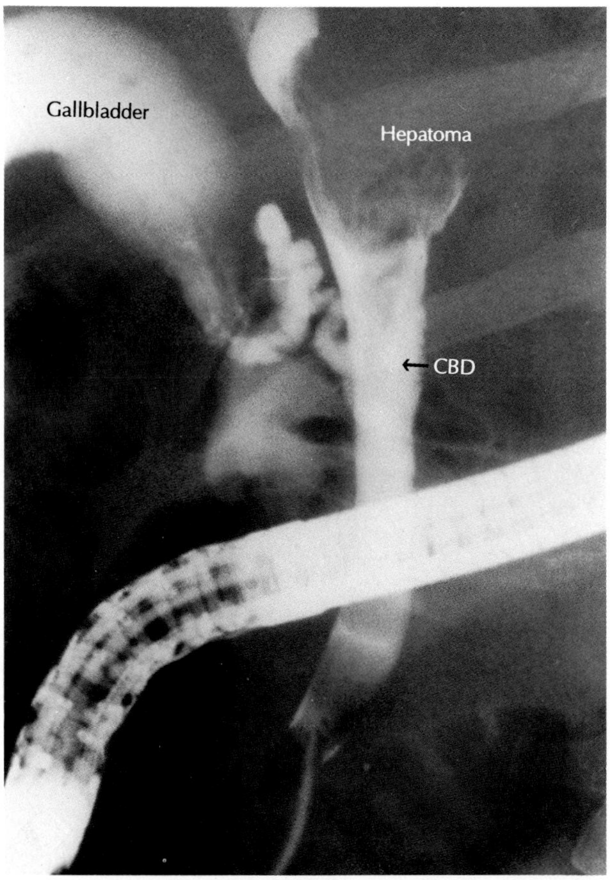

Fig. 1. Cholangiogram showing hepatoma infiltrating the common hepatic duct with luminal extension causing biliary obstruction.

Malignant biliary obstruction

Confirmation of malignancy

Malignant obstructive jaundice is caused by tumours of the ampulla, and carcinoma of the bile ducts, gallbladder, and pancreas, in addition to extrinsic compression by metastatic lymph nodes. In rare cases, hepatocellular carcinoma may infiltrate the bile ducts and cause obstructive jaundice by luminal extension [1•,2•] (Fig. 1). Mucin-secreting villous cholangiocarcinoma is rare and often presents with mucoid biliary obstruction [3•]. Other unusual benign diseases may masquerade as malignancy [4•]. Despite developments in diagnostic imaging, histology is necessary to confirm the underlying diagnosis [5,6•]. In patients with suspicious ampullary lesions, simple biopsy of the papilla provides a firm diagnosis in only 70% of patients in whom an underlying carcinoma is subsequently proven by surgery [7•]. The yield may be increased with biopsy of deeper tissues after sphincterotomy [8]. Peroral choledochoscopy is useful in detecting pathologies within the bile ducts and permits biopsy under direct vision [9•] (Fig. 2). A special sleeved cytology brush with a lead guidewire can be used to obtain specimens while maintaining the track through the bile duct stricture [10•].

Pathophysiology of malignant jaundice

Prolonged biliary obstruction may result in impairment of liver function. The raised intrabiliary pressure may lead to

© Current Science Ltd ISBN 1-870485-32-7 ISSN 0952-6293

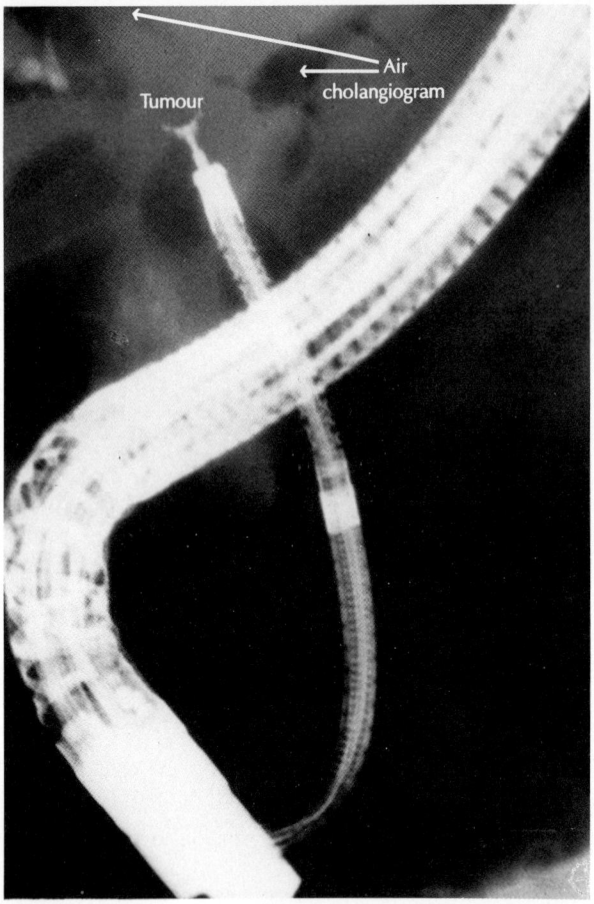

Fig. 2. Radiograph showing the mother and baby scopes with the biopsy forceps opened against a hilar lesion and air cholangiogram.

changes in the bile duct as well as the hepatocytes. Histological studies of the bile duct proximal to the obstruction have revealed extensive denervation changes [11•]. The biliary excretion of immunoglobulins, in particular IgA, which is responsible in part for immunologic defense of the biliary system, is also impaired [12•]. This may favour infection in a contaminated and obstructed biliary system.

Antibiotic prophylaxis for biliary drainage

Despite the use of prophylactic antibiotics, cholangitis and septicaemia are more common in patients with failed or incomplete drainage [13•]. The choice of prophylactic antibiotics depends on the bacteria commonly isolated from bile and also on the method of biliary drainage. Levine *et al.* [14•] showed that there were more Gram-positive organisms isolated from the blood and bile of patients with percutaneous drainage, in contrast to only Gram-negative organisms in patients with endoscopic drainage. We studied the effect of raised intrabiliary pressure on the biliary excretion of antibiotics and showed that there was no antibiotic activity in the bile of patients with complete biliary obstruction despite a 24-hour period of drug therapy. Antibiotics only appeared in bile after establishment of biliary drainage [15••]. The bile level of cefoperazone, an antibiotic with active hepatic excretion, took longer to recover because of impaired liver function compared with ceftazidime, an antibiotic that was passively excreted. The absence of antibiotics in bile no doubt contributes to the high incidence of cholangitis in patients with hilar obstruction and inadequate drainage. The most important steps to prevent biliary infection are to adopt a strict aseptic technique and to use properly disinfected instruments. It is also important to avoid overfilling of the bile ducts until drainage is established.

Palliation of malignant jaundice

The percutaneous approach

Percutaneous transhepatic puncture of the liver was described more than 50 years ago. Percutaneous therapy has been an important treatment modality for biliary diseases over the past decade [16•,17•]. Percutaneous drainage takes the form of external, external/internal catheter drainage and internal stenting. The excessive loss of bile and electrolytes in patients on long-term external drainage may be overcome by creating a biliogastric shunt, as described by Foutch *et al.* [18•]. The technique is now mainly used in patients with failed endoscopic drainage and subsequent stenting performed by the combined procedure [19•]. Two ways of performing the combined procedure have been described, depending on whether the guidewire is introduced by the radiologist percutaneously or by the endoscopist through the endoscope [20•]. In either case, the guidewire that traverses the liver and the endoscope serves as a railway track for stent insertion. Choosing a more peripheral duct during the initial percutaneous puncture and the use of biplane screening may help to prevent malpositioning of stents [21•].

As it is difficult to remove blocked stents, many workers recommend percutaneous stenting only in terminal patients. However, Jackson *et al.* [22•] and Lee *et al.* [23•] have reported a success greater than 50% in exchanging the blocked stents by the percutaneous route.

The endoscopic approach

Endoscopic treatment is a useful alternative to surgery in the palliation of malignant jaundice. In high-risk patients with ampullary carcinoma, endoscopic sphincterotomy offers good palliation for the jaundice [24•]. Shemesh *et al.* [25•] reported the use of endoscopic fulguration and piecemeal removal by polypectomy snare for treating tumour recurrence at the papilla after surgery.

For patients with distal common duct obstruction, endoscopic stenting is superior to percutaneous stenting in terms of the 30-day mortality and associated morbidity [26]. The success of endoscopic stenting is close to 90% for distal and mid common duct obstruction [27••] (Fig. 3). Success with stenting of hilar obstruction is

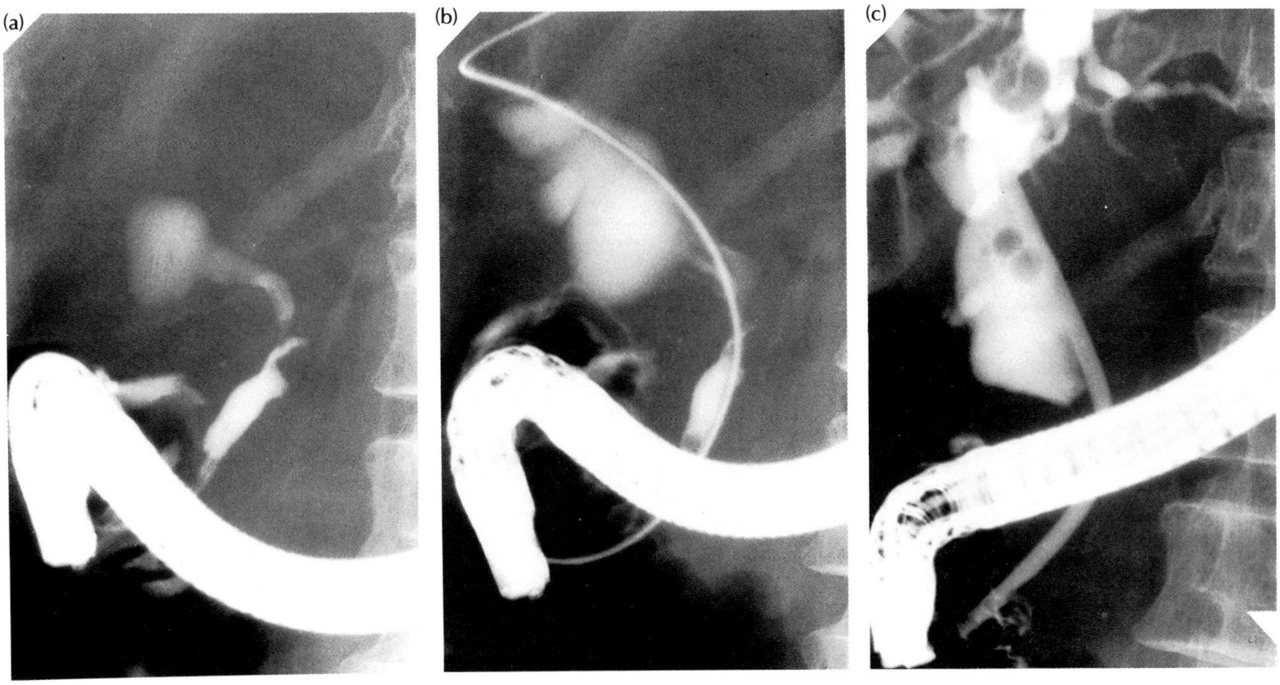

Fig. 3. (a) Distal commom duct stricture caused by carcinoma of the head of pancreas. (b) Guidewire and guiding catheter inserted into the dilated proximal commom duct. (c) 10 F stent inserted into the contrast filled proximal bile duct.

lower at around 80% because of the tightness of strictures and often multiple segment involvement [8]. Successful drainage of both right and left systems by double stents is achieved in only 20% of cases [13•]. The study by Polydorou *et al.* [28] in 151 patients with type II and III strictures showed that drainage of both lobes of the liver was not necessary provided 25% of the liver volume was drained by a single stent. Although the anatomy of the main hepatic ducts favours drainage of the left system, no significant difference was found in the overall results and survival between patients with drainage of either system.

Additional therapy

Siegel and colleagues [29•] used a high-dose-rate remote after-loading device introduced through a 10 French (F) nasobiliary catheter. This allowed high-dose irradiation to be delivered to the lesion in a short period of time and avoided the risk of conventional intracavitary radiation. Percutaneous transhepatic choledochoscopic guided laser therapy was used to treat proximal and mild common duct obstruction in 10 patients [30•]. Good results were obtained with recanalization of the tumour and five out of 10 patients did not require additional stenting for drainage. Indeed, late cholangitis was more common in the other five patients with indwelling stents due to stent blockage.

Stenting versus surgery

Most of the reported studies have been retrospective analyses of single-centre experience. The significance of these studies is limited because they are often nonrandomized and sometimes biased by patient selection [31•,32•]. Two reported randomized studies [33,34] involving small numbers of patients compared endoscopic stenting with bypass surgery. The results showed trends towards an advantage for endoscopic management in the short-term, which, however, was eroded by a higher incidence of readmission due to recurrent jaundice and cholangitis because of stent blockage. However, these studies were too small to allow any meaningful statistical conclusions. A recently completed randomized study comparing endoscopic stenting and surgical bypass involving more than 200 patients with distal common bile duct obstruction was reported by the Middlesex group [35]. The results showed a higher success rate with fewer initial complications and a lower 30-day mortality for endoscopic drainage compared with surgery. However, with extended follow-up, there were more readmissions for recurrent jaundice due to stent blockage and a higher incidence of duodenal obstruction requiring surgical bypass in the endoscopy group [27••]. Although endoscopic stenting offers good palliation for elderly high-risk patients with limited survival, surgical bypass is a better alternative for relatively young and fit patients with unresectable lesions [36•].

The problem of stent clogging

Clogging is the most important complication affecting endoscopic and percutaneous stents. Previous studies have revealed the presence of a bacterial biofilm and bile pigment blocking the lumen of the stent [37] (Fig. 4a).

Groen *et al.* [38] have postulated that blockage is initiated by the adsorption of a 'sticky protein' on the stent surface. They demonstrated the presence of a protein with a molecular weight of 13–16 kD closely adherent to the stent. However, the nature of this protein was uncertain, and they failed to identify the corresponding protein in the patient's bile. We have shown that live bacteria are important in the initiation of stent blockage through adherence and formation of a biofilm [39] (Fig. 4b, c). Both deposition of bacterial mucoprotein and bacterial enzymatic activity may contribute to biliary sludge formation [40•]. The 'sticky protein' may represent part of the bacterial cell wall or mucoprotein.

Possible solutions for stent clogging

Different methods to prevent stent blockage have been studied, including the use of long-term oral antibiotics and mucolytic agents, with little success [41]. We tested the effect of surface modification on bacterial adherence using a silver-coated plastic. In a study *in vitro*, we demonstrated a 100-fold reduction in the number of adherent bacteria compared with the control plastic [42]. The benefit of silver coating in the prevention of stent blockage is currently being tested in a controlled clinical study.

Coene *et al.* [44••], in a separate study, confirmed our previous observation [43] that flow through a stent was affected by its design and configuration, and the presence of side holes improved drainage. They demonstrated that the formation of bacterial biofilm was maximum around the side holes (probably in relation to the rough surface and turbulent flow). Results of a subsequent controlled clinical study showed that stents without side holes had a decreased incidence of clogging. They concluded by recommending the use of a straight tube without side holes for internal drainage. This is perhaps not an ideal solution, as blockage of the endhole by tumour extension stent malposition or sludge will render the stent completely useless.

The position of the stent may affect the rate of clogging. Currently, most of the stents are placed such that their distal tip remains in the duodenum for ease of retrieval in the event of clogging. As the papilla of Vater serves as a natural gateway to prevent entry of bacteria into the biliary system [45••], stents traversing the papilla allow reflux of duodenal contents including food (and especially vegetable fibres) and bacteria up the stent. The significance of reflux is demonstrated by an experiment in which cats with surgically implanted biliary stents that traverse the papilla with the distal tip left in the duodenum have a more rapid onset of cholangitis due to stent clogging compared with those with stents placed entirely within the bile duct (Sung, Leung, Costerton *et al.*, unpublished data).

Management of stent clogging

The current treatment for stent clogging is endoscopic or percutaneous removal of the blocked stent using forceps, baskets or balloon catheters [46•] and replacement with a new stent. This is successful in over 90% of cases. Occasional failures may result from difficulty in recannulating an angulated or long and tortuous stricture. The use of a special stent retriever that goes over a guidewire inserted through the blocked stent maintains the track through the stricture and facilitates subsequent stent replacement (Soehendra, personal communication). This, however, carries a risk of dislodging bacteria from the blocked stent thereby causing cholangitis. Similar risk of precipitating cholangitis or septicaemia existed in unblocking clogged stents with guidewires and forceps [47•]. Although the 5.5 mm duodenoscope allows insertion of large 14 F stents, this requires more skill, and perforation of the bile duct has also been reported with this large stiff stent [48]. Szauter *et al.* [49•] reported the use of an indwelling nasobiliary catheter placed alongside the endoscopic stent for irrigation to prevent stent clogging. To minimize discomfort, the nasobiliary catheter was rerouted through a percutaneous gastrostomy converting it into a gastrosto-biliary catheter flushing system.

Self-expandable metal stents

The self-expandable metal wire mesh stents have become popular for percutaneous or endoscopic drainage over the past 2 years [50,51•]. This stent is delivered in a compressed form using a special applicator system. When fully expanded, the stent has a length of 6.7 cm and a diameter of 1 cm. Delivery and positioning of the stent has to be very accurate as it cannot be moved or removed once it has expanded to its final shape and position. The initial results with this technique are very encouraging. The, stent however, is very expensive. Although clogging is uncommon, the risk of tumour infiltration through the wire mesh remains a potential disadvantage. Indeed, Cremer *et al.* [52•] described two patients with stent blockage due to tumour ingrowth after 4 months. They used a sleeve with a diathermic tip to bore through the tumour to recanalize the obstructed lumen. Because of the fixed length of the stent, 'understenting', as suggested by Gillams *et al.* [53•], has accounted for seven out of 19 of cholangitis in their series. More clinical data with longer follow-up studies are required to establish the benefit of this technique. If clogging does not occur, this stent may be useful for long-term stenting in the treatment of benign biliary strictures.

Benign biliary strictures and bile leaks

Biliary fistulae

A biliary fistula may develop as a complication of cholecystectomy, retained common duct stone or inadvertent surgical trauma to the bile ducts, or is rarely related to blunt abdominal trauma. Spontaneous biliary fistulae such as cholecystocolic fistula [54•] or a bronchobiliary fistula [55•] may form secondary to long-standing calculous diseases. Unusual communications reported in-

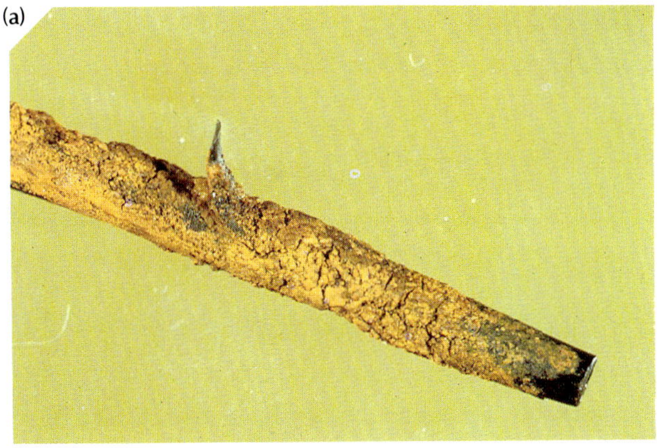

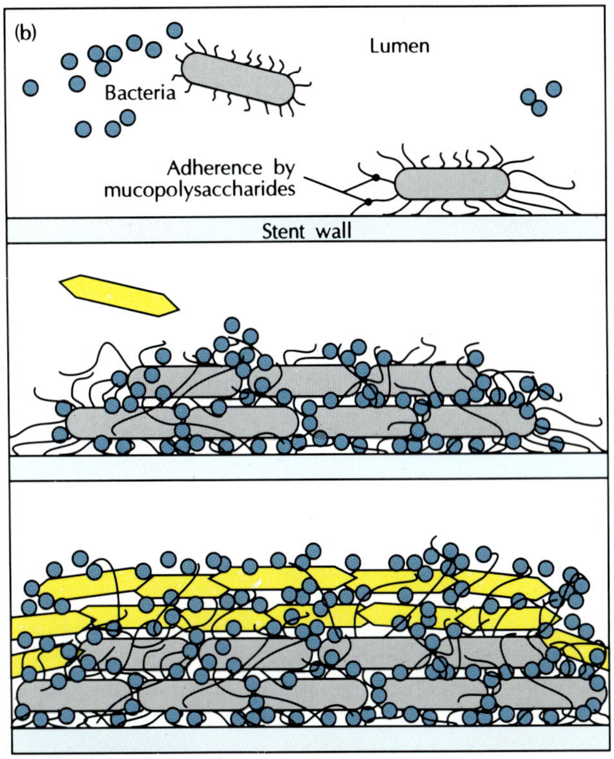

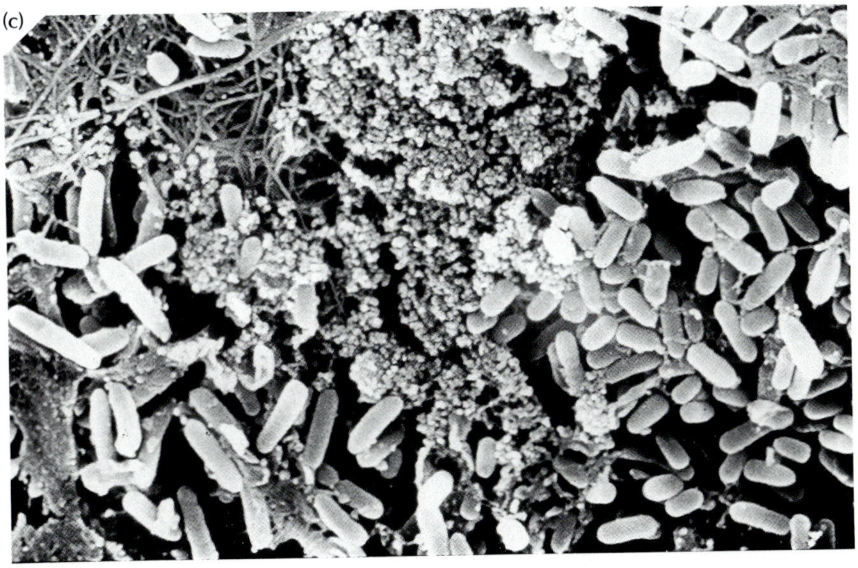

Fig. 4. (a) A blocked biliary stent showing the bile-stained sludge adhering to the outside of the stent, also blocking the side hole at the proximal flap. (b) Diagrammatic representation of biofilm formation showing attachment of bacteria on a surface with trapping of crystals and serving as a foreign surface for further bacterial adherence. (c) Scanning electron micrography showing a bacterial biofilm with the amorphous crystals of calcium bilirubinate mixed with the bacteria.

cluded a pancreaticobiliary fistula complicating ^{125}I interstitial implants for pancreatic cancer [56•]. In the absence of organic obstruction, a bile leak may persist because of the relative resistance to bile flow at the biliary sphincter. Symptoms will depend on the size of the fistula and any subhepatic or subphrenic collection. Although a small leak may not be clinically obvious, a large collection will give rise to clinical symptoms [57]. Whereas abdominal ultrasonography can only demonstrate a subhepatic or subphrenic collection, an HIDA scan is more specific in confirming the bile leak [58]. The presence of bacterial infection may further complicate the bile leak [59•].

Biliary fistulae and bile leaks are difficult to manage surgically. Non-operative management should include diagnostic endoscopic retrograde cholangiopancreatography (ERCP) to define the exact site of leakage, and percutaneous drainage may be required for a sizable fluid collection. Relief of the obstruction to reduce the intrabiliary pressure will promote healing of the fistula [57]. Successful treatment of bile leaks by endoscopic sphincterotomy has been reported. External decompression by a nasobiliary catheter will lead to rapid resolution of the bile leak but is associated with loss of fluid and electrolytes [60] (Fig. 5). Goldin *et al.* [61•] have advocated the use of a large indwelling stent to ensure complete emptying of the biliary system (Fig. 6). Hoffman *et al.* [62•] showed that a small-calibre stent achieved similar results. Berger *et al.* [63] reported a percutaneous method to deliver a spring coil through the fistulous tract to occlude a leaking cystic duct. Another novel approach to obliterate the fistulous tract has involved endoscopic transcatheter embolization of the leaking bile duct with an Ivalon pledget [64•].

Benign biliary strictures

Benign strictures often develop as a result of surgical trauma, after a complicated cholecystectomy or a stenosed bilioenteric anastomosis. Sclerosing cholangitis accounts for a fair proportion of benign strictures in western countries. In the East, benign strictures are a well known complication of intrahepatic stones, which are prevalent in Korea, Japan, Taiwan, Hong Kong and southern China. The aetiopathogenesis of biliary strictures associated with intrahepatic stones remains uncertain. It may be related in part to parasitic infestations with for example, ascariasis or clonorchiasis [65•]. These strictures may predispose to stasis and bacterial infection, and result ultimately in intrahepatic stone formation.

Management of biliary strictures

Conventional treatment for biliary strictures involves surgical repair. Good results have been reported from experienced centers. In a retrospective analysis of 42 patients, Pitt *et al.* [66] have shown that surgical repair of benign strictures achieved a higher success rate (80 versus 55%) and a lower morbidity (4 versus 20%) than balloon dilatation. They recommended that balloon dilatation should only be used for high-risk patients who refused surgery.

Balloon dilatation and stenting for benign strictures

Non-operative management consists of dilatation of strictures with different types of dilators, the most popular being the balloon dilator. This can be inserted percutaneously [67•] or endoscopically [68•] (Fig. 7) under ultrasound or fluoroscopic guidance, or directly under cholangioscopic control. In experienced hands, the procedure is safe with no mortality and a low morbidity. However, in patients with underlying cirrhosis and portal hypertension, massive haemobilia has been reported requiring blood transfusion and angiographic embolization to control the bleeding. The percutaneous approach is particularly useful in patients with previous gas-

(a) (b)

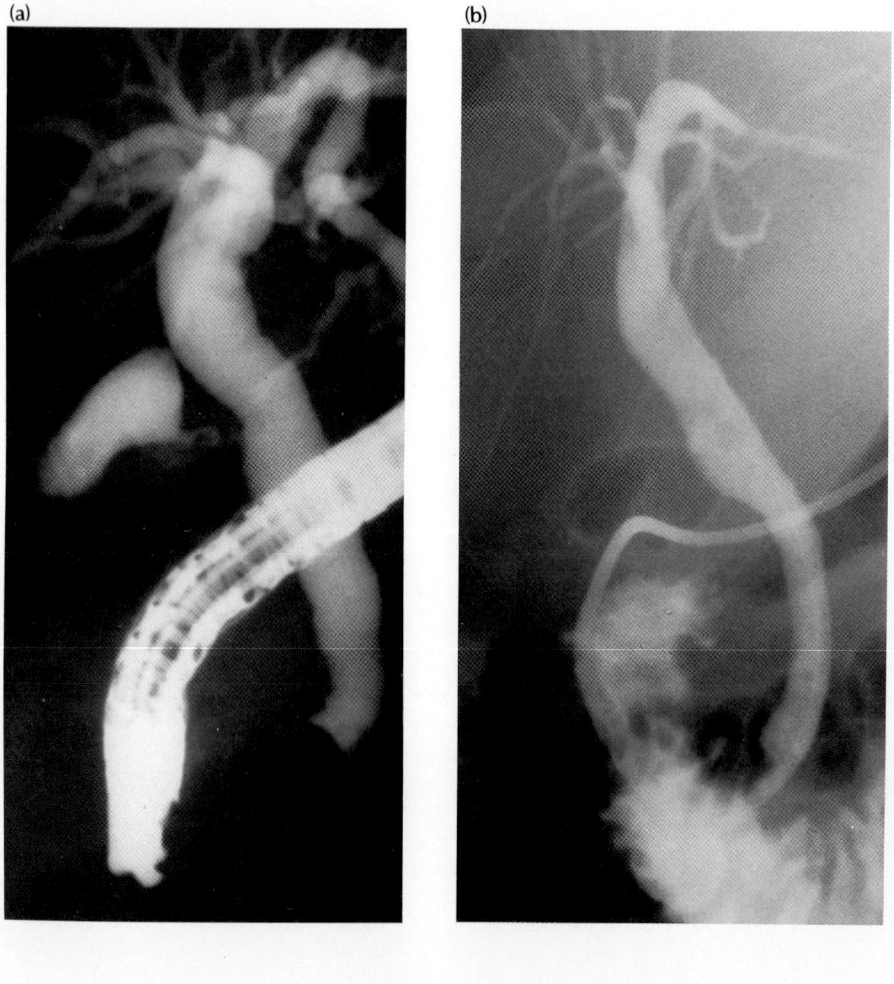

Fig. 5. (a) Occlusion cholangiogram after stone extraction showing leakage of contrast at the level of the cystic duct stump. (b) Pernasal cholangiogram after 3 days, showing that the fistula has healed with no more leakage of contrast.

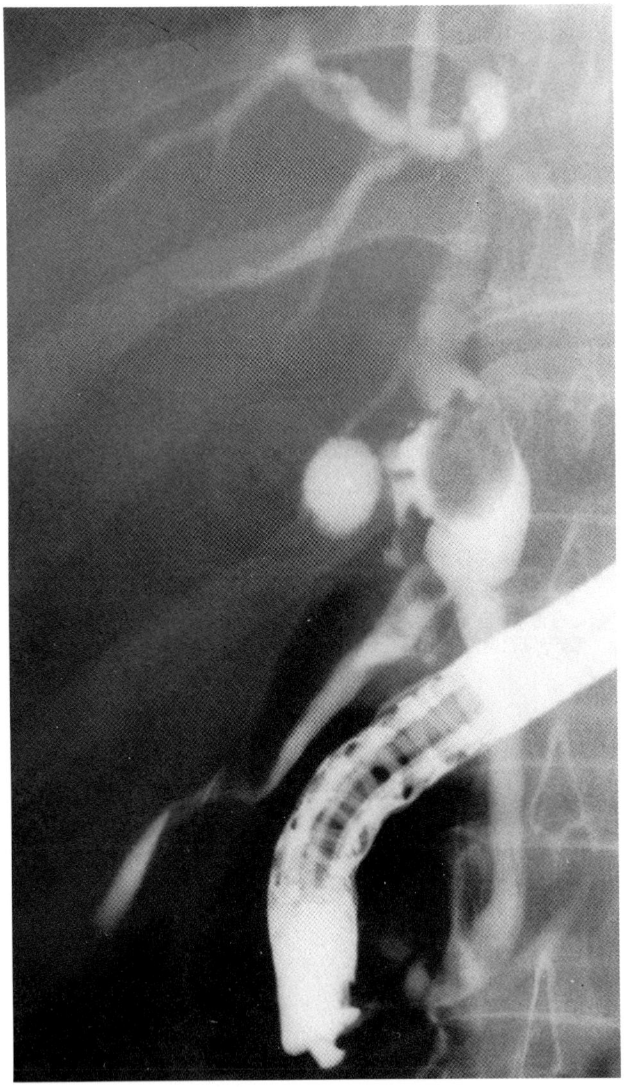

Fig. 6. Spontaneous perforation of the bile duct with leakage of contrast: a stone was demonstrated above the leak, the gall bladder was contracted.

tric surgery or a hepaticojejunostomy that renders the endoscopic approach more difficult [67•].

Simple balloon dilatation may not be sufficient to maintain patency of the lumen. In a series of 63 patients with post-operative biliary strictures, Huibregtse *et al.* [69] used a combination of dilatation with graded catheter dilators and balloons followed by insertion of one or more 10 French stents. The success rate was 86% (54 out of 63) with rapid clearance of the jaundice or cholangitis. The mean follow-up was 32.5 months. Elective stent exchange was performed regularly to prevent clogging and cholangitis. The authors recommended stenting for up to 1 year to ensure that the stricture remained open after removal of the splinting stent. This paper highlighted the difficulties and controversies associated with endoscopic treatment of benign biliary strictures. Similar good results have been reported by Geenen *et al.* [70] in a series of 23 patients with benign strictures undergoing endoscopic balloon dilatation. Stenting was performed in 78% of patients. The success rate was 88% with a mean follow-up of 4 years.

Rossi *et al.* [71•] reported on the use of a self-expandable metal stent inserted percutaneously for stenting biliary strictures. Single or multiple stents have been used but the major limitation was dislocation of the stent either above or below the stricture. The wire mesh self-expandable metal stent has also been used for treating benign strictures.

Benign strictures may also complicate liver transplantation. The incidence of bile leaks is high in series reported from the USA. However, the British experience from the King's College/Cambridge group that used the donor's gallbladder as a conduit has reported a high incidence of strictures formation both at the anastomosis site between the donor's bile duct and gallbladder as well as in the intrahepatic ducts above the anastomosis. The anastomotic stricture was attributed to ischaemia. The intrahepatic strictures which were thought to be related to a long intrahepatic limb of the T-tube resolved soon after the T-tube was removed [72•].

Strictures and intrahepatic stones

Patients with benign strictures complicating intrahepatic stones are difficult to manage. Successful percutaneous balloon dilatation of the strictures and stone extraction has been reported [73•], although complete ductal clearance is often difficult [74]. Success with the peroral endoscopic approach is even lower, with a ductal clearance rate of only 20% (Leung, personal experience). There is also a potential danger of cholangiocarcinoma developing in strictures associated with intrahepatic stones.

Non-operative management of benign biliary strictures using balloon dilatation and temporary stenting achieves good short and intermediate- term-results. However, extended follow-up is required to assess the long-term effects, particularly the recurrence rate after stent removal, before the role of non-operative management can be firmly established.

Conclusion

There is an ever growing armamentarium of instruments and techniques for non-operative management of biliary diseases. One needs to consider the different options on an individual patient basis. Randomized controlled studies would help to define the relative benefits of individual procedures, such as surgery versus endoscopic therapy, but it must be remembered that results often reflect the experience of one particular centre in a selected group of patients under special circumstances. The best approach to the management of patients with biliary problems, especially for difficult cases, is the team approach

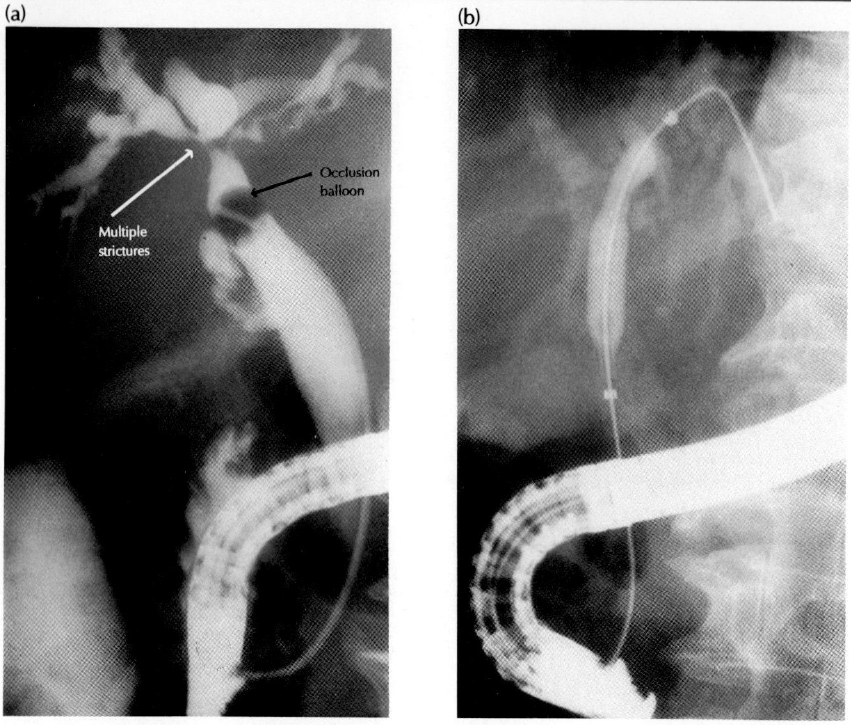

Fig. 7. (a) Cholangiogram showing benign strictures at the liver hilum with multiple segments involvement secondary to surgical trauma of the common hepatic duct. (b) Balloon dilatation of a segmental stricture.

by the gastrointestinal surgeon, the interventional radiologist and the endoscopist. The best available treatment option or combination therapy should be offered to the patient [75•].

References and recommended reading

Papers of special interest, published within the annual period of review, have been highlighted as:

- • Of interest
- •• Of outstanding interest

1. SCHULTZE K, HENTSCHEL R, DUFEK W: **Malignant Bile Duct Obstruction by Tumour Embolism.** *Endoscopy* 1990, 22:197–198. •
An unusual cause of malignant jaundice due to direct infiltration and luminal extension of a primary hepatocellular carcinoma.

2. LAU WY, LEUNG JWC, LI AKC: **Management of Patients with Hepatocellular Carcinoma Presenting as Obstructive Jaundice.** *Am J Surg* 1990, **160**:280–282. •
Eleven out of 340 patients with hepatocellular carcinoma presented with obstructive jaundice. Three were due to direct tumour invasion of the hepatic ducts with luminal extension.

3. HEIT P, MCKINLEY M, JAVORS B: **Mucoid Biliary Obstruction: Direct Endoscopic Visualization of Mucine-hypersecreting Bile Duct Tumor.** *Gastrointest Endosc* 1990, **36**:164–166. •
Recurrent biliary obstruction and cholangitis caused by the mucin produced by a mucin-hypersecreting villous cholangiocarcinoma.

4. ROSENGART TK, ROTTERDAM H, RANSON JHC: **Eosinophilic Cholangitis: A Self-limited Cause of Extrahepatic Biliary Obstruction.** *Am J Gastroenterol* 1990, **85**:582–585. •
An unusual benign disease masquerading as malignant biliary obstruction.

5. HIDEO Y, ITAI Y, MINAMI M, KOKUBO T, OHTOMO K, KURODA A: **Biliary malignancies occurring in choledochal cysts.** *Radiology* 1989, **173**:389–392.

6. TARTAR VM, BALFE DM: **Lymphoma in the Wall of the Bile Ducts: Radiologic Imaging.** *Gastrointest Radiol* 1990, **15**:53–57. •
Three unusual cases of extranodal lymphoma involving the bile ducts and gallbladder presenting as malignant biliary strictures.

7. YAMAGUCHI K, ENJOJI M, KITAMURA K: **Endoscopic biopsy has limited accuracy in diagnosis of ampullary tumors.** *Gastrointest Endosc* 1990, **36**:588–592. •
Endoscopic biopsy of tumors of the ampulla only detected 70% (51 out of 73) of the carcinoma subsequently proven at surgery. Biopsy diagnosis of an adenoma does not rule out the possibility of deeper carcinoma in ampullary tumors.

8. HUIBREGTSE K, TYTGAT GNJ: **Carcinoma of the Ampulla of Vater: The Endoscopic Approach.** *Endoscopy* 1988, 20:223–226.

9. PUA SC, FUJI T, AIBE T, AKIYAMA T, NOGUCHI T, TANAKA S, HARIMA K, SASAKI T, KONDON S, ADACHI K, TANAKA H, OKITA K: **Hepatocellular Carcinoma with Invasion of the Right Intrahepatic Bile Duct Observed by Peroral Cholangioscopy.** *Dig Endosc* 1990, 2:329–334. •
Malignant jaundice owing to direct infiltration of the biliary system by a primary hepatoma.

10. FOUTCH PG, KERR DM, HARLAN JR, MANNE RK, KUMMET TD, SANOWSKI RA: **Endoscopic Retrograde Wire-guided brush Cytology for Diagnosis of Patients with Malignant Obstruction of the Bile Duct.** *Am J Gastroenterol* 1990, **85**:791–795. •
A wire-guided cytology brush was used for cytological sampling from potentially malignant strictures in 34 patients. The diagnostic yield was highest for cholangiocarcinoma and lowest for metastatic disease. The accuracy of the test was 72%.

11. LYGIDAKIS NJ, CARLEI F: **Structural and Functional Biliary Tree Changes Secondary to Extrahepatic Biliary Obstruction.** *Endoscopy* 1990, 21:321–323. •
A histopathological study of surgically resected bile ducts showing a reduced innervation and morphological changes in the proximal bile duct and liver above the level of obstruction, probably a result of raised intrabiliary pressure.

12. OHSHIO G, MANABE T, TAMURA K, KUDO H, YOSHIOKA H, TOBE T: **Effects of Percutaneous Transhepatic Biliary Drainage on Blood–Bile Permeability and Selective IgA Transport in Patients with Biliary Obstruction.** *Ann Surg* 1990, 211:428–432. •
Biliary obstruction led to an increase in permeability between blood and bile and a decrease in immunoglobulin IgA transport into bile. This

may have an adverse effect on the immune defence mechanism of the biliary system.

13. Huibregtse K: **Endoscopic Palliation in Malignant Bile Duct • Strictures: The Amsterdam Experience.** *Dig Endosc* 1990, 2:203–206.
A large personal experience of endoscopic stenting for malignant jaundice.

14. Levine GJ, Botet J, Kurtz RC: **Microbiological Analysis of • Sepsis Complicating Non-surgical Biliary Drainage in Malignant Obstruction.** *Gastrointest Endosc* 1990, **36**:364–368.
Significantly more Gram-positive organisms were isolated from blood and bile cultures of patients with malignant jaundice undergoing percutaneous rather than endoscopic drainage.

15. Leung JWC, Chan RCY, Cheung SW, Sung JY, Chung SCS, •• French GL: **The Effect of Obstruction on Biliary Excretion of Cefoperazone and Ceftazidime.** *J Antimicrob Chemother* 1990, **25**:399–406.
Biliary excretion of antibiotic is impaired in the presence of a raised intrabiliary pressure associated with complete bile duct obstruction.

16. Akiyama H, Okazaki T, Takashima I, Satoh S, Ryan T, Iwamori • S, Hidaka T, Morio K, Okuhara T: **Percutaneous Treatments for Biliary Diseases.** *Radiology* 1990, **176**:25–30.
A review of 173 patients with different biliary pathologies treated by percutaneous transhepatic drainage or choledochoscopy-assisted procedures, including lithotripsy, dilatation of stricture and internal stenting.

17. Kauffmann GW, Roeren T, Friedl P, Brambs HJ, Richter GM: • **Interventional Radiological Treatment of Malignant Biliary Obstruction.** *Eur J Surg Oncol* 1990, **16**:397–403.
An overview of the percutaneous transhepatic procedures in the management of malignant biliary obstruction.

18. Foutch PG, Sawyer RL, Sanowski RA: **The Biliograstric Shunt: • A Method for Simultaneous Internal Diversion of Bile and Enteric Feeding in Patients with Cancer.** *Gastrointest Endosc* 1990, **36**:440–443.
Internal diversion of bile by connecting an external biliary drain to a PEG prevents excessive loss of bile.

19. Hall RI, Denyer ME, Chapman AH: **Percutaneous-endo- • scopic Placement of Endoprostheses for Relief of Jaundice Caused by Inoperable Bile Duct Strictures.** *Surgery* 1990, **107**:224–227.
Stenting by the combined procedure was performed in 53 patients with unresectable malignant biliary strictures with a success rate of 94%. The 30-day mortality was 30%, being higher for patients with hilar obstruction probably related to cholangitis. Single stent provided adequate palliation for bifurcation obstruction.

20. Jacobs M: **Endoscopic Biliary Decompression Aided by a • Different Technique of Percutaneous Transhepatic Access.** *Gastrointest Endosc* 1990, **36**:503–505.
A modification of the existing technique of combined procedure for stenting.

21. Tam PC, Lai ESC, Hui WM, Chan SCH: **Pitfalls of • Percutaneous-endoscopic Biliary Stent Placement.** *Am J Gastroenterol* 1990, **85**:207–209.
Avoidance of central puncture during percutaneous transhepatic drainage and checking with biplane screening may prevent malposition of the stent inserted by the combined procedure.

22. Jackson JE, Roddie ME, Yeung YC, Benjamin IS, Adam A: • **Biliary Endoprosthesis Dysfunction in Patients with Malignant Hilar Tumors: Successful Treatment by Percutaneous Replacement of the Stent.** *AJR* 1990, **155**:391–395.
Blocked percutaneous stents can be successfully removed and replaced by the percutaneous approach.

23. Lee MJ, Mueller PR, Saini S, Morrison MC, Brink JA, Hahn • PF: **Occlusion of Biliary Endoprostheses: Presentation and Management.** *Radiology* 1990, **176**:531–534.
As blocked percutaneous stents can also be removed and replaced percutaneously, stent blockage should not be considered a terminal event in patients with malignant jaundice.

24. Bickerstaff KI, Berry AR, Chapman RW, Britton BJ: **Endo- • scopic Sphincterotomy and Ampullary Carcinoma.** *Br J Surg* 1990, 77:160–162.
Endoscopic sphincterotomy provided good palliation of the malignant jaundice in 17 patients with inoperable carcinoma of the ampulla, with a low mortality of only 6%.

25. Shemesh E, Nass S, Czerniak A: **Endoscopic Sphincterotomy • and Endoscopic Fulguration in the Management of Adenoma of the Papilla of Vater.** *Surg Gynecol Obstet* 1990, **169**:445–448.
Endoscopic sphincterotomy is effective in relieving biliary obstruction caused by ampullary lesions. Diathermic fulguration and tumour polypectomy may be a useful alternative to surgical treatment in high-risk patients.

26. Speer A, Cotton PB, Russell RCG, *et al.*: **Randomized Trial of Endoscopic Versus Percutaneous Stent Insertion in Malignant Obstructive Jaundice.** *Lancet* 1987, ii:57–62.

27. Cotton PB: **Management of Malignant Bile Duct Obstruc- •• tion.** *J Gastroenterol Hepatol* 1990, Suppl 1:63–77.
An excellent review with masterly comments on the different options for treating patients with malignant obstructive jaundice.

28. Polydorou AA, Chisholm EM, Romanos AA, Dowsett SF, Cotton PB, Hatfield AR, Russel RC: **A Comparison of Right Versus Left Hepatic Duct Endoprosthesis Insertion in Malignant Hilar Biliary Obstruction.** *Endoscopy* 1989, **21**:266–271.

29. Urban MS, Siegel JH, Pavlou W, Tuvia J, Gelb AM, Vikram B, • Aubrey R: **Treatment of Malignant Biliary Obstruction with a High-dose Rate Remote Afterloading Device Using a 10 F Nasobiliary Tube.** *Gastrointest Endosc* 1990, **36**:292–296.
A new and quick method of local radiotherapy for malignant bile duct lesions, with a shorter treatment time and hospitalization.

30. Kubota Y, Seki T, Junieda K, Nakahashi Y, Yamaguchi T, • Tateiwa J, Mizuno T, Shiozaki Y, Sameshima Y: **Long Term Efficacy of Percutaneous Transhepatic Choledochoscopic YAG Laser Therapy for Malignant Biliary Obstruction.** *Dig Endosc* 1990, 2:156–163.
Choledoscope-guided neodymium-YAG laser therapy is effective in recanalized malignant biliary strictures and offers good drainage without stenting.

31. Hyoty MK, Nordback IH: **Biliary Stent or Surgical Bypass in • Unresectable Pancreatic Cancer with Obstructive Jaundice.** *Acta Chir Scand* 1990, **156**:301–396.
A respective review of 188 patients treated by surgical bypass, percutaneous or endoscopic stenting for malignant obstructive jaundice. There was no difference in the mortality, 30-day complication and hospital stay but there were more cases of late recurrent jaundice and cholangitis in the group with stenting.

32. Finch MD, Butler JA: **Palliation for Non-pancreatic Malig- • nant Obstruction of the Biliary Tract.** *Surg Gynecol Obstet* 1990, **170**:437–440.
A retrospective analysis of 36 patients with unresectable tumors causing malignant jaundice managed by surgical bypass, stenting or conservative treatment. Surgical bypass was effective in palliating the jaundice with minimal septic complication.

33. Shepherd HA, Royle G, Ross APR, Diba A, Arthur M, Colin-Jones D: **Endoscopic Biliary Prosthesis in the Palliation of Malignant Obstruction of the Distal Common Bile Duct: A Randomized Trial.** *Br J Surg* 1988, **75**:1166–1168.

34. Andersen JR, Sorensen SM, Kruse A, Rokkjaer M, Matzen P: **Randomized Trial of Endoscopic Endoprosthesis Versus Operative Bypass in Malignant Obstructive Jaundice.** *Gut* 1989, **30**:1132–1135.

35. Dowsett JF, Russell RCG, Hatfield ARW, *et al.*: **Malignant Obstructive Jaundice, a Prospective Randomized Trial of**

Bypass Surgery Versus Endoscopic Stenting. *Gastroenterology* 1989, 6:A128.

36. HATFIELD ARW: **Palliation of Malignant Obstructive Jaundice**
• **— Surgery or Stent?** *Gut* 1990, 31:1339–1340.
A leading article commenting on the relative merits of surgery and endoscopic palliation for malignant jaundice.

37. SPEER AG, COTTON PB, RODE J, SEDDON AM, NEAL CR, HOLTON J, COSTERTON JW: **Biliary Stent Blockage with Bacterial Biofilm: A Light and Electron Microscopy Study.** *Ann Intern Med* 1988, 108:546–553.

38. GROEN AK, OUT T, HUIBREGTSE K, *ET AL.*: **Characterization of the Content of Occluded Biliary Endoprosthesis.** *Endoscopy* 1987, 19:57–59.

39. LEUNG JWC, LING TKW, KUNG JLS, VALLANCE OWEN J: **The Role of Bacteria in the Blockage of Biliary Stents.** *Gastrointest Endosc* 1988, 34:19–22.

40. LEUNG JWC, BANEZ VP: **Clogging of Biliary Stents: Mecha-**
• **nisms and Possible Solution.** *Dig Endosc* 1990, 2:97–104.
Bacteria are important in the initiation of stent clogging through biofilm formation. Surface modification with antibiotics, biocides or heavy metal may reduce bacterial adherence and have a potential benefit in preventing stent blockage.

41. SMIT JM, OUT J, GROEN AK, HUIBREGTSE K, JANSEN PL, VAN-MARLE J, TYTGAT GNJ: **A Placebo Controlled Study on the Efficacy of Aspirin and Doxycycline in Preventing Clogging in Biliary Endoprostheses.** *Gastrointest Endosc* 1989, 35:485–489.

42. LEUNG JWC, BANEZ VP, LAM K, COTTON PB, COSTERTON JW: **Mechanisms of Clogging and the Role of Biocide Impregnation in Preventing Stent Clogging.** *Gastrointest Endosc* 1990, 36:160 (abstract).

43. LEUNG JWC, DEL FAVERO G, COTTON PB: **Endoscopic Biliary Prostheses: A Comparison of Materials.** *Gastrointest Endosc* 1985, 31:93–95.

44. COENE PPLO, GROEN AK, CHENG J, OUT MMJ, TYTGAT GNJ,
•• HUIBREGTSE K: **Cloning of Biliary Endoprotheses: A New Perspective.** *Gut* 1990, 31:913–917.
The flow of bile is affected by the configuration of the stent. The absence of side holes is associated with less biliary sludge or biofilm formation and may be beneficial in maintaining stent patency.

45. SUNG JY, OLSEN ME, LEUNG JWC, LUNDBERG MS, COSTERTON JW:
•• **Microbial Flora of the Gastrointestinal and Biliary System in Cats.** *Microbial Ecol Health Dis* 1990, 3:199–207.
A morphological and bacteriological study in cats demonstrated that the intact papilla of Vater served as a natural gateway preventing the migration of bacteria from the duodenum into the biliary system.

46. WENGROWER D, GOLDIN E: **Balloon Retrieval of Biliary Stents.**
• *Gastrointest Endosc* 1990, 36:639–640.
Endoscopic balloon retrieval of a migrated stent.

47. HSU D: **Recanalization of Clogged Biliary Stent.** *Gastrointest*
• *Endosc* 1990, 36:322–323.
Successful recanalization of three clogged biliary stents by traversing the lumen of the stent with catheters and forceps. The risk of dislodging bacteria into the obstructed system with cholangitis is high.

48. COHEN ME, GOLDBERG RI, BARKIN JS, PHILIPS RRS: **Bile Duct Perforation: A Complication of Larger Calibre Endoprosthesis.** *Gastrointest Endosc* 1989, 35:456–458.

49. SZAUTER KM, MULLEN KD, MARSHALL JB: **Gastrosto-biliary Irri-**
• **gation for Maintenance of Stent Patency.** *Gastrointest Endosc* 1990, 36:597–598.
A modified catheter irrigation system through a percutaneous gastrostomy to maintain patency of an indwelling biliary stent.

50. HUIBREGTSE K, CHEUNG J, COENE PPLO, FOCKENS P, TYTGAT GNJ: **Endoscopic Placement of Expandable Metal Stents for Biliary Strictures — A Preliminary Report on Experience with 33 Patients.** *Endoscopy* 1989, 21:280–282.

51. DOMSCHKE W, FOERSTER E: **Endoscopic Implantation of Large**
• **Bore Self-expanding Biliary Mesh Stent.** *Gastrointest Endosc* 1990, 36:55–57.
A case report using the self-expanding metal stent for obstructive jaundice caused by pancreatic carcinoma.

52. CREMER M, DEVIERE J, SUGAI B, BAIZE M: **Expandable Biliary**
• **Metal Stents for Malignancies: Endoscopic Insertion and Diathermic Cleaning for Tumor Ingrowth.** *Gastrointest Endosc* 1990, 36:451–457.
Although stent clogging by biliary sludge is uncommon in the self-expandable metal stents, tumor infiltration through the wire mesh with occlusion of the lumen is a potential disadvantage.

53. GILLAMS A, DICK R, DOOLEY JS, WALLSTEN H, EL-DIN A: **Self-ex-**
• **pandable Stainless Steel Braided Endoprosthesis for Biliary Strictures.** *Radiology* 1990, 174:137–140.
Percutaneously inserted self-expandable metal stents are effective in palliating malignant biliary obstruction. The fixed, but short, length of the stent, may have accounted for the recurrent jaundice and cholangitis because of inadequate drainage.

54. MARSHALL T, KAMALVAND K, CAIRNS SR: **Endoscopic Treatment**
• **of Biliary Enteric Fistula.** *Br Med J* 1990, 300:1176.
A case of cholecystocolic fistula presented with profuse diarrhoea successfully treated by endoscopic stenting.

55. BREM H, GIBBONS GD, COBB G, EDGIN RA, ELLISON EG, CAREY
• LC: **The Use of Endoscopy to Treat Bronchobiliary Fistula Caused by Choledocholithiasis.** *Gastroenterology* 1990, 98:490–492.
An unusual case of bronchobiliary fistula secondary to multiple common duct stones treated by endoscopic sphincterotomy.

56. LEBOVICS E, MITTELMAN A, DEL GUERCIO LRM, HILARIS B,
• MOORTHY C, PUCCIO C, ROSENTHAL WS: **Pancreaticobiliary Fistula and Obstructive Jaundice Complicating ^{125}I Interstitial Implants for Pancreatic Cancer: Endoscopic Diagnosis and Management.** *Gastrointest Endosc* 1990, 36:610–611.
An unusual case of a pancreaticobiliary fistula probably related to local radiotherapy, treated successfully by endoscopic stenting.

57. PONCHON T, GALLEZ JDF, VALETTE PJ, CHAVAILLON A, BORY R: **Endoscopic Treatment of Biliary Tract Fistula.** *Gastrointest Endosc* 1989, 35:490–498.

58. RAYTER Z, TONGE C, BENNETT CE, ROBINSON PS, THOMAS MH: **Bile Leaks After Simple Cholecystectomy.** *Br J Surg* 1989, 76:1046–1048.

59. ANDERSSON R, TRANHERG KG, BENGMARK S: **Role of Bile and**
• **Bacteria in Biliary Peritonitis.** *Br J Surg* 1990, 77:36–39.
An animal experiment demonstrating the detrimental effect of a combination of bile and bacteria in biliary peritonitis.

60. LEUNG JWC, CHUNG SCS, SUNG JY, METREWELI C: **Endoscopic Management of Postoperative Biliary Fistula.** *Surg Endosc* 1988, 2:190–193.

61. GOLDIN E, KATZ E, WENGROWER D, KLUGER Y, KASKEL L, SHILONI
• E, LIBSON E: **Treatment of Fistulas of the Biliary Tract by Endoscopic Insertion of Endoprostheses.** *Surg Gynecol Obstet* 1990, 170:418–423.
Successful treatment of five biliary fistula using endoscopic transpapillary insertion of large biliary stents.

62. HOFFMAN BJ, CUNNINGHAM JT, MARSH WH: **Endoscopic Man-**
• **agement of Biliary Fistulas with Small Calibre Stents.** *Am J Gastroenterol* 1990, 85:705–707.
The use of single small-calibre stent with or without sphincterotomy was effective in treating seven patients with biliary fistula.

63. BERGER H, WEINZIERL M, NEVEILLE ES, PRATSCHKE E: **Percutaneous Transcatheter Occlusion of Cystic Duct Stump in**

Postcholecystectomy Bile Leakage. *Gastrointest Radiol* 1989, **14**:334–336.

64. KRIGE JEJ, BORNMAN PC, BENINGFIELD SJ, NIEUWOULDT JHM,
• TERBLANCHE J: **Endoscopic Embolization of External Biliary Fistula.** *Br J Surg* 1990, 77:581–583.

A novel approach with endoscopic transcatheter embolization of a leaking bile duct to control a biliary fistula.

65. LEUNG JWC, BANEZ VP, SUNG JY, WU ZM, AGAS FV, CHUNG
• SCS: **Endoscopic Cholangiopancreatography in Hepatic Clonorchiasis — a Follow-up Study.** *Gastrointest Endosc* 1990, **36**:

A follow-up ERCP study of hepatic clonorchiasis after anthelminthic therapy showing persistence of strictures of the intrahepatic bile ducts despite eradication of the parasitic infestation.

66. PITT HA, KAUFMAN SL, COLEMAN J, WHITE RI, CAMERON JL: **Benign Postoperative Biliary Strictures: Operate or Dilate?** *Ann Surg* 1989, **210**:417–427.

67. GYA D, SALI A, HENNESSY O, KUNE GA: **Balloon Dilatation of**
• **Biliary Strictures: Experience and Review of the Literature.** *Aust NZ J Surg* 1990, **60**:361–364.

Percutaneous transhepatic balloon dilatation is an effective and useful alternative to surgery in treating patients with recurrent biliary strictures and stenosed bilioenteric anastomosis.

68. RAO KJM, BLAKE H, THOEDOSSI A: **Use of a Modified Angio-**
• **plasty Balloon Catheter in the Dilatation of Tight Biliary Strictures.** *Gut* 1990, **31**:565–567.

Special angioplasty balloons are better than the standard dilating catheter or pneumatic balloon in dilating tight strictures.

69. HUIBREGTSE K, CHENG J, RAUWS EAJ, TYTGAT GNJ: **Postoperative Biliary Strictures: The Endoscopic Approach.** *Scand J Gastroenterol* 1989, **24** (suppl 171):50–56.

70. GEENEN DJ, GEENEN JE, HOGAN WJ, SCHENCK J, VENU RP, JOHNSON GK, JACKSON A: **Endoscopic Therapy for Benign Bile Duct Strictures.** *Gastrointest Endosc* 1989, **35**:367–371.

71. ROSSI P, BEZZI M, SALATORI FM, MACCIONI F, PORCARO ML:
• **Recurrent Benign Biliary Strictures: Management with Self-expanding Metallic Stents.** *Radiology* 1990, **175**:661–665.

Percutaneous transhepatic self-expanding metallic stents were placed in 17 patients with recurrent biliary strictures. The success rate was 82.4%. Present limitations included a fixed length of the stent, failure to expand and a risk of dislocation.

72. EVANS RA, RABY ND, O'GRADY JG, KARANI JB, NUNNERLEY HB,
• CALNE RY, WILLIAMS R: **Biliary Complications Following Orthotopic Liver Transplantation.** *Clin Radiol* 1990, **41**:190–194.

Sixty-three out of 76 patients with liver transplant had abnormal cholangiogram showing biliary strictures, inspissate bile formation causing biliary obstruction, bile leak and T-tube malposition. Balloon dilatation and stenting was of limited use in this series.

73. JENG KS, YANG FS, OHRTA I, CHIANG HJ: **Dilatation of Intra-**
• **hepatic Biliary Strictures in Patients with Hepatolithiasis.** *World J Surg* 1990, **14**:587–593.

Percutaneous drainage and dilatation of intrahepatic strictures is an effective method for removing intrahepatic stones with a low recurrence rate.

74. JENG KS, CHIANG HJ, SHIH SC: **Limitation of Percutaneous Transhepatic Cholangioscopy in the Removal of Complicated Biliary Calculi.** *World J Surg* 1989, **13**:603–610.

75. LIGUORY C, VITALE GC: **Biliary Perestroika.** *Am J Surg* 1990,
• **160**:237–238.

An editorial favouring a collaborative team approach between interventional radiologist, gastroenterologist and surgeon in managing patients with biliary diseases.

Laparoscopy

H. W. Boyce Jr

University of South Florida, Division of Digestive Disease and Nutrition, College of Medicine, Tampa, Florida, USA

Laparoscopy has never received the recognition and respect it deserves from clinicians of all specialties. New therapeutic applications have captured the interest of abdominal surgeons. Instruments for laparoscopic surgery are being developed at a rapid pace. The vast literature on diagnostic laparoscopy awaits review and study by the new medical and surgical enthusiasts. The articles published in 1990, and reviewed here, reflect increasing interest in laparoscopic diagnosis and unparalleled attention to new techniques for laparoscopic therapy.

Introduction

Laparoscopy has gained remarkable prominence during the past year with the continuing evolution and acceptance of it's therapeutic potential. Surgeons who have totally ignored the accuracy and safety of diagnostic laparoscopy over the past several decades now have an avid interest in laparoscopic cholecystectomy and have adopted this method contrary to their old adage about diagnostic laparoscopy — 'why look through the keyhole when you can open the door?' It is hoped that this new interest in therapy will result in a resurgence of enthusiasm, training and clinical application of diagnostic laparoscopy. Published reports do not yet reflect such a trend, but the better training programs in gastroenterology and surgery are certain to develop expertise in basic laparoscopic techniques that will serve to enhance both the diagnostic and therapeutic applications. The vast amount of literature published over the past 40 years on all aspects of diagnostic laparoscopy by gastroenterologists, along with a few surgeons, and therapeutic laparoscopy by gynecologists, awaits discovery by a new generation of surgeon enthusiasts. This review presents most of the 1990 reports on diagnostic laparoscopy and laparoscopic surgery. Additional discussion of laparoscopic surgical techniques may be found in other sections of this text.

Laparoscopy training

The major issues in training for laparoscopy in 1990 relate to the meteoric rise in popularity and performance of laparoscopic surgery, primarily cholecystectomy. Despite the advice and admonitions of those with long experience in diagnostic laparoscopy, the new breed of surgeons suddenly interested in laparoscopy have proceeded full speed to laparoscopic cholecystectomy with few stops on the way. Some have attended short courses and paused briefly in the animal laboratory to perform the technique on several pigs. Others have invoked conceived innate technical abilities as sufficient to proceed with their only training limited to didactic instruction or self-study alone. Hospitals are permitting laparoscopic cholecystectomy with no established credentialing requirements and patients are suffering some complications of both basic laparoscopic technique and cholecystectomy that probably would be preventable with proper training of the operators. We must anticipate that another type of 'complication' will also occur, i.e. complications of omission or failure to appreciate the subtleties of intra-abdominal diseases due to failure to regularly perform a full abdominal and pelvic laparoscopic exploration prior to cholecystectomy. The most likely will be failure to detect small lesions such as metastases and tuberculous granulomas that may readily be seen by the observer trained in diagnostic laparoscopy. Editorials by responsible and experienced surgeons are emphasizing the need for proper training with modern equipment as well as the importance of prospective studies of technique and instrumentation [1•, 2••, 3••]. They have provided initial guidelines for proper training and granting of privileges that should be developed by professional organizations and adopted as appropriate by every hospital before performance of laparoscopic cholecystectomy in the institution. They also suggest that those 'trained' in short courses be proctored in performance of several procedures before being given privileges to perform cholecystectomy alone. Certainly, most of us would consider this a requisite before laparoscopic removal of our gallbladders!

Laparoscopic technique

Re-evaluation of time-honored practices is important for progress, even if the practice under review has proven safe and effective. Jarrett [4•] has done just this by evaluating a technique of directly inserting the laparoscope trocar without establishing a previous pneumoperitoneum as performed with classical laparoscopic technique. He reports a series of 1002 patients examined

© Current Science Ltd ISBN 1-8 70485-32-7 ISSN 0952-6293

for gynecologic indications using a Surgeport Disposable Trocar with a shield that is believed to enhance safety of the method. Jarrett challenges the tenet that insufflation before trocar insertion is safer. He states that the genesis of this notion is unclear and that documentation for it is lacking. He emphasizes that gas insufflation via the needle is not risk-free and, as a consequence, he cites the several maneuvers that are regularly used to be certain the needle is properly positioned. Despite these maneuvers, Jarret maintains that several of the major and minor complications of laparoscopy are still related to production of pneumoperitoneum. The no-pneumoperitoneum technique he used was similar to the trocar introduction method used by most gynecologists through a 1 cm infraumbilical skin incision. The abdominal wall was elevated by grasping with a 4 × 4 inch sponge in one hand and the trocar passed with steady pressure through each detectable tissue plane in an axis toward the pelvic cavity. Insufflation was carried out after trocar removal and passage of the laparoscope under direct vision to ensure proper position in the free abdominal cavity. Jarrett reports that the time saved is significant with this procedural variation. Furthermore, he also points out that abdominal distention secondary to insufflation necessitates increased force to achieve trocar insertion. This suggestion is not true for the patient who is not under general anesthesia and is able to cooperate by forcefully producing extra tension in the abdominal wall by a Valsalva maneuver. Basically, the technique he describes may be easy, quick and safe under general anesthesia, but it would probably be an undesirable experience for both physician and patient if performed under the sedative-analgesia used for diagnostic laparoscopy. There seems little reason for those who perform time-honored diagnostic laparoscopy to consider using this gynecologic approach for trocar insertion without prior pneumoperitoneum.

Complications

Peritoneal adhesions

The potential risks of adhesion-related complications during laparoscopy performed on patients with previous abdominal or pelvic surgery are a justifiable concern. Both large series of laparoscopy experience and studies in postoperative adhesion frequency have provided some reassurance about these risks. Surgeons have recommended minilaparotomy instead of laparoscopy because of this concern. Earlier studies have used laparoscopy to assess the frequency of peritoneal adhesions in patients with and without prior abdominal surgery. Less than 5% of patients without prior surgery will have significant adhesions. Szigetvari *et al.* [5•] found significant adhesions in only 2.7% (19 out of 692) of patients without previous surgery, while 23% (61 of 263) with prior surgery had adhesions. They had no major complications, once again demonstrating the safety of laparoscopy in patients with and without adhesions when the proper technique is used.

Laparoscopy-related metastases

Laparoscopists have been concerned for years over the possibility of the spread of carcinoma from liver and peritoneal metastases to the site of abdominal wall puncture following biopsy. Cava *et al.* [6] report on one of these exceedingly rare instances of metastasis from malignant ascites to the site of introduction of the laparoscope. Although they found only two other cases of similar abdominal wall metastasis reported in the literature, it is fair to say that most laparoscopists with long experience will probably have seen at least one such case. Their patient had a primary adenocarcinoma of the gastroesophageal junction and the two cases found by literature review were due to ovarian carcinoma. The remarkable aspect of this report was the short interval of only 7 days between laparoscopy and the appearance of swelling from the metastasis that was initially thought to be a wound infection.

Pneumoperitoneum

Significant complications from the pneumoperitoneum required for laparoscopy are rare. These usually result from errors in technique enhanced by other factors such as unusual anatomical features, improper site selection for pneumoperitoneum, obesity, and an uncooperative patient. At least two of these factors were probably involved in the report of Pascual *et al.* [7]. They reported a subcutaneous emphysema, pneumoperitoneum, bilateral pneumothorax, and pneumopericardium in an obese, uncooperative patient. This problem usually results from incomplete penetration of the abdominal wall into free peritoneal space. In a very obese patient, penetration of the pneumoperitoneum needle into the typically large, redundant, and sometimes displaced, round ligament allows direct introduction of gas into the extraperitoneal space and potentially immediate passage of gas into pleural spaces and mediastinum. Pneumopericardium is less likely to occur. In this report, the initial placement of the pneumoperitoneum needle was related to prompt appearance of subcutaneous emphysema. The gas introduced at this initial puncture probably led to the extensive spread elsewhere as only pneumoomentum was noted on later successful laparoscopy after successful replacement of the pneumoperitoneum needle at a different site. The authors do not report the precise technical details of the procedure so further analysis of this complication is not possible. As the pneumoperitoneum needle was reinserted at a second site, it is possible that extraperitoneal gas leak under pressure through the first puncture site aggravated the extent of the original subcutaneous emphysema. In any event, the patient did well and the ectopic gas resolved spontaneously.

Post-biopsy septicemia

Serious infections after liver biopsy have been estimated to have an incidence range between 0.03–0.36% with transient bacteremia occurring after 2.9–13.5% of percutanous liver biopsies. Domingo *et al.* [8•] report two cases of septicemia following biopsies taken under laparoscopic control (2 out of 238 laparoscopic biopsies or 0.37% of the liver biopsies and 0.84% of the laparoscopic examinations). The causative organisms were Klebsiella pneumoniae and beta hemolytic streptococcus. There was no evidence of pre-existing cholangitis in either patient. A 27-year-old woman with cirrhosis died with *Klebsiella pneumoniae* septicemia, septic shock and disseminated intravascular coagulation unresponsive to therapy. A 67-year-old male with alcoholic cirrhosis developed septicemia due to both *Klebsiella pneumoniae* and beta hemolytic streptococcus and recovered with antibiotic therapy.

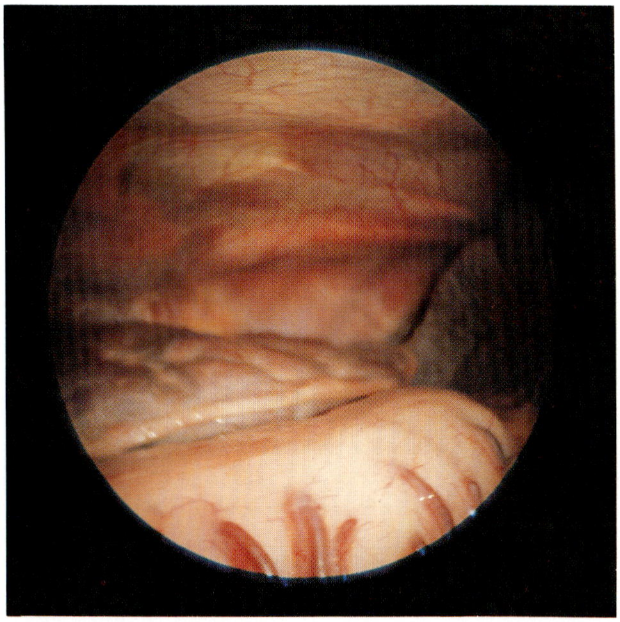

Fig. 1. This laparoscopic view of the left hepatic lobe reveals a lumpy, macronodular surface in a patient from Puerto Rico with hepatic *Schistosoma mansoni* and portal hypertension. The enlarged gastroepiploic veins along the greater curvature of the stomach typical of portal hypertension are shown in the lower margin of the photograph.

Diagnostic laparoscopy
Hepatic schistosomiasis

Schistosoma mansoni infection of the liver with resultant fibrosis and a cirrhotic-like change is reported to be the most common worldwide cause of 'cirrhosis' and portal hypertension. It is estimated that 200 million people are infected, and that 10% of these develop hepatic and splenic involvement. Reports of the anatomic features of hepatic schistosomiasis observed by laparoscopy are uncommon. Contractor *et al.* [9•] report on laparoscopy in 45 patients with liver disease in an area highly endemic for schistosomiasis. In 20 patients, histologic confirmation of hepatic schistosomiasis was obtained. Nine out of 20 patients had generalized hepatomegaly. Size of the liver lobes was variable; the right lobe was markedly shrunken in about one-third and, as noted with other causes of right lobe atrophy, there was compensatory enlargement of the left lobe. Mild uniform irregularity of the liver surface was seen in most cases. Other changes included macronodularity, lumpy surface, tiny white tubercles, white patchy discoloration and perihepatic adhesions of varying thickness (Fig. 1).

Histopathological examination revealed features diagnostic of schistosomiasis in all, with ova demonstrated in six out of 20 patients. An important point made by Contractor *et al.* is the value of direct inspection of the liver plus guided biopsy in their 50 patients with suspected liver disease at high-risk of being related to schistosomiasis. A suspected diagnosis of malignancy was confirmed in three cases and peritoneial tuberculosis in one. Ascites was found in three patients not suspected by clinical examination. When there is a need to clearly define the type and extent of liver and peritoneal disease, laparoscopy with guided biopsy remain the methods *par excellance* for accurate diagnosis.

Chronic pelvic pain

Vercellini *et al.* [10••] confirmed the value of laparoscopy for evaluation of chronic pelvic pain that is defined as constant or intermittent, cyclic or acyclic pain that persists for 6 months or more and includes dysmenorrhea, deep dyspareunia and intermenstrual pain. Laparoscopy in 47 patients between 11–19 years of age revealed no abnormalities in 40.4%, but nearly 60% had treatable pelvic disease. Endometriosis was found in 38.3% of patients, partially obstructive genital tract malformations in 8.4% and other disease in 12.8%. This chronic pelvic pain syndrome can be incapacitating to the adolescent female and sadly, its cause often is not determined despite a thorough examination including extensive laboratory testing, radiographic studies and ulstrasonography. Many clinicians fail to consider laparoscopy but instead wrongly recommend psychiatric evaluation or prescribe medical therapy that includes the risk of chronic analgesic use. When the initial evaluation and appropriate follow-up suggest the patient has real abdominal or pelvic pain, diagnostic laparoscopy should be recommended.

Kaposi sarcoma of liver

The acquired immune deficiency syndrome (AIDS) has resulted in a myriad of unusual clinical disorders due both to bizarre presentations of common diseases and previously unknown presentations of rare diseases. Hasan *et al.* [11•] report on a case of Kaposi sarcoma presenting first in the liver without evidence of prior extrahepatic lesions. All reported cases of hepatic Kaposi sarcoma have had extrahepatic lesions detected before hepatic lesions were found. Their patient presented with abdominal pain, hepatosplenomegaly and rising serum alkaline phosphatase. Laparoscopy revealed multiple 2–3 mm purplish nodules in the liver surface, a large firm liver and a small amount of ascites. Skin lesions of Kaposi sarcoma appeared 6 weeks later.

Peritoneal mesothelioma

A series of 19 (14%) cases of malignant peritoneal mesothelioma among a total of 144 cases of malignant mesothelioma over a 23-year period were reported by van Gelder *et al.* [12]. Seventy-four per cent of the 19 cases had occupational exposure to asbestos with a 44.7 year interval between exposure and diagnosis of the disease. Several important observations relative to diagnosis are discussed. In 12 out of 19 patients, the diagnosis could not be confirmed by cytology of the ascitic fluid. Unfortunately laparoscopy was carried out in only three out of 19 cases as they report laparoscopy was 'not a usual procedure in the past' at their institution. This is surprising as laparoscopy has been widely performed in Europe for over 50 years. Although diagnosis was confirmed in 16 (84%) of the 19 patients by laparotomy in the early years, the authors recommend that laparotomy be avoided and conclude that laparoscopy with directed biopsies should be the diagnostic procedure of choice for suspected cases (Fig.2).

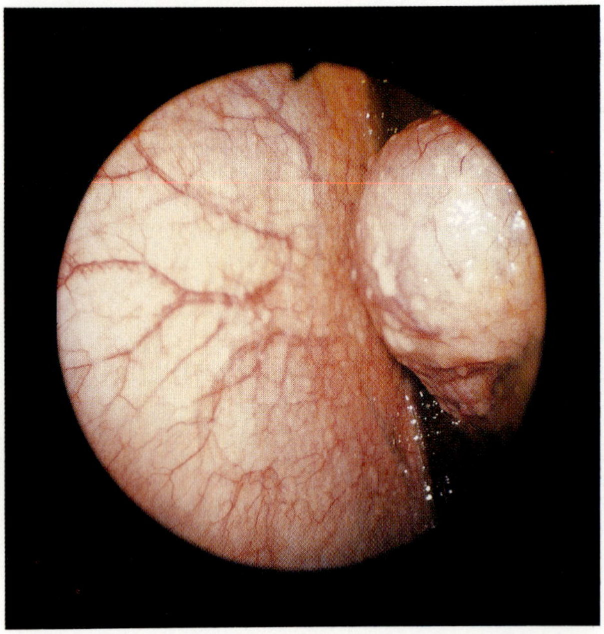

Fig. 2. This view of the right lateral abdomen reveals prominent vasculature of the parietal peritoneum and multiple tiny metastases on the visceral peritoneum of a segment of intestine. Multiple parietal peritoneal metastases also were found, but are so small they are not seen in this view. Biopsy is necessary to differentiate such lesions from other malignancies and tubercular peritonitis. Ascitic fluid is seen at the bottom on both sides of the bowel loop. By courtesy of H. Juergen Nord, University of South Florida College of Medicine, Tampa, Florida, USA.

Laparoscopy has long been shown to be the most accurate method for diagnosis of all types of ascites and it remains so.

Abdominal tuberculosis

Abdominal tuberculosis is most reliably diagnosed by laparoscopy and guided biopsy. Only surgical exploration and post-mortem examination can compete for accuracy but these latter methods are obviously undesirable! Tuberculous peritonitis remains a difficult condition to diagnose because it is not often suspected. In a report by Al-Hadeedi *et al.* [13•] from Kuwait the clinical diagnosis in 42 cases seen between 1984 and 1988 was correct for tuberculosis in only 35% of cases. Laparoscopy was used in only seven out of 42 cases but was diagnostic in all. Laparoscopy should be available for regular use in all clinics and hospitals where abdominal tuberculosis is seen. It is clearly the best diagnostic method for this occult disease that is well treated by anti-tuberculous drugs.

Hepatic candidiasis

Focal hepatic candidiasis is often not recognized antemortem but a report by Gordon *et al.* [14••] suggests the benefit of laparoscopic diagnosis in patients undergoing chemotherapy for acute leukemia. The authors reported two immunosuppressed patients who presented with fever, cholestasis, and neutropenia following chemotherapy. Computed tomography scans were negative in both cases, but laparoscopy revealed diffuse studding of the liver surface with white plaques 0.2–0.5 cm in diameter. Cultures of the biopsy specimens were negative but direct immunofluorescence stains of deparaffinized sections of the biopsies confirmed candidiasis. Repeat laparoscopy in both cases revealed persistent disease that justified continuation of amphotericin B or alternative anti-fungal drugs. The repeat laparoscopy in one case revealed residual white plaques, some of which had evolved into depressed stellate white scars. In the second case, repeat laparoscopy after 2 months revealed filamentous adhesions between most of the white fungal plaques and the parietal peritoneum. As eradication of hepatic candidiasis is difficult and prolonged therapy with amphotericin B carries considerable risk, both accurate initial diagnosis and later proof of post-therapy residual disease are essential for proper therapeutic decisions. These authors also emphasize the safety of laparoscopic visualization with guided pinch biopsies over blind biopsies in patients with blood dyscrasias and thrombocytopenia.

Cirrhosis of the liver

The prognostic value of laparoscopic findings in patients with hepatic cirrhosis was evaluated by Tameda *et al.* [15••]. The anatomic parameters used included the degree of development and size of regenerating nodules, presence of reddish markings and small lymphatic vesicles, the presence or absence of patchy markings, the size of the right and left hepatic lobes, and the degree of splenomegaly. The cumulative survival rate was compared with these anatomic parameters. Statistically significant differences were observed in the cumulative survival rate with respect to the degree of development of regenerating nodules, the size of the right hepatic lobe, the formation of small lymphatic vesicles in the liver surface, and the degree of splenomegaly.

The results of this study indicated that the development of regenerating nodules is the most useful predictor of outcome in patients with cirrhosis, followed by appearance of surface lymphatic vesicles and splenomegaly. Although regenerating nodules also are a pathognomonic sign of hepatic cirrhosis, they are often missed because of sampling error inherent in blind percutaneous liver biopsy but easily identified by direct inspection during laparoscopy. Another interesting observation was that the larger the right lobe, the more favorable the outcome. Left lobe enlargement tended to be associated with a less favorable prognosis probably because it frequently appeared to occur as a compensatory response to right lobe atrophy.

The important question to be asked here is whether these variables in hepatic anatomy and splenomegaly have any practical clinical applications that may benefit the patient. Only careful serial laparoscopic studies of the natural history of hepatic cirrhosis with photographic documentation and biopsy correlation may provide the answer.

Earlier reports have found a widely variable concordance between liver biopsy and laparoscopic diagnosis of cirrhosis. Orlando *et al.* [16••] have reviewed the reasons for this variation including biopsy technique, the pathologist's knowledge of the laparoscopic findings, the histologic and macroscopic criteria used and the degree of nodularity on the liver surface at the time of diagnosis. In a retrospective analysis of 411 patients with cirrhosis, Orlando *et al.* found concordance between guided liver biopsy and laparoscopy in only 57.2%. This is surprising when compared with other reports and makes one wonder about the validity of their laparoscopic criteria [17,18]. When the two methods were evaluated separately, a final diagnosis was possible by guided liver biopsy in 78.8% and by laparoscopy in 78.4% of cases. By doing both procedures there was a reduction in the false-negatives for both procedures resulting in a diagnostic accuracy of 97.7%.

There is little question that laparoscopy with guided biopsy is by far the most accurate approach for the diagnosis of cirrhosis of the liver. The laparoscopic approach is indicated in patients for whom confirmation or exclusion of the diagnosis of cirrhosis is necessary for planning therapy or for prognosis.

Fatty liver

Inui *et al.* [19•] used laparoscopy and the statistical method of multiple regression analysis to evaluate the etiologies of fatty liver and the presence or absence of fibrotic changes in biopsy specimens. Under laparoscopic observation the coloration of the liver surface was classified into three types: 'spotty' yellow color type, 'diffuse' yellow color type, and without yellow color type. The first two types are further defined: the term 'spotty' means a brownish red network with the margins of yellow color areas sharply defined; 'diffuse' means that the network pattern was obscure and the margins of the yellow color spots were not clear. The major possible etiologies considered were alcoholic fatty liver, obesity and diabetes mellitus; their criteria for each of these three etiologies are presented. Biopsies were used to calculate the amount of deposited lipid in terms of the area occupied by the lipid droplets as a percentage of the whole area of each biopsy specimen. Intralobular distribution of the fat droplets was divided into four types and droplet size was classified as small, medium, large and mixed. Evaluation of the factors related to the presence of yellow color and the 'spoty' or 'diffuse' appearance of the yellow color was performed by multiple regression analysis.

The data derived from this study suggest that the amount of lipid deposited was responsible for the presence of yellow color on the liver surface both with and without fibrotic change. The presence of yellow color and whether the liver appeared 'spotty' or 'diffuse' were unexpectedly independent of the intralobular distribution and size of the lipid droplets. The authors also found that the coexistence of fibrotic change was a major factor for giving the yellow colored liver a 'diffuse' appearance. This is explained by the fact that the normal brownish red color of the portal areas at laparoscopy is obscured by the presence of fibrosis. Fibrotic change in the portal areas resulted in a yellowish white color that blended with the lobular fat deposition to produce the 'diffuse' yellow appearance of the surface. Thickening of the hepatic capsule owing to inflammation was found to make the differentiation of all of these fatty liver patterns difficult.

Neonatal cholestasis

Transabdominal ultrasonography can accurately rule out biliary artesia in many children with neonatal cholestasis. Laparoscopy is considered justified when the diagnosis is uncertain because it is safe, less traumatic than laparotomy, and diagnostically accurate. In a report of 36 children with neonatal cholestasis who had laparoscopy, 12 eventually underwent laparotomy because of biliary artesia [20•]. The authors concluded that in the evaluation of neonatal cholestasis, laparoscopy helps avoid unnecessary laparotomies and that its diagnostic accuracy is equal to laparotomy.

Staging laparoscopy

Laparoscopy is the procedure *par excellance* for preoperative staging of pancreatic cancer. Small or widely scattered hepatic metastases and most peritoneal metastases are not detectable by non-invasive scanning techniques. Laparoscopy permits visual detection and biopsy confirmation of metastases in liver and in peritoneum that are as small as 1–2 mm. Although the efficacy of diagnostic laparoscopy for staging has been clearly proven for decades, nearly all surgeons who treat pancreatic cancer have refused to use laparoscopy for this purpose. Their rationale for omitting laparoscopy in the staging sequence is not understandable. However, enlightened surgical groups are now emphasizing the vital role of laparoscopy in pancreatic cancer thereby avoiding needless laparotomy with its attendant discomfort, cost and complications.

Carcinoma of the pancreas

Warshaw *et al.* [21••] have once again provided important information on the place of laparoscopy in staging pancreatic cancer. They studied 88 consecutive surgical candidates prospectively by computed tomography, magnetic resonance imaging, angiography and laparoscopy. Resectabillity was proved in 16 (29%) out of 55 patients for cancer of the pancreatic head, one (6%) out of 17 for body and tail, and 14 (88%) out of 16 for the ampulla. Ninety per cent of unresectable tumors were identified. Seventy-eight per cent of pancreatic head cancers were resectable when all test results were negative versus 5% (2 out of 37) when any test result was positive. Small liver and peritoneal metastases were found in 15 (27%) out of 55 cancers of the head of the pancreas, 11 (65%) out of 17 cancers of the body and tail, and 1 (6%) out of 16 cancers of the ampulla. Computed tomography missed all but two of these metastases but laparoscopy with biopsy identified 22 (96%) out of 23 instances. Isn't it about time preoperative staging laparoscopy is accepted and applied in order to obviate unnecessary laparotomy in these unfortunate patients who do not deserve anything that further increases their suffering?

There seems little question that the long-term practice of many surgeons to routinely explore the majority of patients with pancreatic cancer to determine resectability can no longer be justified (Fig. 3).

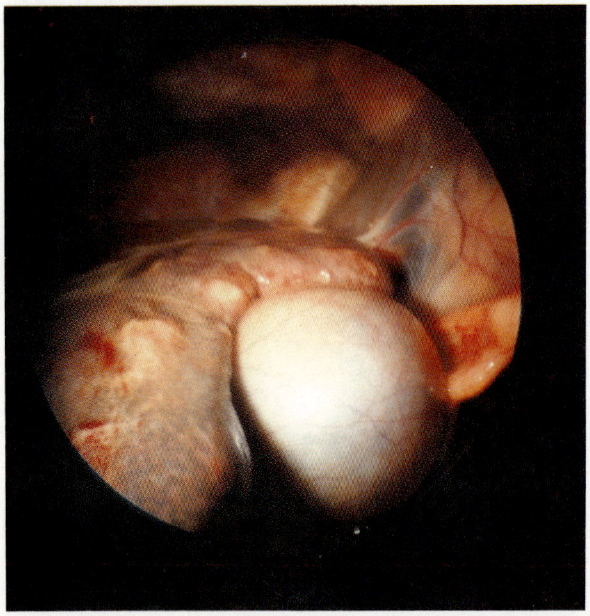

Fig. 3. View of medial aspect of right hepatic lobe and gallbladder in a patient with common bile duct obstruction due to pancreatic cancer. Note the dark green mottling of the liver surface typical of cholestasis. Multiple pale yellow metastases 3–6 mm diameter (not detected by computed tomography or abdominal ultrasound) are scattered over the liver surface just above the distended and tense gallbladder. The falciform ligament is shown along the right upper and right center margin. In such a patient, the best palliation is a common bile duct stent placed during ERCP rather than laparotomy with biliary by-pass.

This is clearly true because non-surgical palliation of bile duct obstruction is possible with bile duct stents placed during endoscopic retrograde cholangiopancreatography (ERCP) or transhepatically by radiologic methods. Integration of laparoscopy into the preoperative staging scheme improves accuracy, permits a reduction in unnecessary operations and allows appropriate patient referral and tailoring of indicated operations to specific needs based on data obtained by staging.

Carcinoma of the ovary

The use and efficacy of laparoscopy for 'second-look' examination in the follow-up of ovarian cancer has been previously confirmed. Marti-Vicente *et al.* [22•] report laparoscopy for this purpose in 205 (7%) of a total of 3088 laparoscopies performed during the period of 1980-1987. There were 72 laparoscopic explorations in 52 patients who were in complete clinical remission after surgery and chemotherapy. Of the 72 examinations, 44 were second-look and 28 third-look laparoscopies. In 35 (48.6%) laparoscopies residual cancer was found and a second-look laparotomy thereby avoided. Although a positive laparoscopy eliminates the need for surgical exploration in many cases, it must be recognized that a negative laparoscopy does not eliminate the need for further investigation. In patients who had a negative second-look laparoscopy, a second-look laparotomy revealed persistent cancer in four out of 13 (31%) patients.

Therapeutic laparoscopy peritoneal dialysis catheters

Repositioning of blocked peritoneal dialysis catheters continues to be a reliable technique performed under laparoscopic control. Gibson *et al.* [23] report five patients in whom they successfully used this method. They indicated their report was the first account for this purpose, however, numerous cases describing this application have been reported over the past 20 years.

Adnexal torsion

The leaders in laparoscopic surgery for the past two decades have been our gynecology colleagues. They have clearly shown the efficacy and safety of pelvic surgery by this route and continue to develop new techniques. Laparoscopy has been useful in the diagnosis of adnexal torsion that is most common in women of childbearing age. Mage *et al.* [24•] reported their results of complete management by laparoscopy in 27 out of 35 cases. This conservative therapy by laparoscopy was successful in these 77% of cases with only one recurrence. When gangrenous adnexa, organic ovarian cyst and unusual ovarian attachment are detected by laparoscopy, the ability to make an early decision for definitive therapy through laparotomy enhances the patient's chances for optimum treatment.

Laparoscopic surgery

During 1990 the first book devoted primarily to laparoscopy for surgeons was published [25••]. Salky has been a proponent of the clinical value of diagnostic laparoscopy during the past decade — one of the few abdominal surgeons to do so. It is proper and fitting that he has joined Berci in the United States, Cuschieri of Scotland, and Perissat and Dubois of France to encourage proper training for and application of the technique of laparoscopic cholecystectomy and other laparoscopic surgical procedures [1•,26••]. The pioneers in laparoscopic abdominal surgery are emphasizing appropriate rational guidelines for training and practice that hopefully will be implemented before misadventures by untrained surgeons and others result in a measure of disrepute for the procedure.

The main subjects covered in Salky's text are instrumentation and technique, abdominal pain, abdominal masses, liver disease, ascites, therapeutic laparoscopy, abscess/cyst damage, appendectomy, lysis of adhesions, clearing obstruction and repositioning peritoneal dialysis catheters, laparoscopic cholecystectomy, and a chapter on emergency laparoscopy by George Berci.

New developments in laparoscopic surgery are presently limited only by the initiative of surgeons and the availability of suitable instruments. Reports of laparoscopic surgery being developed in animals that may prove applicable for common conditions in humans are discussed below. It is hoped these methods will be extensively evaluated and instruments perfected before subjecting humans to the insults of technique development. With cholecystectomy and appendectomy leading the way can herniorrhaphy, vagotomy, pyloroplasty, antireflux procedures and bowel resection be far behind?

Cholecystectomy

Perissat *et al.* [27••], one of the pioneers in laparoscopic cholecystostomy and cholecystectomy, reported the results of treatment in 42 patients. The technique involves use of an intracorporal ultrasonic lithotripter for gallstone fragmentation and removal followed by cholecystostomy in 17 cases or cholescystectomy in 25 cases with good results. The same group had earlier reported the results in 40 of these cases in another journal. Most laparoscopic cholecystectomies carried out in the USA do not employ intracorporeal ultrasonic lithotripsy.

Developments in technique to enhance the safety and efficiency of laparoscopic surgery are necessary and are evolving. Nathanson and Cuschieri [28•] have provided a brief report on their method for improving visualization of the subhepatic area and specifically the cystic duct pedicle. As diagnostic laparoscopists have recognized for years, the falciform ligament in obese persons may be very large and hangs down to interfere with good visualization of the midhepatic area. The technique described is simple and consists of a transabdominal heavy suture placed through the abdominal wall on one side, pulled under the round and falciform ligaments and passed up through the abdominal wall on the other side. Moderate traction applied to both sutures pulls the round and falciform ligaments up to the anterior abdominal wall, the two ends are tied and later released after the cholecystectomy.

The new 'catch' term for laparoscopic surgery is 'minimal access surgery'. Two of the pioneers in these methods have provided an overview with emphasis on recommendations related to laparoscopic cholecystectomy in their recent editorial [2••]. Cuschieri and Terblanche tell us that minimal access surgery techniques are developing along three lines: laparoscopic surgery, endoluminal surgery (sleeve resections of the rectum) and endoscopic extraluminal dissection (visually controlled dissection of the esophagus). The authors are appealing that proper prospective clinical trials on laparoscopic cholecystectomy should be carried out before the indiscriminate and widespead use of the procedure make it impossible for us to undertake such an assessment. Unfortunately, the time for this has passed. For the most part, this is the result of training courses given by some pioneers in the field to many other surgeons, most of whom had no prior experience with diagnostic laparoscopy technique. Those who develop new methods should assume responsibility for prospective trials before they publicize and teach such procedures to others. The rush to start laparoscopic cholecystectomy by poorly trained surgeons is resulting in unnecessary complications and the potential for forcing this technique into undeserved disrepute. These authors' review their valid concerns about the training required, unresolved technical questions, indications and the possibility of mass abuse of proven surgical principles and doctrines in the rush to perform laparoscopic cholecystectomy. Their advice and caveats should be accepted but we all know that will probably not happen — sadly for their patients!

Cuschieri and Terblanche are also appropriately concerned that laparoscopic cholecystectomy will be used to remove asymptomatic gallstones, a practice they label as clearly unacceptable. They urge initiation of studies to resolve issues such as the best procedure for cholangiography, management of ductal calculi, optimal methods for dissection of the gallbladder, and improved instrumentation.

Appendectomy

Gotz *et al.* [29••] has pointed out that Semm, the pioneer in operative endoscopy in the pelvis and originator of laparoscopic appendectomy technique, was able to avoid almost 80% of all laparotomies in his field through the use of laparoscopic techniques. Gotz *et al.* began laparoscopic appendectomy in 1987 and reported their experience with 388 patients. There were 31 other patients in whom appendectomy via conventional laparotomy was performed for the following reasons: patient was very obese; no surgeon with adequate experience in laparoscopic appendectomy was available; or the patient refused the laparoscopic approach. The article describes their technique in some detail. There was no operative mortality but early in their experience various problems forced them to abandon the laparoscopic approach and use conventional surgery in 3% of the cases. Remarkably, the operation time measured from skin incision to closure was 15–20 minutes! Uncontrollable bleeding occurred in three cases early in their experience and post-laparoscopy abscess formation occurred in two patients with perforated appendices, all of whom required laparotomy.

New instruments now make laparoscopic appendectomy feasible in obese patients, offering them significant advantages over appendectomy via laparotomy. In most cases, food intake was possible on the first post-operative day when intestinal function was restored. Patients were discharged usually about 1 week after the procedure but this duration will probably be reduced in the near future.

Inguinal hernia repair

Ger *et al.* [30] reported their experience with a technique for management of indirect inguinal hernias through the laparoscope using metal clips to close the neck of the sac. The hernias were clinically cured in 14 out of 15 beagle dogs and in two humans. In 1982 the validity for the efficacy of this approach was established by Ger when coincidental hernias present in 13 patients during an intra-abdominal procedure were treated effectively by closure of the internal hernial opening with metal clips [31•]. This internal approach to hernia repair has several advantages and minimal disadvantages but long-term follow-up will be required to determine its lasting effect.

Popp [32•] reports a patch repair of a direct inguinal hernia in a 27-year-old female using a laparoscopic technique. Previous experience with equipment and laparoscopic surgery had been gained with gynecologic laparoscopy. Two trocar sheaths, one 5 mm and one 11 mm diameter, were required for the instruments needed. After three sutures were used to close the hernia defect a 4 × 5 cm oval patch of dehydrated dura mater was applied over the repair to prevent development of intra-abdominal adhesions at the repair site. The author states that other abdominal wall defects may be diagnosed and repaired using endoscopic surgery.

Jejunostomy

O'Regan and Scarrow [33•] reported on their experience with laparoscopic jejunostomy in a single patient. The procedure was considered indicated because of failure of percutaneous endoscopic jejunostomy in a patient with severe accident trauma treated over a protracted course. The jejunostomy was accomplished through three access sites that permitted visualization, placement of a probe and use of a needle holder via the third site. Two sutures were placed through the proximal jejunal wall just beyond the duodeno-jejunal junction to allow fixation of the bowel for scissors incision and intralumenal placement of a Foley catheter under direct vision. A third suture was placed to obliterate the opening around the catheter to prevent leakage. The jejunal wall was approximated to the parietal peritoneum at the site by tieing the three sutures over gauze bolsters on the skin. The inflated Foley catheter balloon was pulled and fixed to further ensure fixation of jejunum to anterior parietal peritoneum. There is every reason to expect that this technique can be further perfected in animals with development of better instruments and will be accepted as a safe and effective alternative to standard percutaneous gastrojejunostomy and surgical jejunostomy in selected patients.

Gynecologic laparoscopy

Our gynecologist colleagues, though relatively late entering the field of diagnostic laparoscopy compared with gastroenterologists, and a few general surgeons, have been the leaders in the development of laparoscopic surgery over the past two decades. The American Association of Gynecologic Laparoscopists (AAGL) has been the primary organization responsible for guiding gynecologic laparoscopy effectively through its evolution. This organization reported results of 1,151 surveys received from a mailing to their 4,832 members [34•]. The questionnaire included questions about operative laparoscopies performed by AAGL members only during the 1988 calendar year.

Significantly this AAGL survey reported more operative laparoscopies (36928) than sterilization procedures (30480) in 1988. The authors emphasized the change in orientation by its members and the new need to study all types of complications and their prevention. Their concluding statement is important for all who perform laparoscopy, especially those just beginning laparoscopic surgery: 'The lessons learned in the 1970's are now applicable to the complications of operative procedures in the 1980's and 90's: Understanding etiology, planning management and understanding prevention.'

Laparoscopy in research prevention of adhesions

Interceed (TC7) (Johnson and Johnson Patient Care, Inc.), an absorbable fabric specially designed to reduce post-surgical adhesions, was used in a multicenter, prospective, randomized clinical trial to evaluate its efficacy in reducing adhesions in humans [35•]. Patients being evaluated for infertility who had bilateral pelvic adhesions found at laparotomy were studied at laparotomy and second look laparoscopy to determine Interceed's effectiveness in reducing reformation of adhesions. After removal of adhesions at laparotomy the deperitonealized area of one pelvic sidewall was covered with Interceed. The contralateral sidewall served as the control. A second-look laparoscopy was performed 10 days to 14 weeks after the laparotomy. Pelvic sidewalls covered with Interceed had a 90% improvement over control sidewalls in preventing adhesion formation. The investigators concluded that Interceed significantly reduced incidence, extent, and severity of post-surgical pelvic adhesions. This application proves to be another ideal way to use laparoscopy in research on responses to some types of intra-abdominal therapies.

Pancreatic biopsy

Pancreatic biopsy during laparoscopy was performed by Hanafusa *et al.* [36•] in seven patients newly diagnosed with Type 1 (insulin-dependent) diabetes mellitus. The purpose was to obtain tissue to evaluate immunopathological changes of the pancreatic islets that may lead to selection of patients for immunotherapy. Standard laparoscopic technique under local anesthesia was used. As Type I diabetics usually have minimal intra-abdominal fat deposition the pancreatic body was easily viewed through the thin gastrohepatic or lesser omentum after the left hepatic lobe was elevated by a palpating probe passed via a second puncture. A biopsy forceps was used to puncture the pancreas through the lesser omentum and the site observed for 10 minutes for bleeding. There were no complications of this biopsy method. An inhibitor of pancreatic enzymes was infused prophylactically for 24 hours after biopsy during which time the serum amylase and lipase were measured every 6 hours.

Chemical cholecystectomy

Cuschieri *et al.* [37•] reported a new experimental approach to treating gallbladder disease — chemical cholecystectomy under laparoscopic guidance. The procedure entails creation of percutaneous cholecystectomy for gallstone removal or fragmentation. After endoscopic occlusion of the cystic duct, the alkali corrosive sodium carbonate was instilled into the gallbladder for 10–15 minutes in 11 animals. There were three deaths due to technical errors. In five out of the eight survivors, histology confirmed complete destruction of the gallbladder without damage to the rest of the biliary tract or liver parenchyma. What will be next in 1991?

References and recommended reading

Papers of special interest published within the annual period of review, have been highlighted as:
- • Of interest
- •• Of outstanding interest

1. CUSCHIERI A, BERCI G, MCSHERRY CK: **Laparoscopic Cholecystectomy.** *Am J Surg* 1990, **159**:273.
• An important, rational and responsible assessment of the importance of proper training, development and clinical application of laparoscopic cholecystectomy.

2. CUSCHIERI A, TERBLANCHE J: **Laparoscopic Cholecystectomy: Evolution, Not Revolution.** *Surg Endosc* 1990, **4**:125–126.
•• The authors stress the need for restraint in use of laparoscopic cholecystectomy and the importance of training and prospective studies to assure efficacy.

3. AIRAN MC: **Letter to the Editor. Laparoscopic Cholecystectomy.** *Am J Surg* 1990, **159**:619.
•• A letter of caution regarding the need for training and proper use of laparoscopic cholecystectomy. Recommendations for a minimally acceptable laparoscopic cholecystectomy training course are presented.

4. JARRETT JC II: **Laparoscopy: Direct Trocar Insertion Without Pneumoperitoneum.** *Obstet Gynecol* 1990, **75**:725–727.
• Report of a modification of trocar insertion that appears to have applicability only to the patient under general anesthesia.

5. SCZIGETVARI I, FEINMAN M, BARAD D, BARTFAI G, KAALI SG: **Association of Previous Abdominal Surgery and Significant Adhesions in Laparoscopic Sterilization Patients.** *J Reprod Med* 1989, **34**:465–466.
• Emphasizes the low frequency of peritoneal adhesions that prove to be a hindrance or increased risk for laparoscopy.

6. CAVA A, ROMAN J, QUINTELA AG, MARTIN F, ARAMBURO P: **Subcutaneous Metastasis Following Laparoscopy In Gastric Adenocarcinoma.** *Eur J Surg Oncol* 1990, **16**:63–67.

7. PASCUAL JB, BARANDA MM, TARRERO MT, GUTIERREZ MFM, GARRIDO IM, ERRASTI CA: **Subcutaneous Emphysema, Pneumomediastinum, Bilateral Pneumothorax and Pneumopericardium After Laparoscopy.** *Endoscopy* 1990, **22**:59.

8. DOMINGO M, GRAU J, VAZQUEZ A, DIEZ A, COLL J, VIVANCOS J: **Septic Shock and Bacteremia Associated with Laparoscopic Guided Liver Biopsy, Report on Two Cases.** *Endoscopy* 1989, **21**:240–241.
• Two cases of rare septic sequelae of laparoscopic liver biopsy are presented.

9. CONTRACTOR QQ, BENSON L, CONTRACTOR TQ, KHER YR: **Laparoscopic Appearance of the Liver in *Schistosoma Mansoni* Infection.** *Endoscopy* 1990, **22**:137–139.
• The macroscopic pathology of the hepatic alterations caused by hepatic *Schistosoma mansoni* are presented by description and photographs.

10. VERCELLINI P, FEDELE L, ARCAINI L, BIANCHI S, ROGNONI MT, CANDIANI GB: **Laparoscopy in the Diagnosis of Chronic Pelvic Pain in Adolescent Women.** *J Reprod Med* 1989, **34**:827–830.
•• Laparoscopy again is shown to be an excellent method for differential diagnosis and treatment of chronic pelvic pain.

11. HASAN FA, JEFFERS LJ, WELSH SW, REDDY KR, SCHIFF ER: **Hepatic Involvement as the Primary Manifestation of Kaposi's Sarcoma in the Acquired Immune Deficiency Syndrome.** *Am J Gastroenterol* 1989, **84**:1449–1451.
• An atypical presentation of malignancy in acquired immunodeficiency syndrome is presented.

12. VAN GELDER T, HOOGSTEDEN HC, VERSNEL MA, DE BEER PH, VANDENBROUCKE JP, PLANTEYDT HT: **Malignant Peritoneal Mesothelioma: A Series of 19 Cases.** *Digestion* 1989, **43**:222–227.
•• Appropriate emphasis is placed on the difficulties of mesothelioma and the preference of laparoscopy over laparotomy for diagnosis.

13. AL-HADEEDI S, WALIA HS, AL-SAYER HM: **Abdominal Tuberculosis.** *CJS* 1990, **33**:233–237.
• The long-recognized benefit of laparoscopy for diagnosis of peritoneal tuberculosis is again reported.

14. GORDON SC, WATTS JC, VENERI RJ, CHANDLER FW: **Focal Hepatic Candidiasis with Perihepatic Adhesions: Laparoscopic and Immunohistologic diagnosis.** *Gastroenterology* 1990, **98**:214–217.
•• Laparoscopy has a role in both diagnosis and subsequent evaluation for post-therapeutic persistence of hepatic candidiasis.

15. TAMEDA Y, YOSHIZAWA N, TAKASE K, NAKANO T, KOSAKA Y: **Prognostic Value of Peritoneoscopic Findings in Cirrhosis of the Liver.** *Gastroinstest Endosc* 1990, **36**:34–38.
•• Several anatomical findings associated with cirrhosis appear to have a statistically significant correlation with prognosis for survival.

16. ORLANDO R, LIRUSSI F, OKOLICSANYI L: **Laparoscopy and Liver Biopsy: Further Evidence That the Two Procedures Improve the Diagnosis of Liver Cirrhosis.** *J Clin Gastroenterol* 1990, **12**:47–52.
••

Surprisingly low correlation between laparoscopic visual diagnosis and guided liver biopsy is reported. Both procedures on the same patient rarely will miss the diagnosis of cirrhosis.

17. NORD HJ: **Biopsy Diagnosis of Cirrhosis: Blind Percutaneous Versus Guided Direct Vision Techniques:** A Review. *Gastrointest Endosc* 1982, **28**:102.

18. DAGNINI G: Laparoscopy in Cirrhosis and Portal Hypertension; in *Gastroenterologic Endoscopy* (1st Edition), Sivak MV ed., WB Saunders Company, Philadelphia, 1987, 1080–1108.

19. • INUI Y, KAWATA S, TARUI S: **Laparoscopic Findings of Fatty Liver Using Multiple Regression Analysis.** *Endoscopy* 1990, 22:27–30.

The authors report a detailed analysis of a comparison between color changes in the hepatic surface and biopsy findings.

20. • SCHIER F, WALDSCHMIDT J: **Experience with Laparoscopy for the Evaluation of Cholestasis in Newborns.** *Surg Endosc* 1990, 4:13–14.

Laparoscopy can eliminate the need for diagnostic laparotomy in many newborns with cholestasis.

21. •• WARSHAW AL, GU Z, WITTENBERG J, WALTMAN AC: **Preoperative Staging and Assessment of Resectability of Pancreatic Cancer.** *Arch Surg* 1990, **125**:230–233.

An update on a 1986 report reconfirms the value of preoperative laparoscopy in staging and for therapeutic decision making.

22. • MARTI VICENTE A, SAINZ S, SORIANO G, OJEDA B, MENDEZ C, ALONSO C, CUSSO X: **Utilidad de la Laparoscopia Cómo Metodo de Second-look En Las Neoplasias de Ovario.** *Rev Esp Enf Digest* 1990, 77:275–278.

Laparoscopy remains the best initial second-look procedure to re-stage carcinoma of the ovary.

23. GIBSON DH, HEASLEY RN, PRICE JH, DOHERTY CC, DOUGLAS JF: **Laparoscopic Repositioning of Blocked Peritoneal Dialysis Catheters in Patients on CAPD.** *Clinical Nephrol* 1990, 33:208.

24. • MAGE G, CANIS M, MANHES H, POULY J-L, BRUHAT M-A: **Laparoscopic Management of Adnexal Torsion. A Review of 35 Cases.** *J Reprod Med* 1989, **34**:520–524.

Adnexal torsion is effectively treated and differential diagnosis confirmed by laparoscopy which obviates the need for laparotomy.

25. •• SALKY BA: **Laparoscopic Cholecystectomy.** In *Laparoscopy for Surgeons.* Igaku-Shoin., New York, p 136.

This textbook-atlas provides a good update on basic diagnostic laparoscopy and is the first to provide details of technique and illustrations on laparoscopic abdominal surgery.

26. •• DUBOIS F, BERTHELOT G, LEVARD H: **Cholecystectomy Under Celioscopy.** *Ann Chir* 1990, **44**:206.

A report on technique and results of laparoscopic cholecystectomy by one of the groups who pioneered in its development.

27. •• PERISSAT J, COLLET D, BELLIARD R: **Gallstones: Laparoscopic Treatment — Cholecystectomy, Cholecystostomy, and Lithotripsy.** *Surg Endosc* 1990, 4:1–5.

An update on laparoscopic cholecystostomy and cholecystectomy by a group who are pioneers in the method that uses intracorporal ultrasonic lithotripsy.

28. • NATHANSON LK, CUSCHIERI A: **The Falciform Lift: A Simple Method for Retraction of the Falciform Ligament During Laparoscopic Cholecystectomy.** *Surg Endosc* 1990, 4:186.

A simple accessory procedure to improve visualization of the right upper quadrant during laparoscopic cholecystectomy is described.

29. •• GOTZ F, PIER A, BACHER C: **Modified Laparoscopic Appendectomy in Surgery. A Report on 388 Operations.** *Surg Endosc* 1990, 4:6–9.

Technique and results of a large series of laparoscopic appendectomies are reviewed.

30. GER R: **The Management of Certain Abdominal Herniae by Intra-abdominal Closure of the Neck of the Sac.** *Ann R Coll Surg Engl* 1982, **64**:342–344.

31. • GER R, MONROE K, DUVIVIER R, MISHRICK A: **Management of Indirect Inguinal Hernias by Laparoscopic Closure of the Neck of the Sac.** *Am J Surg* 1990, **159**:370–373.

An update on animal research to develop laparoscopic herniorrhaphy and a report on results in two patients using the technique.

32. • POPP LW: **Endoscopic Patch Repair of Inguinal Hernia in a Female Patient.** *Surg Endosc* 1990, 4:10–12.

Report of laparoscopic hernia repair using a dehydrated dura mater patch.

33. • O'REGAN PJ, SCARROW GD: **Laparoscopic Jejunostomy.** *Endoscopy* 1990, 22:39–40.

Another technique performed successfully by laparoscopy that may prove beneficial in selected patients who require long-term enteral feeding.

34. • PETERSON HB, HULKA JF, PHILLIPS JM: **American Association of Gynecologic Laparoscopists' 1988 Membership Survey on Operative Laparoscopy.** *J Reprod Med* 1990, **35**:587–589.

A survey of a large number of laparoscopies performed by gynecologists with emphasis on complications and their prevention.

35. • COHEN SM, FRANKLIN RR, HANEY AF, ET AL.: **Prevention of Postsurgical Adhesions by INTERCEED(TC7), an Absorbable Adhesion Barrier: A Prospective, Randomized Multicenter Clinical Study.** *Fertil and Steril* 1989, **51**:933–938.

A report on recent laparoscopy research on the efficacy of an absorbable cellulose fabric designed to act as a barrier for postoperative adhesion formation.

36. • HANAFUSA T, MIYAZAKI A, MIYAGAWA J, ET AL: **Examination of Islets in the Pancreas Biopsy Specimens from Newly Diagnosed Type 1 (Insulin-dependent) Diabetic Patients.** *Diabetologia* 1990, **33**:105–111.

Laparoscopy was used to obtain pancreatic biopsies for research purposes in newly diagnosed patients with insulin-dependent diabetes mellitus with no complications.

37. • CUSCHIERI A, ABD EL GHANY AA, HOLLEY MP: **Successful Chemical Cholecystectomy: A Laparoscopic Guided Technique.** *Gut* 1989, **30**:1786–1794.

This fascinating innovation for treatment of a diseased gallbladder is provocative, but far from being ready for use in humans.

Endoscopic instrumentation

M.B. Kimmey and R.W. Martin

Department of Medicine, University of Washington, Seattle, Washington, USA

Although there were no revolutionary innovations in the field of endoscopic instrumentation in 1990, several modifications have improved fiberoptic and video endoscopes, endoscopic ultrasound devices, and accessory equipment.

Introduction

The literature describing the development and clinical testing of new endoscopic instruments often lags behind the availability of these instruments. In an effort to make this chapter more useful to the practising endoscopist, we discuss the instruments introduced in 1990 by the major manufacturers of endoscopic equipment. The current medical literature pertaining to these devices is also reviewed when available. In many cases, however, we have relied upon the information provided to us by the manufacturers, with a focus on the technical specifications rather than on the marketing hyperbole. Manufacturers are acknowledged with regard to each device in order to aid the reader who would like to obtain more information. However, this acknowledgement is not intended as an advertisement or endorsement of a specific product.

Several new fiberoptic and video endoscopes were introduced in 1990. A greater range of instrument sizes, channel sizes, and double-channel instruments is now available in both fiberoptic and video format. Computers are also being applied more frequently in the endoscopy unit to connect procedure rooms, store and manipulate data, and generate reports.

Several new developments have also occurred in the field of endoscopic ultrasound. Ultrasound colonoscopes and duodenoscopes have been introduced. A new ultrasound upper endoscope can be used as an accessory with a versatile ultrasound processor that accepts other transducers for transcutaneous ultrasound. This system also has color Doppler capability and should expand the role of ultrasonographers in the field of endoscopic ultrasound.

Finally, new endoscopic accessories have been introduced for the treatment of variceal bleeding, for use at endoscopic retrograde cholangiopancreatography (ERCP), and for miscellaneous uses. Most of these are modifications of existing technology but may result in better results of several endoscopic therapies.

Endoscopes

Fiberoptic endoscopes

Although most new endoscope developments have occurred in the video area, it is notable that new fiberoptic scopes are still being introduced. Many of the new fiberoptic scopes emphasize areas where fiberoptics are still superior to video endoscopes: for the diagnosis and treatment of gastrointestinal bleeding and for screening endoscopy without sedation using small-caliber instruments.

A 13 mm outer diameter gastroscope that contains channels of 3.7 and 2.8 mm has been introduced (Olympus GIF-2T20, Olympus Corp., Lake Success, New York, USA). This instrument allows use of a thermal or injection device through one channel without significant loss of suction capability. Another potentially useful feature of this instrument is an elevator attached to the smaller channel for directing auxiliary devices placed through the channel.

The degree of further suction provided by additional large channels is worth discussing. In addition to being able to suction larger clots and debris, the speed of suction of any liquid increases with the fourth power of the radius of the channel size according to Poiseuille's equation:

$$Q = \frac{P\pi r^4}{8\nu L}$$

This equation states that when a pressure (P) is applied across a tube of length (L) and inside radius (r) then a fluid with a viscosity (ν) will flow at rate of Q. Figure 1 shows calculated flows for several endoscope channel sizes to demonstrate the dramatic increase in suction rates achieved with larger channel sizes.

Fiberoptic scopes are available in smaller outside diameters than video endoscopes, the diameter of which is limited by the size of currently available charge coupled devices or 'chips'. These smaller endoscopes are better tolerated by patients, especially when no sedation is used. Fiberoptic and video endoscopes of several diameters have been recently redesigned by one manufacturer (Series 7, Fujinon Inc., Wayne, New Jersey, USA), emphasizing lighter weights, smaller handles, and better valves.

Video endoscopes

Video endoscopy provides many advantages over fiberoptic endoscopy, including the following: higher resolu-

© Current Science Ltd ISBN 1-870485-32-7 ISSN 0952-6293

Channel diameter (mm)	Flow of water at 37°C (cm^3/s)	Flow of blood at 37°C (cm^3/s)
2.0	7.5	1.6
2.8	29.0	6.2
3.2	49.4	10.5
3.7	88.3	18.8
4.1	147.0	31.2

*Assumes a 100 cm channel length with 100 mmHg applied suction pressure.

Fig. 1. Fluid flow through endoscopic channels* (based on Poiseuille's equation).

tion; brighter images; more comfortable use; better documentation; easier teaching; a greater role for the endoscopy assistant; and the potential for more durable instruments [1•]. It should not be assumed, however, that diagnostic accuracy is an improvement over conventional fiberoptic endoscopy. No difference in the accuracy of diagnosing common upper gastrointestinal mucosal diseases was found in a recent randomized comparison of fiberoptic and video examinations [2]. This may reflect the current rather primitive state of the art of endoscopic diagnosis; more studies are needed using high-resolution video instruments to see whether the enhanced resolution of these endoscopes can lead to further diagnostic refinements.

No significant progress has been made in the controversy over whether the simultaneous or sequential color generating systems provide the best overall image. The sequential systems emphasize image resolution, while the simultaneous systems emphasize the loss of artifacts caused by motion. A recent review of video endoscopy [1•] points out that it takes 50 ms to build up a color image with the sequential system; if endoscope or patient movement occurs during this time period, the image will be blurred.

A number of new video endoscopes were introduced last year. Several of these have large channels for greater application of larger biopsy forceps and therapeutic devices. These instruments include a colonoscope and side-viewing duodenoscope, both with 4.2 mm diameter channels (CF-1T100 and TJF-100, Olympus Corp., Lake Success, New York, USA), and a two-channel gastroscope and colonoscope (EG-3800T and EC-3800TL, Pentax Precision Corp., Orangeburg, New York, USA).

A video enteroscope has also been introduced (ESI-P2000, Pentax Precision Instrument Corp., Orangeburg, New York, USA). This is a sonde-type instrument that passes through the small bowel by peristalsis. It is 6.5 mm in diameter and 400 cm long, and has a 2.0 mm channel.

Computer systems for the endoscopy unit

Computer technology is being used in the gastrointestinal endoscopy suite for several applications. Endoscopic video systems in multiple-procedure rooms can be connected to a central computer to facilitate the following: patient data entry; image manipulation and storage; image recording on videotape, computer disk, or video printer. This centralization reduces the need for duplicate recording and image storage equipment in several procedure rooms.

Endoscopy reports can be generated electronically in several formats. An abbreviated report that emphasizes images can be made using a 4 on 1 format and a video printer. Fluoroscopic images from ERCP can also be included in these mini-reports [3]. Longer reports can be made with various wordprocessing software or on standard report programs such as those developed by the American Society of Gastrointestinal Endoscopy. A recently introduced endoscopy report generator uses voice recognition technology along with preprogrammed standard phrases and instructions to generate a report (Endospeak, Olympus Corp., Lake Success, New York, USA).

Endoscopic unit management can also be facilitated by computers in several ways. Lists of patients that are to be recalled for follow-up examinations can be generated, along with the appropriate letters for these patients if desired. Software has also been written to aid compliance with quality assurance requirements (PV-ERBD, Pentax Precision Instrument Corp., Orangeburg, New York, USA).

A microcomputer-based system that captures and stores endoscopic images and combines them with other patient data was recently described [4]. An understanding of how this system works requires some knowledge of how images are generated, captured, displayed, and stored. It also requires some knowledge of computer language and the difference between analog and digital information. In analog format, the value of the voltage in an electronic device is directly related to the value of the parameter of information it represents. In digital format, the voltage in the device takes on only one of two values: either low or high. The value of the variable is represented in a code composed of these low or high states (often called bits). For example, the numbers 0–3 are represented in two bits of information as follow: 0 = low low, 1 = low high, 2 = high low, and 3 = high high (based on the standard binary method). Higher numbers require a greater length of sequences or more bits. This coded information is stored or manipulated in electronic devices in either a single circuit, switching to various high or low states at various sequential points in time, or several circuits in the device at the same point in time.

Information is handled in either analog or digital format, depending on the type of electronic device. Some devices function better in one mode than the other. For example, video cameras and image monitors are predominantly analog, whereas current computers are digital. As a consequence, in a video endoscopy system, information has to be converted back and forth between analog and digital formats. This is accomplished by using an analog to digital converter or digital to analog converter. Information can be degraded or lost in this process, and so conversion should be minimized within a system.

Another important factor in image quality is the resolution of the image. Most digital image manipulation devices divide the image display into grids such as 512 divisions horizontally and 480 divisions vertically. At each point in this grid, the subtlety of gray or color is controlled by the number of bits used. A 512 × 480 displayed image is the same as broadcast quality and is considered to be of fairly high quality. However, for X-ray images and images where one wishes to magnify a region in the image for further study, a 512 × 480 display may be insufficient.

Many of the high-quality imaging display devices are now being offered in 1028 × 1024 divisions per image or higher. Again, the value of higher-resolution display device is dependent on whether the original video camera produces information that also has such high resolution. If not, little is gained unless several images will be combined onto one display.

The methods of storing information by electronic means is continually changing, with the trend being from analog towards more digital methods. Historically, methods for storing images have used analog video tape. It has been easier and more information could be stored on the same amount of tape. With the increasing availability of devices that will store images in digital format in a very compact form, digital methods increase in attractiveness. Digital information is preserved more accurately and is easy to blend together with other types of information (for example, endoscopic images and patient information), and information is more easily acquired and manipulated with the computer.

Endoscopic ultrasound

An ultrasound duodenoscope (JF-UM3) and colonoscope (CF-UM3) have been introduced by the Olympus company (Olympus Corp., Lake Success, New York, USA) for use with the standard EU-M3 endoscopic ultrasound system. Both instruments are available in either 7.5 or 12 MHz frequencies but are not switchable between these frequencies like the upper ultrasound endoscope (GF-UM3) that is used with this system. The duodenoscope has side-viewing optics and is 10.4 mm in outside diameter, which should allow easier insertion into the descending duodenum for imaging the ampulla and pancreatic head.

The ultrasound colonoscope has been constructed to allow forward endoscopic viewing by reducing the ultrasound sector to 300°. The endoscopic fibers and biopsy channel shield the ultrasound image where they cross the ultrasound beam emitted from the rotating transducer mounted just proximal to the endoscope's tip. Preliminary clinical use of prototypes of this instrument in imaging colonic neoplasms, subepithelial masses, and inflammatory bowel disease has been recently published [5,6•]. Images are similar to those obtained with rigid transrectal ultrasound probes. Use of this ultrasound colonoscope is unlikely to change the management of most patients with colonic neoplasms, who will still have surgical resection of the neoplasm. The technique may be useful in a select group of postoperative patients with a rising carcinoembryonic antigen level, where recurrent carcinoma is suspected but cannot be found using conventional imaging techniques. Ultrasound may also prove to be useful in guiding endoscopic ablative therapy in patients unfit for surgery.

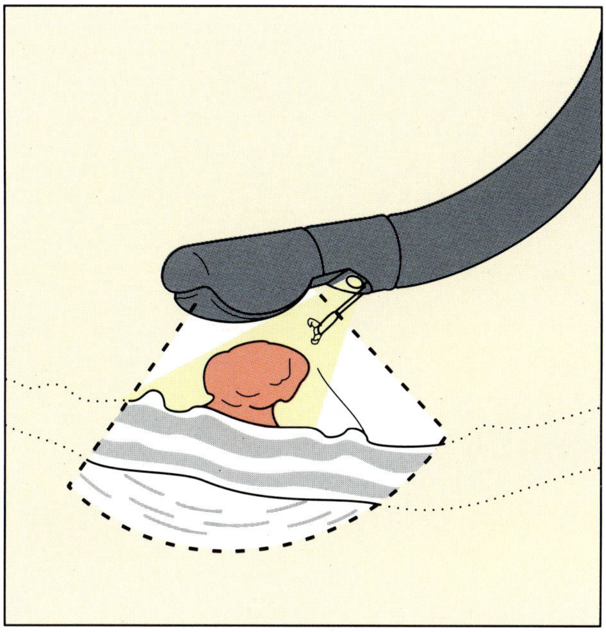

Fig. 2. The Pentax FG-32UA ultrasound endoscopes utilize an ultrasound transducer moved mechanically in a 100° sector parallel to the long axis of the endoscope. The endoscope's optics and channel are oriented toward the area of tissue being imaged.

A new endoscopic ultrasound system has been introduced by Pentax (Pentax Precision Instrument Corp., Orangeburg, New York, USA). This ultrasound endoscope (FG-32UA) obtains a 100° mechanical sector scan in the same plane as the endoscope's tip (Fig. 2). The endoscope's optics are forward oblique, with the lens and biopsy channel mounted proximal to the ultrasound transducer to allow endoscopic viewing of the area being imaged and to facilitate ultrasound directed biopsy or aspiration. This configuration is conducive to imaging of endoscopically visible lesions within or just outside the gastrointestinal wall, but will not allow comprehensive scanning of the pancreas and other paraintestinal structures. A major advantage of this instrument is that it can be used as an accessory with a Hitachi ultrasound unit that has other transducers available for conventional transcutaneous ultrasonography. This flexibility should make endoscopic ultrasonography more economically feasible by allowing sharing of instrument costs between endoscopy and ultrasound departments. This system has switchable frequencies of 5 and 7.5 MHz, and has color Doppler capability.

Ultrasound probes

Initial experience with a 7.5 MHz, 3.7 mm diameter radial ultrasound probe (Olympus Optical, Tokyo, Japan) suggests that it can be used to image within strictures not passable by conventional ultrasound endoscopes [7]. Limited ultrasound penetration and a narrow focal zone have not allowed optimal images to be obtained with this device. The physical limitations imposed by small-diameter ultrasound transducers are discussed below.

Preliminary *in vitro* experience with a 20 MHz radial probe (Boston Scientific Corp., Watertown, Massachusetts, USA) originally designed for imaging within arteries has been described [8]. This probe was used to image the bile duct through the papilla in two dogs at laparotomy and duodenotomy. The bile duct wall was imaged as a 1.4 mm thick structure but little detail of the wall structure can be discriminated in these images.

Further experience has been obtained with a 20 MHz mechanical linear probe (Sonoprobe, Fujinon Inc., Wayne, New Jersey, USA). High-resolution images of mucosal and subepithelial lesions can be made [9]. A 15 MHz linear probe is also now available with this system to increase tissue penetration without a significant loss of resolution. A limited tissue area is scanned with this probe, confining its use to endoscopically visible or diffuse diseases of the gastrointestinal wall.

The relationship of ultrasound frequency and transducer size to image resolution should be discussed. The degree of structural detail that one sees in an ultrasound image is defined by the resolution of the ultrasound transducer system. This resolution is divided into axial resolution (the resolution in the direction of the ultrasound beam) and lateral resolution (the resolution transverse to the direction of the ultrasound beam). Axial resolution is generally related to ultrasound frequency; if all other things are equal, then the higher the frequency, the better the axial resolution. Lateral resolution has two components if the transducer is not a disk type, but for simplicity we will only consider the resolution associated with a disk transducer.

An electric voltage applied to ultrasound transducer material (piezoelectric material) will cause it to expand or contract depending on the polarity of the voltage. The expansion or contraction sets up an acoustic wave that propagates away from the transducer along an axis that lies perpendicular to the face of the transducer. Initially, the lateral diameter of this wave (lateral resolution) is approximately the same as the diameter (aperture) of the disk. This diameter gradually reduces as the wave propagates until it reaches the point known as the near–far field transition point. At this point the diameter of the wave may be approximately 40% of the aperture size of the disk. As the wave propagates beyond this point it begins to spread and the lateral resolution progressively becomes worse as the beam grows in size. The rate at which this grows and the point at which the near–far field transition occurs are both related to the size of the aperture and the ultrasonic frequency used. This principle is illustrated in Fig. 3 for a 2 mm diameter disk transducer operated at 7.5 MHz and at 20 MHz. The lateral resolution is better over a greater distance with the higher frequency.

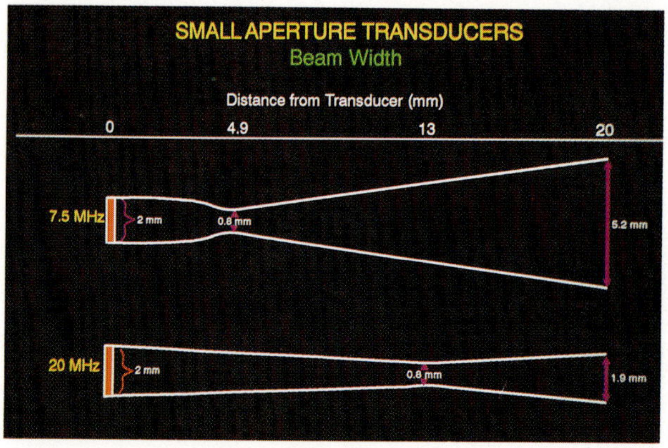

Fig. 3. The ultrasound beam width or lateral resolution is plotted as a function of distance from a 2 mm diameter transducer. The best resolution (0.8 mm) is achieved at the near–far field transition point of 4.9 mm from the transducer with the 7.5 MHz system and at 13 mm from the transducer with the 20 MHz system. Note that the higher frequency system has a better lateral resolution over a greater distance.

Doppler probes

A continuous-wave endoscopic Doppler probe (Olympus Keymed, Essex, England) was evaluated in 22 patients with recent ulcer bleeding [10••]. These 22 patients were selected from a group of 56 patients with active bleeding, visible vessels, or adherent clot that could not be washed away. The ulcer was not accessible to the probe in five other cases. Seven of the eight patients with a positive Doppler signal rebled and eight of the nine patients with an endoscopically visible vessel had a positive Doppler signal. All ulcers that rebled had either a visible vessel or a positive Doppler signal. This series suggests that use of a Doppler probe adds little to visual assessment in determining rebleeding risk for most patients with bleeding ulcers.

This continuous-wave Doppler probe has the disadvantage over pulsed Doppler probes in that it does not discriminate large deep vessels, such as the aorta, and its major branches from the smaller vessels that are the cause of ulcer bleeding. The continuous-wave type usually uses two transducer elements, one for transmission and one for reception. Energy is continuously transmitted and the scattered energy is continuously received. The electronic circuity is simple and the signal quality is high with most continuous wave units. The disadvantage of the continuous method is that the Doppler signal may arise from any place within the tissue where the transmitting and receiving beams intersect. This can occur at more than one place in the tissues; in practice, a Doppler signal from a deeper vessel may falsely suggest the presence of a more superficial vessel.

Pulsed Doppler probes use brief bursts of ultrasonic energy that are transmitted in a repetitive manner; received energy is processed to detect Doppler shifted information only between these bursts of transmitted energy. Only one transducer is needed to both transmit and receive the signal. Furthermore, it is possible to preset an electronic time window after energy transmission so that only the signals that have been scattered from a certain depth of the tissue are processed. This time of signal sampling can be adjusted to exclude or include Doppler signals from vessels at various depths.

Another principle worth considering is the angle that the ultrasound propagates with respect to the way the blood vessel is oriented. The best Doppler signal occurs when the beam is oriented along the axis of the blood vessel, whereas the worst case is when it is oriented perpendicular to the axis of the blood vessel. Probe designs that easily transmit obliquely into the wall of the blood vessel have an advantage in detecting blood vessels that flow parallel to the mucosal surface.

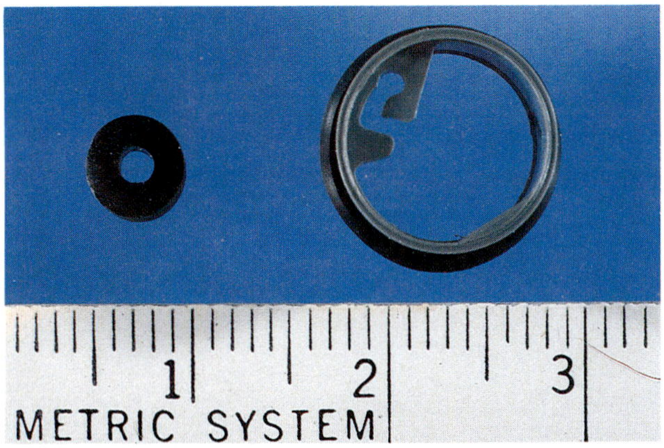

Fig. 4. A rubber O-ring is prestretched onto a plastic cylinder (right) for use with the Stiegmann-Goff variceal ligator. When the ring is released onto a varix it contracts to a few millimeters in diameter (left).

Endoscopic accessories

Variceal ligator

A banding device that attaches to endoscopes and is used to ligate esophageal varices was initially described in 1986. After several other preliminary reports and device modifications, the Stiegmann-Goff variceal ligator was introduced commercially in 1990 (C.R. Bard Inc., Billerica, Massachusetts, USA). This device uses a semi-flexible ring that is held by friction onto the distal tip of any endoscope. A stretched rubber band is fitted into this distal ring prior to passing the endoscope (Fig. 4). Following suction of a varix into the ring on the end of the endoscope, the band is released by pulling on a trip wire that runs through the endoscope's channel. A shortened overtube is provided with the ligating set to facilitate the repeated intubations required for ligation of multiple varices. The band and encaptured varix sloughs after several days, leaving a shallow ulcer. Ultimately, varices are obliterated through the associated inflammatory reaction.

The initial report of a multicenter randomized comparison of this variceal ligator with endoscopic sclerotherapy in patients with esophageal variceal bleeding suggests equal efficacy in stopping bleeding with fewer inflammatory complications such as esophageal ulcers and strictures [11•]. The technique was also reported to be useful in 12 in whom patients endoscopic sclerotherapy had failed (defined as rebleeding, eradication failure, or the production of deep ulcers or strictures) [12]. The banding techniques may ultimately prove to be most useful in stopping variceal bleeding in the patients awaiting liver transplantation. The deep ulcers produced by sclerotherapy can lead to serious infectious complications in the immunosuppressed patient following transplantation.

A novel use for the variceal ligation kit has been recently described [13]. Upper gastrointestinal foreign bodies are suctioned into the ring on the endoscope's distal tip. The foreign body is then removed by pulling it along with the endoscope out through the overtube.

Biopsy forceps

Several modifications of endoscopic biopsy forceps have been introduced recently. A rotatable forceps (FB-24KR, FB-25KR, Olympus Corp., Lake Success, New York, USA) may be useful for obtaining biopsies from the esophagus and other difficult locations but is currently only available with standard-sized cups. Another forceps with teeth on each forceps cup has been introduced as a disposable product (Radial Jaw Forceps, Microvasive Watertown, Massachusetts, USA). These 2.2 mm diameter forceps are advertised to provide better sample sizes. Unfortunately, no good comparative data are available to assess the adequacy of mucosal biopsies that are achievable with the various types of forceps. A recent study [14] of 249 biopsies in 30 patients showed that a disposable forceps with plastic cups (Singular forceps, C.R. Bard Inc., Billerica, Massachusetts, USA) obtained biopsies that were shallower and about one-third smaller in surface area than a reusable, fenestrated, needle forceps with a similar diameter. The one reliable way to increase the size of mucosal biopsies is to use a forceps with large-diameter cups through a therapeutic endoscope. Larger biopsies are assumed to provide more diagnostically useful information; however, this assertion has never been adequately tested.

Gallstone lithotriptors

A newly designed mechanical lithotriptor (BML-3Q and BML-4Q, Olympus Corp., Lake Success, New York, USA) should allow more successful retrieval of large common bile duct stones. The basket is designed to be used through either a 3.2 (BML-4Q) or 4.2 mm (BML-3Q) channel and allows up to approximately 85 pounds of force to be applied to stones captured in the lithotripsy basket. The specially designed baskets maintain an octagonal shape when opened, allowing easier stone capture (Fig. 5). These features are a significant advantage over other mechanical lithotriptors that require endoscope removal prior to use or whose baskets incompletely expand.

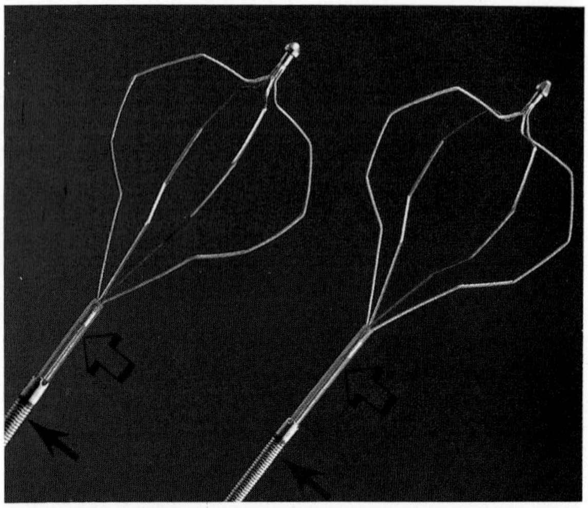

Fig. 5. The mechanical lithotriptors recently introduced by the Olympus company have an octagonal wire basket that opens from a Teflon inner sheath (open arrows) for easy bile duct cannulation. A metal coil (closed arrows) is then advanced to the base of the basket containing the stone prior to closing the basket and fragmenting the stone. By courtesy of Olympus Corp., Lake Success, New York, USA.

Prototypes of the larger mechanical lithotriptor (BML-3Q) were used in a series of 26 patients with common duct stones that could not be removed after endoscopic sphincterotomy [15••]. Forty-three out of 45 stones between 13 and 35 mm in diameter were broken and removed. One large impacted stone and another 4 cm stone could not be captured by the basket.

Another technique for fragmenting large common duct stones is the use of a tunable dye laser. Successful stone fragmentation and duct clearance were achieved in 20 out of 25 difficult patients with this device [16]. The tunable dye laser is not readily available to most endoscopists and usually requires a special delivery system ('mother – baby' scope combination) to allow stone targeting.

Papillotomes

Smaller-diameter, more flexible papillotomes have been introduced for placement over a guidewire. These double-lumen papillotomes are now available in 5.5 F (Microvasive, Watertown, Massachusetts, USA) and 6 F (Wilson-Cook Medical Surgical, Winston-Salem, North Carolina, USA) for use over a 0.035 inch guidewire. A 5-F instrument can be used over a 0.021 inch guidewire (Wilson-Cook Medical Inc., Winston-Salem, North Carolina, USA). These papillotomes are easier to place into the bile duct over guidewires than the older and stiffer 7 F double-lumen papillotomes. Another convenient use for these double-lumen papillotomes is in cannulating the bile duct when a sharp cephalad angle is needed. Contrast can be injected through the tip of the papillotome without leaking into the duodenum where the cutting wire exits the catheter.

Guidewires

Two new types of guidewires have been introduced for use at ERCP. A 0.035 inch diameter Teflon-coated wire with a tapered tip appears to be more rotatable than standard guidewires and is constructed to prevent kinking (Geenen Endotorque guidewire, Microvasive, Watertown, Massachusetts, USA).

Another wire that has been extensively used by interventional radiologists was introduced in a longer, 260 cm length for use at ERCP. The wire (Guidewire, Microvasive, Watertown, Massachusetts, USA) can be directed through the papilla as well as through tight and eccentric stenoses with little friction because of a special hydrophilic coating that becomes very slippery after water immersion. This reduced friction design also allows more rotational control of the wire tip, which is flexible in comparison to the proximal portion of the wire.

This guidewire was used to access areas of the biliary tree that were not accessible by conventional techniques in a series of 44 patients [17••]. Selective cannulation of the papilla was achieved in 10 out of 13 cases; biliary strictures were negotiated in 12 out of 12 cases; and the valves of Heister were passed, allowing gallbladder access, in 16 out of 19 attempts. These results suggest that this wire will significantly improve ERCP success rate and may lead to further endoscopic treatments of gallbladder diseases.

Stents

Modifications of conventional straight biliary stents have been made and more experience has been obtained with expandable metal stents. A stent retrieval device (Soehendra stent retriever, Wilson-Cook Medical, Winston-Salem, North Carolina, USA) has been designed to allow exchange of conventional straight stents without losing access through the stricture. This device uses a stainless steel cable that is placed over a guidewire introduced through the old stent.

The cable is then advanced and torqued to engage the stent, which is then removed along with the cable; the wire remains through the stricture to guide placement of the new stent. This device may prove to be useful for stents placed through eccentric strictures and should allow stent exchange with a single passage of the endoscope.

Examination of biliary stents that have been removed reveals an excess of debris at rough edges as on side holes. A recent study [18] confirmed this finding *in vitro* and then *in vivo* in a series of 20 patients who had placement of either a conventional straight stent or one without side holes. There was no difference between the two groups in relief of jaundice. When removed after 2 months, the stents without holes had significantly less debris than the stents with side holes. These results suggest that straight biliary stents should be redesigned with attention to producing fewer rough edges.

Additional clinical experience has been obtained with use of expandable metal stents for malignant biliary strictures. Two reports of endoscopic placement of Wallstents (Medinvent SA, Lausanne, Switzerland) in a total of 18 patients suggest a high technical success rate [19,20•]. However, despite the ability to expand up to 30 F, two patients had recurrent jaundice 4 months following stent insertion due to tumor ingrowth through the stent mesh. These patients required stent recanalization with a modified electrocautery device to maintain stent patency. Further experience and comparative clinical trials with conventional straight stents are needed.

Cytology brushes

Brushes placed over a guidewire have variable success in obtaining adequate specimens for confirming the malignant cause of strictures. Foutch *et al.* [21•] described the use of a standard cytology brush (Mill-Rose Laboratories, Mentor, Ohio) placed over a 0.025 inch guidewire in 39 strictures. A positive brushing was obtained in all strictures caused by cholangiocarcinoma, 60% of biliary strictures due to pancreatic cancer, and only 20% of strictures caused by metastases. Only two of the four malignant pancreatic duct strictures yielded a positive brushing.

Similar diagnostic results were achieved using another pancreaticobiliary brush cytology system in 53 patients [22]. This system uses a brush mounted 3 cm proximal to the distal tip of a wire that is placed through an outer catheter (Wilson-Cook Medical, Winston-Salem, North Carolina, USA). After the stricture is brushed, the brush is withdrawn into the catheter and the entire assembly withdrawn through the endoscope. This system has the potential disadvantage of losing guidewire access through the stricture.

Esophageal stents

Expandable wire stents (Wallstent, Medivent SA, Lausanne, Switzerland) were used to palliate dysphagia in a patient with a malignant esophageal stricture [23]. Two 5 cm long stents were placed to overlap in the axial direction. After introduction through a 6 mm diameter catheter the stents expanded to 20 mm in diameter. More experience is needed with these promising devices to determine which patients will benefit the most from their placement and to define the importance of tumor ingrowth between the expanded wires.

Achalasia dilating balloons

A randomized trial in 20 patients with achalasia showed that the 35 mm diameter Rigiflex achalasia balloon (Microvasive, Watertown, Massachusetts, USA) was less effective than the Brown–McHardy balloon in relieving dysphagia and promoting esophageal emptying [24]. However, the Rigiflex balloon did result in significant improvement in seven out of 10 patients and was used exclusively by the authors when a dilated and tortuous esophagus was encountered.

Cystoenterostomy device

A new device was described to assist endoscopic drainage of pancreatic pseudocysts [25]. After cutting the gastric or duodenal wall overlying a cyst with a diathermy needle, a 10 F catheter with a metal tip is advanced into the cyst while applying electrocautery current to this tip. After the cyst is entered the catheter can be exchanged over a guidewire for a nasocystic tube or double pigtail stent. Use of this and other devices should allow endoscopists to safely drain more pancreatic pseudocysts in the future.

Bipolar snare

A bipolar electrocautery snare (Everest Medical, Minneapolis, USA) was compared with a monopolar snare in surgically created mucosal elevations in the canine stomach [26]. As expected from theory and from similar experiments with other bipolar devices, the bipolar instrument produced less deep and less extensive surrounding tissue injury than the monopolar snare. This device is proposed to allow safer polypectomy, although this will be difficult to prove as the incidence of polypectomy complications is only approximately 1%.

Conclusions

Several innovations were introduced in 1990, the value of which will be apparent in the next few years. Much has been learned of the value of some devices that were introduced in previous years. We look forward to the new developments that will occur in 1991.

References and recommended reading

Papers of special interest, published within the annual period of review, have been highlighted as:

- • Of interest
- •• Of outstanding interest

1. • De Knyrim K, Seidlitz H, Vakil N, Hagenmuller F, Classen M: **Perspectives in 'Electronic Endoscopy'.** *Endoscopy* 1990, 22:2–8.

Outlines the history of video endoscopy and the difference between the types of color generators.

2. De Reuck M, Ramdani B, Jonas C, *et al.*: **A Randomized Multi-Observer, Comparative Evaluation of Conventional Fiberendoscopy and Videoendoscopy in the Upper GI Tract.** *Endoscopy* 1990, 22:9–12.

3. STROEHLEIN JR, BARROSO A, GLOMBICKI A, SACHS I: **Documentation of Fluoroscopic and Endoscopic Images Using a Color Video Printer.** *Gastrointest Endosc* 1990, 36:392–394.

4. FRANCESCHI D, STELLATO TA: **Microcomputer Image Processing in Gastrointestinal Endoscopy.** *Am Surg* 1990, 56:128–130.

5. RÖSCH T, LORENZ R, SUCHY R, DANCYGIER H, CLASSEN M: **Colonic Endoscopic Ultrasonography: First Results of a New Technique.** *Gastrointest Endosc* 1990, 36:382–386.

6. • SHIMIZU S, TADA M, KAWAI K: **Use of Endoscopic Ultrasonography for the Diagnosis of Colorectal Tumors.** *Endoscopy* 1990, 22:31–34.

The first large series of patients imaged with the ultrasound colonoscope. The types of images that can be obtained are presented.

7. RÖSCH TH, CLASSEN M: **A New Ultrasonic Probe for Endosonographic Imaging of the Upper GI Tract.** *Endoscopy* 1990, 22:41–46.

8. GOLDBERG BB, LIU JB, MERTON DA, KURTZ AB: **Endoluminal US: Experiments with Nonvascular Uses in Animals.** *Radiology* 1990, 175:49–43.

9. KIMMEY MB, MARTIN RW, SILVERSTEIN FE: **Endoscopic Ultrasound Probes.** *Gastrointest Endosc* 1990, 36: (suppl)S40–S46.

10. •• FULLARTON GM, MURRAY WR: **Prediction of Rebleeding in Peptic Ulcers by Visual Stigmata and Endoscopic Doppler Ultrasound Criteria.** *Endoscopy* 1990, 22:68–71.

Study of a continuous wave Doppler probe showing that the endoscopically detected visible vessel usually contains flowing blood and often rebleeds.

11. • STIEGMANN G, GOFF J, MICHALETZ P, KORULA J, LIEBERMAN D, REVEILLE M, SUN J: **Endoscopic Variceal Ligation vs. Sclerotherapy for Rebleeding Esophageal Varices: Early Results of a Prospective Randomized Trial.** *Gastrointest Endosc* 1990, 36:189.

The first report of this randomized study, which will merit careful review once it is published in full form.

12. SAEED ZA, MICHALETZ PA, WINCHESTER CB, *ET AL.*: **Endoscopic Variceal Ligation in Patients Who Have Failed Endoscopic Sclerotherapy.** *Gastrointest Endosc* 1990, 36:572–574.

13. SAEED AZ, MICHALETZ PA, FEINER SD, *ET AL.*: **A New Endoscopic Method for Managing Food Impaction in the Esophagus.** *Endoscopy* 1990, 22:226–228.

14. YANG R, VUITCH F, WRIGHT K,: **Adequacy of Disposable Biopsy Forceps for Gastrointestinal Endoscopy: A Direct Comparison with Reusable Forceps.** *Gastrointest Endosc* 1990, 36:379–381.

15. •• SHAW MJ, DORSHER PJ, VENNES JA: **A New Mechanical Lithotripter for the Treatment of Large Common Bile Duct Stones.** *Am J Gastroenterol* 1990, 85:796–798.

Excellent results in fragmenting large common duct stones were achieved using this mechanical lithotriptor, which can be used while a therapeutic duodenoscope remains in place.

16. COTTON PB, KOZAREK RA, SCHAPIRO RH, *ET AL.*: **Endoscopic Laser Lithotripsy of Large Bile Duct Stones.** *Gastroenterology* 1990, 99:1128–1133.

17. •• MCCARTHY JH, MILLER GL, LAURENCE BH: **Cannulation of the Biliary Tree, Cystic Duct and Gallbladder Using a Hydrophilic Polymer-coated Steerable Guidewire.** *Gastrointest Endosc* 1990, 36:386–391.

A hydrophilic coated guidewire significantly enhanced cannulation of the papilla, cystic duct, and difficult biliary strictures.

18. COENE PP, GROEN AK, CHENG J, OUT MM, TYTGAT GN: **Clogging of Biliary Endoprostheses: A New Perspective.** *Cut* 1990, 31:913–917.

19. DOMSCHKE W, FOERSTER E: **Endoscopic Implantation of Large-bore Self-expanding Biliary Mesh Stent.** *Gastrointest Endosc* 1990, 36:55–57.

20. • CREMER M, DEVIERE J, SUGAI B, *ET AL.*: **Expandable Biliary Metal Stents for Malignancies: Endoscopic Insertion and Diathermic Cleaning for Tumor Ingrowth.** *Gastrointest Endosc* 1990, 36:451–457.

Expandable metal stents can be placed through biliary strictures with a high degree of technical success, although tumor ingrowth can cause late occlusion.

21. • FOUTCH PG, KERR DM, HARLAND JR, MANNE RU, KUMMET TD, SANOWSKI RA: **Endoscopic Retrograde Wire-guided brush Cytology for Diagnosis of Patients with Malignant Obstruction of the Bile Duct.** *Am J Gastroenterol* 1990, 85:791–795.

A brush technique is reported that gives high yields and allows a guidewire to be maintained across the stricture.

22. VENU RP, GEENEN JE, KINI M, HOGAN WJ, PAYNE M, JOHNSON GK, SCHMALZ MJ: **Endoscopic Retrograde Brush Cytology.** *Gastroenterology* 1990, 99:1475–1479.

23. DOMSCHKE W, FOERSTER EC, MATEK W, RODL W: **Self-expanding Mesh Stent for Esophageal Cancer Stenosis.** *Endoscopy* 1990, 22:134–136.

24. STARK GA, CASTELL DO, RICHTER JE, WU WC: **Prospective Randomized Comparison of Brown-McHardy and Microvasive Balloon Dilators in Treatment of Achalasia.** *Am J Gastroenterol* 1990, 85:1322–1326.

25. CREMER M, DEVIERE J, BAIZE M, MATOS C: **New Device for Endoscopic Cystoenterostomy.** *Endoscopy* 1990, 22:76–77.

26. TUCKER RD, PLATZ CE, SIEVERT CE, VENNES JA,. SILVIS SE: ***In vivo* Evaluation of Monopolar Versus Bipolar Electrosurgical Polypectomy Snares.** *Am J Gastroenterol* 1990, 85:1386–1390.

Pediatric endoscopy

K.J. Benkov

Division of Pediatric Gastroenterology and Nutrition, Mount Sinai Medical Center, New York, USA

Pediatric endoscopic articles published during 1990, though few in number, covered a wide range of topics, including peptic ulcer disease, inflammatory bowel disease, gastroesophageal reflux, and the use of endoscopic retrograde cholangiopancreatography (ERCP) in children. Exact details of technique and indications for these procedures remain lacking.

Introduction

During the past year, few new reports have been published concerning pediatric endoscopy. This is probably an aberration that does not reflect a decrease in clinical activity, but rather a decrease in scholarly writing. For the first time ever, board qualifying examinations in pediatric gastroenterology were given in November 1990, and in all likelihood, many extra-clinical endeavors were put on hold in preparation.

As another manifestation of the same phenomenon, the majority of the few papers published were submitted by pediatric surgeons and adult gastroenterologists, who obviously are not required to take these examinations. The question of who is the appropriate physician to perform endoscopic procedures on infants and children is one that will have to be answered in the future. There are obvious differences in anesthesia, technique and management; these depend on the background of the endoscopist. Unfortunately, most of the publications discussed in the present review did not address endoscopic technique.

Use of endoscopic retrograde cholangiopancreatography

Probably the only significant contribution for 1990 was a review on endoscopic retrograde cholangiopancreatography (ERCP) in children by Buckley and Connon [1••]. They performed ERCP in 42 children, ranging in age from 1–19 years, with an average age of 10.5 years. The authors found three major indications for ERCP. The first was for the assessment of suspected or proven pancreatic disorders in 18 children; the next was for the evaluation of the biliary tract in 15 children, and the third for the investigation of unexplained abdominal pain in nine children. Standard adult side-viewing (Olympus JF1T) endoscopes were used in all patients, with intravenous diazepam as a local anesthetic; however, children under 12 were treated under general anesthesia. Buckley and Connon had no endoscopic complications, but two patients had mild post-cannulation pancreatitis, similar to other reported series in adults. The pancreatic diseases documented included familial pancreatitis, lupus, and idiopathic pancreatitis. Hepatobiliary disorders diagnosed were choledocholithiasis, cirrhosis, sclerosing cholangitis, cystic fibrosis, choledochal cysts, intrahepatic cholestasis, hepatoma, and one extrahepatic biliary atresia, the patient having already undergone a Kasai procedure. The group of children with unexplained abdominal pain were poorly detailed. These seemed to include children with underlying illnesses, such as cystic fibrosis, thrombotic thrombocytopenic purpura, vomiting of bile, and congenital hepatic fibrosis, who might be at risk of secondary hepatobiliary or pancreatic disease. The authors commented that ERCP was not particularly helpful in this setting and, further, that the standard adult endoscope was suitable in all children except perhaps those under 6 months of age.

Other reviews of ERCP in children have been published [2,3], along with isolated case reports; however, the report by Buckley and Connon was one of the larger ones. The authors uncovered a fair number of abnormalities, but other than the one case of biliary atresia, they paralleled those found in adults. They did mention additional applications of ERCP in children, namely investigation of biliary atresia and children who have undergone a transplant, but had no such patients in their series. Until additional applications are found in pediatrics, their comment that 'pediatric gastroenterologists are less likely to be familiar with indications for ERCP and less skilled in performance' will prevail. Of children who have undergone a transplant, 60–70% have usually been treated for extrahepatic biliary atresia, making an ERCP impossible [4].

The major indication for ERCP in children may conceivably become the ruling out of extrahepatic biliary atresia in newborns with direct hyperbilirubinemia. These infants usually undergo hepatobiliary scans that often fail to demonstrate excretion, even in intrahepatic cholestasis. Sonograms in this setting are notorious for being erroneous and misleading. The most useful study in these children before the exploratory laparotomy and intraoperative cholangiogram has been the percutaneous liver biopsy. An invasive procedure, percutaneous liver biopsy [5] requires hospital admission and can be inconclusive in 30–40% of cases. If ERCP were readily available, this procedure would supplant the other less useful ones and the need for hospitalization. We have used ERCP in

© Current Science Ltd ISBN 1-870485-32-7 ISSN 0952-6293

three such children, including one who was previously reported [6]. A smaller prototype instrument was used with intravenous sedation, allowing successful cannulation in two of the infants. Buckley and Connon comment that 'there is no need for special pediatric endoscopes' and 'the technique... is no more difficult... once adequate sedation has been obtained.'

These simple comments emphasize the basic disputes in pediatric endoscopy. It is our belief that general anesthesia has no routine role in pediatric endoscopy. Percutaneous gastrostomies have been performed in infants as young as 1 month and esophageal varices have been sclerosed in 18-month-old infants, both without general anesthesia. Small instruments are necessary in young infants when using intravenous sedation as oversized endoscopes tend to occlude the airway; they also angulate, maneurve (and so cannulate) more easily in neonates.

A few isolated reports in the pediatric surgical literature highlighted the use of ERCP. Crombleholme *et al.* [7•] report on two children with mediastinal pseudocysts as a complication of pancreatitis. ERCP was used to document ductal anomalies, enabling the surgeons to plan the appropriate drainage procedure. As an aside, they also comment on the futility of ultrasound in detecting this entity that requires computed tomography or magnetic resonance imaging. The same authors in another paper [8•] reported on the use of a modified Puestow procedure in 10 children with chronic relapsing pancreatitis over a 20-year period. Their recommendation, which is well taken, is that any child with chronic pancreatitis should have his or her ductal anatomy clarified. ERCP is well suited to the determination of duct size and the detection of obstruction, leaks, or origin of pseudocysts.

Obstruction requires drainage either by sphincterotomy or by the Puestow procedure, as was the case in Crombleholme *et al.'s* series. Grosfeld *et al.* [9•] report on the operative drainage of post-traumatic pancreatic pseudocysts after percutaneous drainage failed. ERCP was used to determine transected pancreatic ducts in two of the four patients who were eventually operated on.

The use of upper endoscopy

A novel technique was reported by Borgstein *et al.* [10•] in a 6-month-old infant who had a repaired esophageal atresia and tracheo-esophageal fistula with delayed anastomosis and who developed complete dysphagia. A total stricture at the anastomosis was documented and parenteral nutrition was started with placement of a feeding gastrostomy. Flexible esophagoscopy demonstrated a very small aperture of the stricture that would not allow any dilating instrument to pass. At that point, under general anesthesia, an endoscope was passed through the gastrostomy into the distal esophagus while esophagoscopy was performed. A sclerotherapy needle was passed through the membrane that had formed at the stricture to the distal esophagus under direct vision by the other endoscope. Biopsy forceps were used to open the stricture using the sclerotherapy needle as a guide. Balloon dilatation were then carried out. Over the ensuing months, both balloon dilatation and Tucker retrograde dilatation were performed. The stricture recurred, presumably secondary to reflux. The child eventually underwent an anti-reflux procedure without any recurrence of the stricture. This article makes the excellent point that further surgery of the esophagus should always be avoided even if unorthodox approaches are required. Stricturing at the anastomosis site is not always related to reflux. No mention was made of any medical attempt at treating the reflux prior to surgery. As a technical note, this is another example of the use of general anesthesia. In addition, neither the passage of an endoscope through a gastrostomy nor the navigation through the sharp angulation into the distal esophagus is easily accomplished.

On a different note, a study from Hong Kong on peptic ulcers in 39 children, admitted over a 6-year period [11•], reports that thirty-six of the children were diagnosed by flexible endoscopy, three being diagnosed at the time of surgery. Five children required surgery for complications, including two for obstruction, two for perforation and one for bleeding. Various medical details were given, but endoscopy repeated at 3 months documented total healing in 70% of cases, although 30% required three or more courses of H_2 antagonists. The first point made by Tsang *et al.* [11•], which has been previously expressed elsewhere, was that the seemingly increased incidence of ulcer disease in children is probably related to the improved diagnostic capability of endoscopy [12]. They also pointed out that they found a predominance of duodenal ulcers compared with other series.

A rather interesting study from Sweden [13••], on gastroesophageal reflux in infants, attempted to correlate endoscopically proven esophagitis with pH-proven reflux. A group of 141 consecutively referred infants, average age 7.3 months, were studied. They all had suspected reflux on the basis of 'digestive' or 'extra-digestive' symptoms, including respiratory near-sudden infant death syndrome apnea, and failure to thrive, and all underwent pH studies. Sixty had reflux on the basis of the pH studies, 52% of the digestive group and 24% of the extra-digestive group. One hundred and fifteen infants underwent endoscopy, in which 30% had mild histologic inflammation and only 8% had moderate or severe histologic esophagitis. Absolutely no correlation was found between the presence of esophagitis and pH proven reflux.

Use of colonoscopy

Holmquist *et al.* [14•], in a different area, reported on children with inflammatory bowel disease on the relation of clinical disease activity and colonoscopic assessment of mucosal inflammation. Thirty-six children with ulcerative colitis and 24 children with Crohn's colitis were included, none of whom had any small bowel involvement. Fifteen out of 20 patients with ulcerative colitis had none or questionable clinical activity yet still had moderate or severe endoscopic findings. Nineteen out of 20 patients of the same group had significant histologic inflammatory changes, despite the paucity of clinical symptoms. Of questionable interest were various other manipulations performed with the data, including reporting that 29% of their ulcerative colitis patients with moderate or severe inflammation of the proximal colon showed mild or non-existent changes in rectum. Fifty-six per cent of Crohn's colitis patients with moderate to severe proximal activity had minimal or no rectal findings, but it is unclear why this should be such a revelation. About 30% of these patients were on rectal steroids; this could also explain the findings. Their conclusion, which is not really innovative, suggests that a true correlation between colonoscopic findings and clinical disease does not exist. Moreover, rectal involvement is not always predictive of more proximal inflammation, especially in Crohn's disease.

The major question that remains is whether to treat colonoscopic and histologic inflammation if clinical symptoms do not warrant it. If one is to treat clinical symptoms alone, then the role of colonoscopy in children with inflammatory bowel disease should be drastically curtailed as dysplasia is not a major concern early on in the disease.

Conclusion

The last two studies [13••,14•] highlight one of the major dilemmas in pediatric endoscopy. Gastrointestinal disease in children differs from adults and as a rule does not involve malignancy. Correlation between endoscopic findings and clinical manifestations has been seen to be weak. The indications for endoscopy in children, an invasive and uncomfortable procedure, should clearly be reserved for those cases in which it will affect clinical management. As pediatric gastroenterology becomes a more defined subspeciality, these questions will be answered. It is to be hoped that next year's publications will deal more adequately with these issues.

Annotated references and recommended reading

Papers of special interest, published within the annual period of review, have been highlighted as:
• Of interest
•• Of outstanding interest

1. •• BUCKLEY A, CONNON JJ: **The Role of ERCP in Children and Adolescents.** *Gastrointest Endosc* 1990, 36:369–372.
Discussion of the role and technique of ERCP in pediatric patients, with the range of abnormalities encountered.

2. COTTON PB, LAAGE NJ: **ERCP in Children.** *Arch Dis Child* 1982, **52**:131–136.

3. ALLENDORPH M, WERLIN SL, GEENEN JE, HOGAN WJ, VENU RP, STEWART ET, BLANK EL: **ERCP in Children.** *J Pediatr* 1987, **110**:206–211.

4. BALISTRERI WF: **Neonatal Cholestasis: Medical Progress.** *J Pediatr* 1985, **106**:171–184.

5. ESQUIVEL CO, IWATSUKI S, GORDON RD, MARSH WW, KONERU B, MAKOWKA L, TZAKIS AG, TODO S, STARZL TE: **Indication for Pediatric Liver Transplantation.** *J Pediatr* 1987, **111**:1039–1045.

6. MAUER K, WAYE JD: **A New Pediatric Duodenoscope: Successful Cannulation Without a Cannula Elevator.** *Gastrointest Endosc* 1989, **35**:437–439.

7. • CROMBLEHOLME TM, DELORIMIER AA, ADZICK NS, LONGAKER MT, HARRISON MR, COX KL, HEYMAN MB: **Mediastinal Pancreatic Pseudocysts in Children.** *J Pediatr Surg* 1990, **25**:843–845.
The use of ERCP to demonstrate mediastinal pseudocysts thereby more effectively, facilitating subsequent surgery.

8. • CROMBLEHOLME TM, DELORIMIER AA, WAY LW, ADZICK NS, LONGAKER MT, HARRISON MR: **The Modified Puestow Procedure for Chronic Relapsing Pancreatitis in Children.** *J Pediatr Surg* 1990, **25**:749–753.
The use of ERCP to define ductal anomalies and decide on the necessary drainage procedures in chronic pancreatitis.

9. • RESCORLA FJ, CORY D, VANE DW, WEST KW, GROSFELD JL: **Failure of Percutaneous Drainage in Children with Traumatic Pancreatic Pseudocysts.** *J Pediatr Surg* 1990, **25**:1038–1042.
ERCP was shown to be useful in demonstrating traumatic breaks in the pancreatic duct that require drainage.

10. • BORGSTEIN ES, HUNTER DS, YOUNGSON GG: **Endoscopic Restoration of Esophageal Continuity.** *J Pediatr Surg* 1990, **25**:1222–1223.
Innovative use of endoscopy to prevent the need for re-exploration of an esophageal stricture after a prior repair for esophageal atresia.

11. • TSANG T-M, SAING H, YEUNG C-K: **Peptic Ulcer in Children.** *J Pediatric Surg* 1990, **25**:744–748.
One center's experience with endoscopically documented peptic ulcer disease in children.

12. CAULFIELD ME, WYLLIE R, SIVAK MV, MICHENER WM, STEFFEN RM: **Upper Gastrointestinal Tract Endoscopy in the Pediatric Patient.** *J Pediatr* 1989, **115**:339–345.

13. •• MASILIAH C, GALMICHE J-P, CLOAREC D, GERARD P, CZERNICHOW P, BRULEY DES VARANNES S: **Twenty-four Hour Oesophageal pH Monitoring in Infants with Suspected Gastro-Oesophageal Reflux Disease: Relationships with Symptoms, Endoscopy and Evolution.** *Eur J Gastroenterol Hepatol* 1990, 2:137–142.
Large study showing the poor correlation between pH probe-proven gastroesophageal reflux and histologic esophagitis.

14. • HOLMQUIST L, AHREN C, FALLSTROM SP: **Clinical Disease Activity and Inflammatory Activity in Relation to Mucosal Inflammation Assessed by Colonoscopy: a Study of Children and Adolescents with Chronic Inflammatory Bowel Disease.** *Acta Paediatr Scand* 1990, 79:527–534.
Straightforward analysis of experience using colonoscopy to assess clinical activity in inflammatory bowel disease.

Colonoscopy: polyps and cancer

C.B. Williams

Endoscopy Unit, St Mark's and St Bartholomew's Hospitals, London, UK

The goal of colorectal cancer prevention continues to motivate many reports of colonoscopic polypectomy, particularly at-risk subjects being those with multiple adenomas or a family history of multiple close relatives. Discovery of the relevant gene(s) will improve the efficacy of endoscopic surveillance by pre-identifying high-risk subjects. Careful endoscopy can reveal surprisingly small or flat malignancies and dye-contrast, endosonography and other techniques enhance the accuracy of endoscopic assessment.

Introduction

A massive quadrennial review [1••] on polypology from the endoscopist's point of view under the title 'Management of colorectal polyps: is all the effort worthwhile?' comes to the general conclusion that the results on first presentation are extremely worthwhile. However, there is a danger that, thereafter, lavishing excessive follow-up energy on post-polypectomy patients, who may mostly be at rather low lifetime risk of colorectal cancer after the initial examination, is largely a waste of time compared with the possibilities of identifying other at-risk patients and those at high lifetime risk. The problem is how to identify those at high long-term risk.

Large numbers of adenomas in an individual are known from previous studies to predict higher risk of cancer. This is borne out by patients from a large colonoscopy experience [2•] identified as having five or more polyps, a strikingly high percentage of whom had carcinomas at initial colonoscopy (eight out of 52 patients or 15%), mainly in the caecum. Six of these cancers occurred amongst 25 patients with five or more adenomas, and five were in the caecum; two cancers occurred in 27 patients with three adenomas and other hyperplastic polyps. The main implication of the paper is that the presence of multiple adenomas, regardless of size, should be taken as an indication for careful total colonoscopy.

The risk of cancer is known to be greater in older people, but the reason for this and the exact relationship with age is not understood. Ninety patients over 50 years of age with no known risk factors for colorectal cancer other than their age had stool occult blood tests, double-contrast barium enema (DCBE) and colonoscopy (83 total examinations) [3•]. Twenty-four per cent of the patients had adenomas (mean size 6 mm). No linear association was demonstrated with increasing age in the relatively small numbers studied. As also shown by other literature series, the prevalence of adenomas was double in men (27%) compared with that in women (14%).

A publication from the National Polyp Study in America [4••] gives further details of first-presentation characteristics of their patients with relation to dysplasia grade — and thus cancer risk. Adenomas in the distal colon (rectum, sigmoid and descending colon) were found to be twice as likely to contain severe dysplasia as those proximally, and were also larger, probably because of the (also unexplained) tendency for villous adenomas to occur distally, with characteristically larger size and higher grade of dysplasia. However, the fact that histopathological assessment of dysplasia can be shaky is demonstrated by a comparative histological slide review amongst community histopathologists of forceps biopsies of polyp specimens [5•]. Biopsies from five hyperplastic and five adenomatous polyps were reviewed by 22 pathologists with good agreement on which lesions were neoplastic or not, but considerable disagreement on the degree of dysplasia (atypia) present.

The disputed question of the relevance of hyperplastic polyps to colorectal cancer risk is further muddied by a histopathological description of 110 polyps with dysplastic cells but 'serrated' architecture intermediate between adenomas and hyperplastic polyps (and different from others containing 'mixed' well-defined foci of adenomatous and hyperplastic tissue) [6•]. The fact that only 110 such polyps intermediate between hyperplastic and adenomatous could be found in a review of pathology reports of 18 000 polyps of all types suggests that they are an adenoma variant (the authors describe them as serrated adenomas) that have curiosity value rather than much endoscopic significance (Fig. 1).

A formal Working Group statement from the European Congress in Rome [7•] summarizes the orthodox position on classification and management of adenomas, with particular reference to the correct use of nomenclature and acceptable histological criteria.

Screening or 'case finding': the place of sigmoidoscopy and colonoscopy

A general review of colorectal cancer screening methods, [8], primarily by occult blood testing, notes that flexible sigmoidoscopy could become a viable screening modal-

© Current Science Ltd ISBN 1-870485-32-7 ISSN 0952-6293

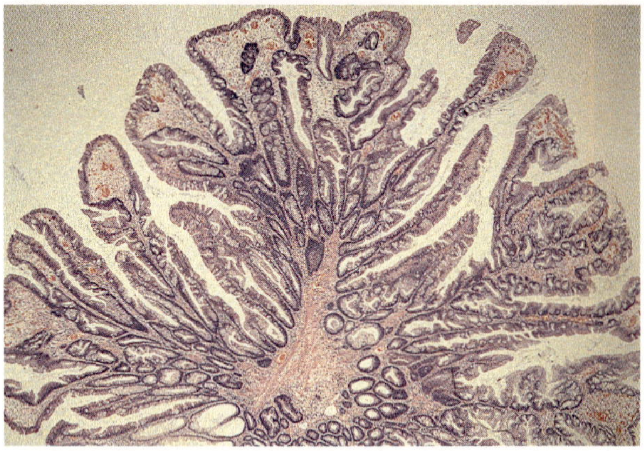

Fig. 1. A 'serrated adenoma' showing histology intermediate between a hyperplastic polyp and an adenoma.By courtesy of I.C Talbot, Pathology Department, St Mark's Hospital, London, UK.

ity if performed by non-medical personnel to reduce the cost, whereas colonoscopy is precluded by its excessive cost, complexity and complication rate. The possibility of achieving up to 45% population compliance to screening flexible sigmoidoscopy is suggested by a careful interview study [9•] of Australian city residents (another 30% of the sample would not even agree to interview). Younger people and those with previous episodes of bleeding were shown by the interview to be more likely to comply, but those with previous experience of sigmoidoscopy were less likely to agree to future repeat examinations — once bitten, twice shy? The use of flexible sigmoidoscopies on 329 asymptomatic patients of 50 years or over yielded evidence of 8% adenomas (size not stated) on first examination, compared with 4% on second and 2% on third examination [10•]. Over half of the small numbers of those with adenomas submitted to total colonoscopy had further adenomas proximally. Perversely, although three pathologists reviewed the histology and classified adenomas by histological subtype (tubular, tubulovillous and villous) and degree of dysplasia (mild, moderate, severe), the authors then fell into the common trap of considering 'dysplasia' as a significant finding, whereas all adenomas show dysplasia by definition. In another portentous, but uncritical, paper endoscopies of uncertain extent were performed on hospital surgical in-patients with a range of indications, yielding evidence of many 'polyps' of uncertain size and 51 cancers [11•]. A single occult blood test, routinely performed before colonoscopy, was negative in 40% of the cancers. On this basis the authors state that 'it is reasonable to make colonoscopy the screening test of choice for colorectal neoplasms' — which is offensively simplistic considering the complexity of the issue and the inadequacy of their data.

Other authors [12••] provocatively calculate that more than half the adenomas detected by occult blood screening may actually be non-bleeding and simply a 'lucky hit'. As a result, they question the need for 'aggressive surveillance' of such patients by colonoscopy thereafter, since they mostly have small adenomas and may therefore not be at high risk, especially because more than half the adenoma-forming population originally surveyed remain unidentified but at risk. An editorial accompanying the article [13•] comments on 'the swing away from the widespread and largely uncritical enthusiasm for colorectal screening', and adds that 'there is good reason for scepticism about the widespread practice of colonoscopic surveillance every 1–3 years in people found to have small adenomas'. A more upbeat attitude [14•] to strategies for management of patients with positive occult blood results or adenoma(s) (possibly hyperplastic polyps, too) found on sigmoidoscopy commends total colonoscopy — but makes no mention of follow-up thereafter. The author hopes that 'ongoing studies' will show whether reduction in colorectal cancer mortality results.

Endoscopy enthusiasts have a tendency to forget some of the less palatable truths about the limitations of colonoscopy (technical difficulty in whole colon examination, 20 times greater complication rate and 10 times greater mortality than DCBE, as well as greater cost, especially in the USA), all of which are strongly emphasized in a radiological conference summary [15•]. Effectively, barium enema takes a midway position between occult blood testing (cheap, safe but relatively inaccurate except for mass-screening purposes) and colonoscopy (which is the gold standard but at a certain cost). The implication for the endoscopist is that professionalism and technical improvements are needed to increase safety and success rates, whilst market forces will inevitably slowly reduce costs. Costs of endoscopy are primarily related to professional charges, the actual institutional and instrumentation costs being only marginally higher than those of barium enema [British Society of Gastroenterology Report: Provision of Gastrointestinal Endoscopy and Related Services,(*Gut* 1991 32:95-105); full version available from BSG, 4 St Andrew's Place, Regent's Park, London NW1].

A slightly heavy Norwegian analysis [16•] of the indications for 1000 colonoscopies, as compared with the endoscopist's prediction of the likely 'benefit' of the examination and the actual endoscopic findings (50% of examinations showed 'clinically significant abnormality'), concludes that bleeding and first examination of cancer patients were the two most significant clinical indications for colonoscopy.

Surveillance of patients with polyps or cancer

The Working Group statement for the Rome European Congress [7•] also admits that practical guidelines on follow-up examinations cannot be formalized until the results of large prospective studies become available. Many literature series agree that an initial colonoscopy in cancer patients is exceedingly worthwhile. A review of the methodology available for cancer patients [17•] suggests that the prime function of colonoscopy is only to diagnose other colonic neoplasms, whereas CEA, ultrasound and clinical assessment are the best methods of diagnosing extra-colonic recurrence, which is much more common than anastomotic recurrence. An Italian series [18•] using colonoscopy and DCBE in 89 patients revealed synchronous carcinoma in 4%, often at an early stage, only half the cancers being shown by the barium enema. Preoperative colonoscopy is strongly recommended by the authors, although in over 25% of their patients it was impossible or impracticable, making postoperative colonoscopy necessary.

The fear has been expressed that the trauma of preoperative colonoscopy might cause spread or seeding of cancer cells. In a comparison of operation findings, recurrence rates and clinical follow-up of two groups of cancer patients respectively endoscoped or not [19•], those endoscoped actually fared better. The pickup of symptomless cancers in 4–7% and adenomas in 30–60%, with modification of surgical procedure in 11–13% of literature series, argues strongly for routine initial colonoscopy in cancer patients. Thereafter, there is a danger of grossly overdoing the frequency of surveillance of cancer patients, with uncertain long-term benefit. One hundred and seventy-four colorectal cancer patients followed postoperatively 'for at least one year', and then by barium enema or colonoscopy 'annually but at different time periods' shows that long-term follow-up can yield a few resectable true metachronous cancers (four in the series), and 3–5% per year of significant-sized polyps; it does not, however, prove that annual colonoscopy is needed — as the accompanying critical comments point out [18].

A study of 100 patients having follow-up colonoscopy 1 year after removal of an adenoma [20•] showed that those who initially had multiple polyps were more likely to have a further adenoma at 1 year. Sixty per cent of follow-up adenomas were in the proximal colon, 90% being under 1 cm and so thought to be new, although the remainder were larger and probably missed initially — justifying 1-year examination in all adenoma patients in the opinion of the authors.

Identifying high-risk genetic factors

The known risk of multiple colonic adenomas with increased cancer risk has been mentioned earlier [2], the classic expression of this being in familial adenomatous polyposis (FAP). However, genetic factors are thought to contribute to the pathogenesis of about 10% of non-polyposis cases of colorectal cancer. The genetic mechanisms are predicted to be worked out in the next 5–10 years, with enormous implications for the endoscopist, who will then be presented with only those patients known to be genetically susceptible. A remarkable marker study illustrating this comes from Salt Lake City [21••], where endoscopy of 51 members of a colorectal cancer family was combined with genotype analysis and genetic linkage studies. Only two members of the family showed adenomatous polyposis, whereas other members had between two and 40 adenomas, but all showed a defect near the characteristic site for FAP on chromosome 5. As so often happens in science, it looks likely that the position about inheritance of adenoma/colorectal cancer risk will become more, rather than less, complicated with greater knowledge. Clearly, there is a possibility for different genetic defects that will result in such intermediate clinical situations between FAP as currently recognized and the bearers of a few 'sporadic' adenomas. Lynch's group [22] suggest that the occurrence of multiple small adenomas (especially if flat) in the proximal colon of patients under 40 years of age should warn of the possibility of hereditary cancer syndrome, indicating the need to take a careful genetic history in other family members, including those with cancers contributing to 'Lynch II' family cancer syndromes: breast, skin, female genital cancer and possibly also pancreatic, small bowel and stomach cancer. They further report that 30% of 44 colorectal cancer family members (mean age 42 years) submitted to colonoscopy had one or more adenomas, of which 18% were proximal to the splenic flexure [23•]. These results were three to four times higher than those in an age-matched control group and double those of other literature series — although the authors admit that their results are skewed by the findings in members of a single multiple-adenoma family.

Too many of the endoscopic series appearing are essentially uncritical and often retrospective, do not have proper genetic input, and include patients with selection bias because of bleeding or symptoms that cause them to become anxious and then to present for 'genetic screening', supposedly because of a known relative with polyps or cancer. One such retrospective review [24•] identified 475 patients colonoscoped 'with the indication that a first or second degree relative had polyps or cancer', yielding neoplasms in 72 (15%). Of these 34 (47%) were malignant (an oddly high yield), one-third of the malignancies being proximal to the splenic flexure. However, another retrospective review [25•] identified 125 patients undergoing total colonoscopy because of family history of colorectal cancer (no details given), with the finding of adenomas in 12%, only 5% above the reach of the flexible sigmoidoscope. This yield is more in line with other series suggesting that colonoscopy is not a particularly worthwhile exercise when only a single first-degree relative is involved. In our own series [26•] patients were selected for colonoscopy on the basis of empiric genetic risk assessment suggesting lifetime cancer risk of 10% or more. The worthwhile results obtained included diagnosis of FAP in two, cancers in five and adenomas in 62 out of 380 patients colonoscoped, although these findings too may have been biased by unrecognized patient self-selection factors. Another Canadian series [27•] found 108 patients, with mainly one or more first-degree relative involved, to have 21% neoplasms including two cancers, 25% of polyps being in the proximal colon. The authors support the principle of colonoscopy even with a single first-degree relative and suggest that screening should ideally start after the age of 40 years but, if negative, follow-up need be at only 3–5 yearly intervals thereafter.

Flat adenomas and 'early' cancers

Japanese authors have a valuable role in emphasizing the importance of fastidious endoscopic and radiological technique to achieve early diagnosis; most self-critical endoscopists readily acknowledge that, through poor bowel preparation and technical limitations of some procedures, it is possible to miss a small percentage of even raised lesions. Seven 'depressed adenomas' less than 3 mm diameter were noted in 1000 Japanese colonoscopies [28•], the dysplastic lesion being in the reddened and roughened central area of the tiny mucosal 'doughnut' ring, more easily seen on deflation of the colon. An Australian series [29•] reported three patients with multiple neoplasms who also had a 6–8 mm flat cancer without residual adenoma, visible to the endoscopist as small plaques with a reddened and/or depressed central area. From another Japanese series of 52 'early colorectal cancers' [30•], including sessile malignant polyps, details were given of eight small, flat ulcer cancers managed surgically (two with lymph nodes), of which six were less than 2 cm and three less than 1 cm in diameter. A further detailed account [31•] of a Japanese experience of 96 'early' invasive carcinomas, and others with focal dysplasia (16 pedunculated/semi-pedunculated, the rest sessile) concludes that surgical management is required for sessile malignant polyps, regardless of apparent completeness of endoscopic excision, because of the lymph-node involvement in 12.5% of their operated cases. The authors unfortunately give insufficient histological data to substantiate this fully.

In spite of Shinya's vast overall experience of colonoscopy and polypectomy, it is a criticism of the realities of American private practice that inadequacies of record-keeping, follow-up and histopathological criteria prevent any analysis of 104 patients [32•] with malignant polyps followed for a mean of 5 years. If anything, the article succeeds only in confusing matters, not least by recommending routine surgery for all polypoid carcinomas, a policy which is not rational providing that such lesions are pedunculated and conform to the accepted criteria for completeness of excision (including poor or moderately-well differentiated tumour, absence of lymphatic invasion and especially 2–3 mm or more margin between invasion and line of endoscopic excision). In contrast, a well-documented Israeli series [33•] of only 58 patients with 66 malignant polyps (mean 4.4 years follow-up), in which all pedunculated polyps had uncomplicated follow-up or no residual cancer if submitted to surgery, convincingly supports the criteria for conservative management of pedunculated polyps. However, the study advises operation on sessile malignant lesions — nine out of 11 such patients in their series submitted to surgery proving to have Duke's B or C staging.

Improved diagnosis: technical means

Experimental studies in the past, including radioisotope uptake with autoradiography, have shown that even normal-looking mucosa of neoplasm-bearing subjects can be shown to be cytologically abnormal on appropriate testing. A relatively simple immunohistochemical staining technique, using a monoclonal antibody to a nucleic acid analogue marker (bromodeoxyuridine) rapidly taken up by biopsy tissue from tissue culture medium, shows the mucosa of adenoma patients to demonstrate abnormal extension of proliferative cells towards the epithelial surface compared with controls [34•]. This technique, known as 'Brdu labelling', a simpler alternative to radio-thymidine uptake, is crude compared with the future potential for DNA probe studies but nonetheless of current interest. Another 'fashionable' assay assesses ornithine decarboxylase enzyme activity, which has been suggested to be greater than normal in the mucosa of patients with benign or malignant neoplasms. However, in a study [35•] of groups of normal subjects (haemorrhoidal bleeding) and others with family history of colorectal cancer, current adenomatous polyps or previously excised colorectal cancer, biopsies from the sigmoid colon showed no difference in levels of ornithine decarboxylase activity between these groups during check total colonoscopy. Discrimination between adenomatous and normal (or hyperplastic) tissue was possible with 94% predictive value using a dye-spray laser light transmitted down a contact quartz fibre, which induced sufficient difference in autofluorescence measurements at the appropriate wavelength [36•].

The 10–20 times magnification obtained with newer-generation videoendoscopes is comparable to that obtained with dissecting microscopes, and raises the possibility that surface staining or colour dye-contrast techniques might also be used to enhance visualization of the mucosal surface in high-risk patients (for instance looking for flat adenomas) or to attempt discrimination between small adenomas and hyperplastic polyps (eliminating the small risk of delayed haemorrhage by unnecessary electrocoagulation of non-neoplastic polyps). Dye-contrast of the mucosal surface (in contradistinction to mucosal staining techniques such as methylene blue, which also colours mucus) can be obtained with an 0.1% solution of indigocarmine. The use of such a non-staining dye has the added advantage that it does not permanently discolour clothing and can be relatively easily washed off hands and so on. A convenient way of obtaining repeated local dye-contrast coloration is by the 'bolus' technique illustrated in Figure 2: the preferred method in instruments having a syringe attachment is to inject the 2 cm^3 bolus into the water system of the instrument, thus avoiding the risk of messy leakage; the alternative method injects the bolus through the instrument channel. In either case the admixture of a small amount of silicone anti-foaming agent reduces surface tension and prevents persistence of air bubbles in the dye contrast. Examples of the results obtained are shown in Figure 3. 'Dye-contrast' seems a preferable term to 'dye-spray' because catheter spray is not essential, the blue dye coating of the mucosa being an endoscopic colour-contrast technique analogous to the radiologists' use of barium-contrast coating.

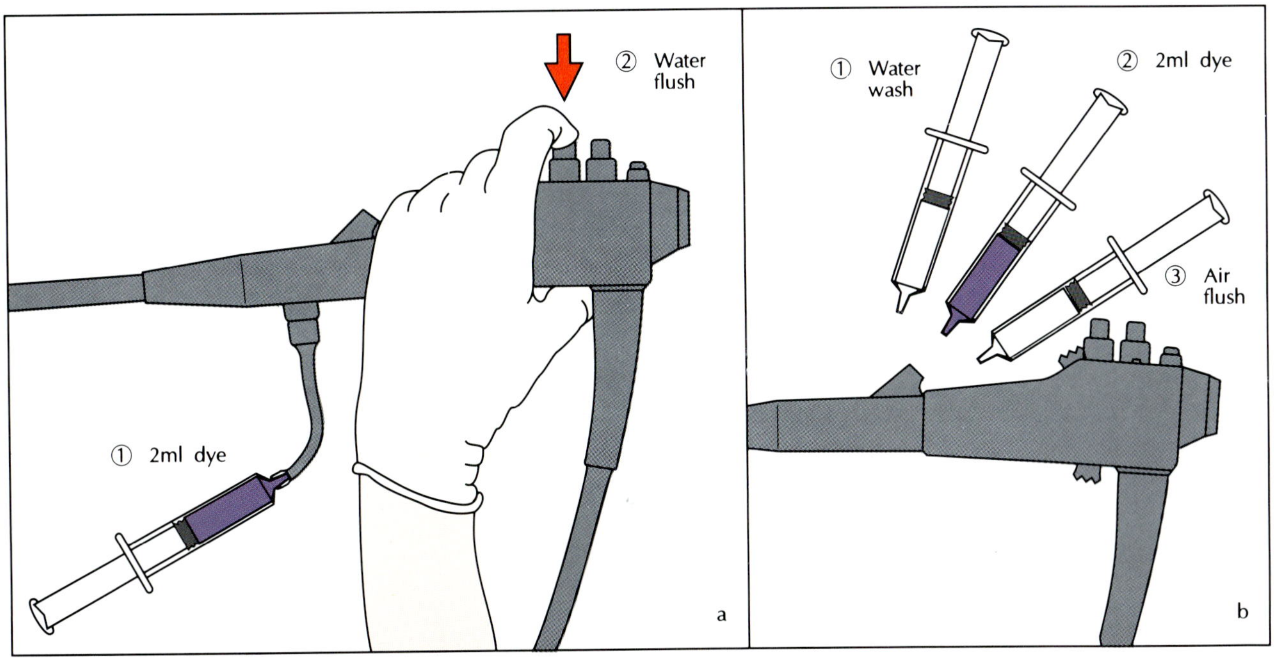

Fig. 2. Bolus dye-contrast techniques (with 1% indigo-carmine): (a) preferred method; using colonoscope washing syringe ;(b) alternative method: through suction/instrumentation channel (more likely to cause spillage)

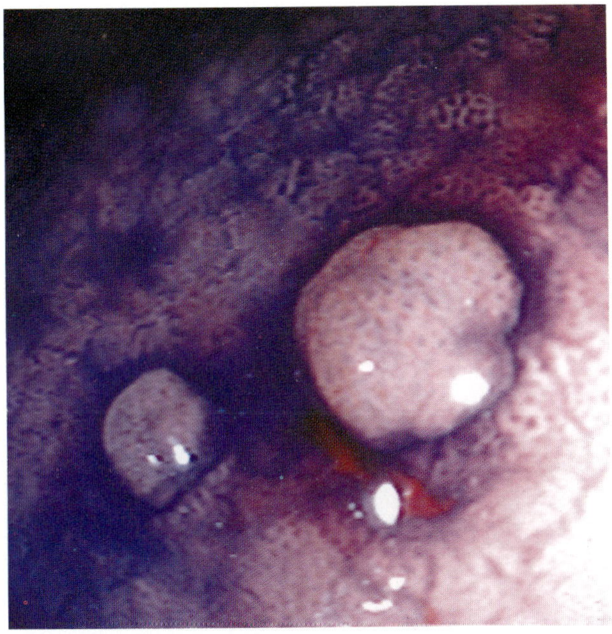

Fig. 3. 1–2 mm tubular adenomas with surface detail shown up by dye-contrast.

Endosonography and scintigraphy in assessment of malignancy

A clear review for the non-initiate of the usefulness of rectal ultrasound in assessing the presence or absence of invasion, recurrence or involved lymph nodes (as dark hyperechoic appearances) estimates that the technique affects management in 30% of rectal cancer patients [37••]. The Munich group [38•] shows that the forward-viewing ultrasound colonoscope, with its inbuilt rotating scanner, can be used for total colonoscopy in spite of its 4 cm rigid tip section. Preliminary experience by this group [39•] (seven large sessile adenomas and 25 carcinomas), with a literature review, suggested that the technique should be rather accurate in differentiating benign from malignant lesions, and probably more accurate than computed tomography in diagnosing early recurrence. However, distant lymph nodes will not be seen and granulation or scar tissue are likely to give false-positive findings in operated subjects. The description of the first commercial prototype of an ultrasound probe for use down the channel of standard colonoscopes [40•] emphasizes that such miniaturized devices (with a 20 MHz transducer) reach only 7 mm through normal tissue and less in fibrous malignant tissue, so significantly limiting usefulness except in extremely flat lesions.

Another approach in the rectum [41•] has used gamma-camera scintigraphy after submucosal injection of 0.1 cm^3 technetium sulfacolloid. This was 76% accurate in predicting presence or absence of lymph node involvement in patients with cancer. The technique is based on the principle that an uninvolved lymph node takes up the technetium whereas an involved one does not. Even in the rectum, with a predictable pattern of lymph-node drainage in 50% of control subjects, interpretation was frequently difficult; it seems likely that application will be more difficult still in excluding early invasive disease in lesions of the proximal colon, which are those of prime interest to endoscopists. Even so, the possibility of injecting marker or contrast material endoscopically to provide specific enhancement for scanning techniques may have great future potential.

Laser and other methods of cancer palliation

In an impressive summary of a French laser experience [42••], mainly with neodymium-YAG palliation of 170 advanced cancer patients, laser coagulation relieved symptoms in 89% of subjects by a mean of 15 days and with 2.5 treatments, the effect lasting over 40 months. Low-power laser coagulation was used (rather than vaporization), resulting in complications in only 3% of patients. The neodymium-YAG laser was used in a heterogeneous group of tumour patients [43•], most on an out-patient basis and requiring an average of 2.75 treatments (three having more than 18), each treatment lasting 45 min. The long-term cost of laser therapy was calculated to be two-thirds that of surgery, although poor-risk patients were spared operation. Use of photosensitizing agents to enhance the effectiveness of laser treatment is an attractive concept, although the haematoporphyrin photodynamic sensitizers currently available are not ideal. Sixteen inoperable cancers of the rectosigmoid were included in an uncontrolled study [44•] of photodynamic therapy in gastrointestinal cancers. The procedure resulted overall in a 22% major complication rate (mainly dilatable stenosis) but gave promising results in terms of tumour regression and negative histology.

Most laser groups attempt prior debulking, normally using an electrosurgical snare, so as to speed up the procedure. In the rectum it is possible to use an aggressive transanal resectoscope approach alone, under 1.5% glycine solution as would be used in the prostatic bed [45•]. Eighty-one patients with benign or malignant rectal lesions managed in this way had a 5% procedure-related mortality and 15% major complication rate, the claimed advantages over laser being cheapness and speed, although the procedure required general anaesthesia. An alternative, even cheaper and less scary, flexible endoscope technique is the use of injected sclerotherapy solution (polidocanol 3%) [46•]. Five inoperable rectal cancer patients, three with impending obstruction, were relieved of symptoms by multiple injections using an 8 mm needle and 15–20 ml solution per session, repeated every few months according to survival. The disadvantage in obstructing patients is that the time taken to local tissue necrosis is up to 48 hours.

Polypoid lesions

Lipomas, or fatty lipomatous enlargements of the ileocaecal valve region, are a not-uncommon chance finding during endoscopy (or contrast radiology) (Fig. 4). In most cases the lipoma has no clinical relevance and should be left alone, although larger lesions can be the cause of intussusception, and surface ulceration (presumably ischaemic) resulting in blood loss has been described. A retrospective review [47•] of a rather disastrous experience of endoscopic management of large lipomas reported major perforation in three out of five lipomas snared. The complications occurred in those 3–5 cm in diameter and broad-based, the authors reasonably concluding that surgery is the procedure of choice for any lipoma over 2 cm in diameter that merits removal clinically. On the other hand, case reports of a lipoma and a lymphangioma [48], both pedunculated and prolapsing through the ileo-caecal valve, resulted in safe and easy removal by snare polypectomy, avoiding the risk of subsequent intussusception. An editorial by Christie [49] discusses these papers, pointing out the technical difficulty in electrocutting lipomatous tissue because of the poor electrical conductivity of fatty tissue, and the 'risky business' of attempting endoscopic transection of sessile lipomas; perhaps needle-knife mucosectomy or use of the laser could also have a place?

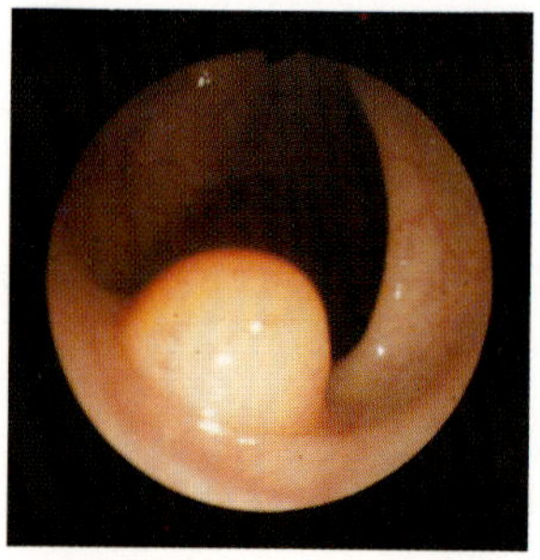

Fig. 4. Lipoma in the ascending colon— a typical rounded shiny-surfaced lesion. There is rarely any indication for snaring.(See also Waye p 151).

Most endoscopists have experience of occasional referral of patients with a known or suspected diagnosis of endometriosis, most commonly because of recurrent bleeding (and, by the vagaries of human nature, usually presenting for the examination at an inappropriate moment in the menstrual cycle). In a clinical review [50] of the characteristics of nine patients with the much rarer presentation of endometriosis causing obstructive symptoms, the endoscopy performed in five patients contributed nothing — showing only an extraluminal mass and yielding normal mucosa on biopsy. The authors conclude that surgery is always needed in obstructing endometriosis, because the deformity is due to unalterable fibrosis and the alternative diagnosis of carcinoma must be absolutely excluded.

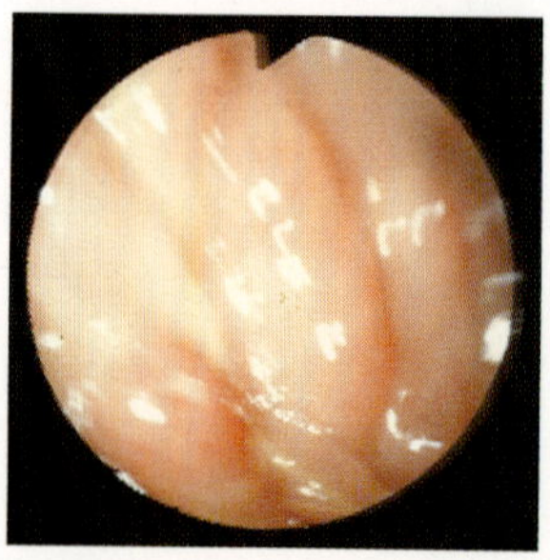

Fig. 5. Small polypoid colonic mucosal elevations in disseminated lymphomatosis. Lymphomatous polys tend to show 'umbilication' with a dimpled apex (see also Schuman p 26).

A case report [51] describes carpeting of the colon with polyps up to 1.5 cm diameter in a patient with 'lymphosarcoma cell leukaemia' (poorly differentiated lymphocytic lymphoma), also involving the upper gastrointestinal tract, bone marrow and prostate, with generalized lymphadenopathy. The endoscopic characteristic of disseminated lymphomatous polyposis is that the mucosal nodules are dimpled or umbilicated on their apex, but it is also characteristic that both ends of the gastrointestinal tract are involved; 'top and tail' endoscopy and a few biopsies make the diagnosis (Fig. 5).

Three cases are reported of obscure mass lesions seen endoscopically but eventually managed surgically. A bleeding ulcerated polypoid mass at the splenic flexure in a 30-year-old man proved to be composed of displaced gastric mucosal and pancreatic tissue [52•]. A semi-necrotic intussuscepting tumour at the splenic flexure was a leiomyosarcoma (there are apparently only 45 in the world literature) [53•]. An ulcerated blue-red dome-like lesion compressing the sigmoid colon of a 16-year-old was the fourth literature case of an angiosarcoma involving the colon [54•].

Conclusion

It is remarkable that complications are now so rarely reported considering the enormous numbers of therapeutic colonoscopy procedures, suggesting that the techniques are 'mature'. On the other hand, there is a dearth of large, well-organized prospective studies giving conclusive evidence on efficacy of colonoscopic surveillance work in cancer prevention; cancers rarely occur in the patients examined, but,are so many examinations needed? At the individual patient level it is warming to know that new techniques such as trans-channel endosonography, scintigraphy, gene-probes and histochemical techniques are evolving to support the efforts of the endoscopist.

References and recommended reading

Papers of special interest, published within the annual period of review, have been highlighted as:
- • Of interest
- •• Of outstanding interest

1. WILLIAMS CB, BEDENNE L: **Quadrennial Review: Management •• of Colonic Polyps — is all The Effort Worthwhile?** *Gastronterol Hepatol* 1990, **5**:144–165.

A massive (160 reference) review of the 1980/90 polypology literature concludes that results on initial presentation polypectomy is well worth it although excessively frequent long-term follow-up may not be.

2. SCHUMAN BM, SIMSEK H, LYONS RC: **The Association of Multi- • ple Colonic Adenomatous Polyps with Cancer of the Colon.** *Am J Gastroenterol* 1990, **85**:846–849.

Fifty-two patients with five or more polyps (identified retrospectively) showed a high percentage of carcinomas, mainly in the caecum.

3. JOHNSON DA, GURNEY MS, VOLPE RJ, JONES DM, VANNESS MM, • CHOBANIAN SJ, AVALOS JC, BUCK JL, KOOYMAN G, CATTAU EL A **Prospective Study of the Prevalence of Colonic Neoplasms in Asymptomatic Patients with an Age-related Risk.** *Am J Gastroenterol* 1990, **85**:969–974.

Ninty patients over 50 years of age without risk factors with colorectal cancer had occult blood testing, DCBE and colonoscopy; 24% had adenomas (mean size 6 mm) with double prevalence in men but no direct association with increasing age.

4. O'BRIEN MJ, WINAWER SJ, ZAUBER AG, GOTTLIEB LS, STERNBERG •• SS, DIAZ B, DICKERSIN GR, EWING S, GELLER S, KASIMIAN D, KOMOROWSKI R, SZORN A: **The National Polyps Study: Patients and Polyp Characteristics Associated with High-grade Dysplasia in Colorectal Adenomas.** *Gastroenterology* 1990, **98**:371–379.

Adenomas in the distal colon (R & S & D) twice as likely to contain severe dysplasia and were larger (because large and villous adenomas occurred there and tended to show high-grade dysplasia).

5. DEMERS RY, NEALE AV, BUDEV H, SCHADE WJ: **Pathologist • Agreement in the Interpretation of Colorectal Polyps.** *Am J Gastronterol* 1990, **85**:417–421.

Review by 22 community pathologists of forceps biopsies from five hyperplastic and five adenomatous polyps gave good agreement as to which were neoplastic, but considerable disagreement on the degree of atypia/dysplasia present.

6. LONGACRE TA, FENOGLIO-PREISER CM: **Mixed Hyperplastic Ade- • nomatous Polyps/Serrated Adenomas. A Distinct form of Colorectal Neoplasia.** *Am J Surg Pathol* 1990, 14:524–537.

A histopathological description of 110 polyps with dysplastic cells but serrated architecture intermediate between adenomas and hyperplastic polyps (and different from others containing 'mixed' foci of adenomatous and hyperplastic tissue).

7. MORSON BC, WILLIAMS CB, FRUHMORGEN P, GRIGIONI W, • KRONBORG O, ATKIN W, WINAWER SJ: **Colorectal Adenomas: Risk of Cancer and Results of Follow-up (Working Team Report — Rome European Congress).** *Gastroenterol Internat* 1990, 3:57–62.

A formal Working Group statement from the 1988 Rome European Congress on the classification and management of adenomas.

8. HARDCASTLE JD, THOMAS WM: **Screening an Asymptomatic • Population for Colorectal Cancer.** *Balliere's Clinical Gastroenterology* 1989, 3:543–566.

A review of colorectal cancer screening methods, principally occult blood mentions flexible sigmoidoscopy as a possible screening modality if performed by non-medial personnel whereas colonoscopy is precluded by cost, complexity and complication rate.

9. AGREZ MV, REDMAN S, SANSON-FISHER R, HENNRIKUS D: **Feasi- • bility of Sigmoidoscopic Screening for Colorectal Cancer in the Hunter Region.** *Dis Colon Rectum* 1990, 33:87–92.

Forty-five per cent possible compliance to screening flexible sigmoidoscopy is suggested by a careful interview study of Australian city residents (30% of the sample would not agree even to interview).

10. RIFF ER, DEHAAN K, GAREWAL GS: **The Role of Sigmoidoscopy • for Asymptomatic Patients. Results of Three Annual Screening Sigmoidoscope, Polypectomy, and Subsequent Surveillance Colonoscopy in a Primary Care Setting.** *Clevel Clin J Med* 1990, **57**:131–136.

Flexible sigmoidoscopies on 329 asymptomatic patients of 50 years or over yielded 8% adenomas on first examination, 4% on second and 2% on a third. Over half of those submitted to colonoscopy had adenomas proximally.

11. REILLY JM, BALLANTYNE GH, FLEMING FX, ZUCKER KA, MODLIN • IM: **Evaluation of the Occult Blood Test in Screening for Colorectal Neoplasms. A Prospective Study Using Flexible Endoscopy.** *Am Surg* 1990, **56**:119–123.

An uncritical study on hospital surgical in-patients yielded many 'polyps' of uncertain size and 51 cancers; a single occult blood test, routinely performed, was negative in 40% of the cancer patients.

12. RANSOHOFF DF, LANG CA: **Small Adenomas Detected During •• Decal Occult Blood Test Screening for Colorectal Cancer. The Impact of Serendipity.** *JAMA* 1990, **264**:76–78.

Provocative paper calculating that over half the adenomas detected on occult blood screening are likely to be non-bleeding and a 'lucky hit', not necessarily justifying subsequent surveillance when any of the not-so-lucky at-risk patients remain unidentified. A counterblast against polyp-hunting hysteria.

13. SIMON JB: **Colonic Polyps, Occult Blood, and Chance.** *JAMA* • 1990, **264**:84–85.

An editorial accompanying Ransohoff and Lang 1990 [12] comments on the'swing away from... uncritical enthusiasm for colorectal screening' and adds that 'there is good reason for scepticism about the widespread practice of colonoscopic surveillance every 1–3 years in people found to have small adenomas' (by chance).

14. LIEBERMAN DA: **Colon Cancer Screening: The Dilemma of**
• **Positive Screening Tests.** *Arch Intern Med* 1990, **150**:740–744.
A commentary on strategies for management of patients with positive occult blood results or adenomas (possibly hyperplastic polyps too) on sigmoidoscopy recommends total colonoscopy and admits that there is no proof that colorectal cancer mortality is reduced as a result.

15. WHALEN E: **Colon Cancer — Diagnosis in an Era of Cost**
• **Containment — ACR Conference, November 8, 1989.** *Am J Roentgenol* 1990, **154**:875–881.
Summary of a radiological conference emphasizing the limitations of colonoscopy (technical difficulty) in whole examination, 20 times complication rate and 10 times mortality of DCBE as well as greater cost. Some of the points made are very reasonable, but some bigoted.

16. BRENNA E, SKREDEN K, WALDUM HL, MARVIK R, DYBDAHL
• JH, KLEVELAND PM, SANDVIK AK, HALVORSEN T, MYRVOLD HE, PETERSEN H: **The Benefit of Colonoscopy.** *Scand J Gastroenterol* 1990, **25**:81–88.
Analysis of the indications for 1000 colonoscopies, compared with the endoscopist's prediction of likely 'benefit' of examination and eventual findings (50% had 'clinically significant abnormality'), concludes that bleeding and first examination of cancer patients were the two most significant clinical indications.

17. FANTINI GA, DECOSSE JJ: **Surveillance Strategies after Resec-**
• **tion of Carcinoma of the Colon and Rectum.** *Surg Gynecol Obstet* 1990, **171**:267–273.
A review of the methodology available for cancer patients suggests colonoscopy to diagnose other colon neoplasms but using CEA, ultrasound and clinical assessment to diagnose extracolonic recurrence subsequently

18. JUHL G, LARSON GM, MULLINS R, BOND S, ROLK HC: **Six-year**
• **Results of Annual Colonoscopy After Resection of Colorectal Cancer.** *World J Surg* 1990, **14**:255–261.
One-hundred and seventy-four colorectal cancer patients followed postoperatively 'for at least one year' and then at different time periods shows that longterm follow-up yields metachronous cancers (four) and 3–5% per year of significant-sized polyps. It does not prove the authors suggestion that annual colonoscopy is needed — as the accompanying comments point out.

19. HOWARD ML, GREENE PL: **The Effect of Preoperative En-**
• **doscopy on Recurrence and Survival Following Surgery for Colorectal Carcinoma.** *Am Surg* 1990, **56**:124–127.
New evidence that the trauma of preoperative colonoscopy causes spread or seeding of cancer cells in a comparison of operation findings, recurrence rates or clinical follow-up of 239 cancer patients endoscoped or not endoscoped (those endoscoped actually fared better).

20. WOOLFSON IK, ECKHOLDT GJ, WETZEL CR, GATHRIGHT JB, RAY
• JE, HICKS TC, TIMMCKE AE, FERRARI BT: **Usefulness of Performing Colonoscopy One Year After Endoscopic Polypectomy.** *Dis Colon Rectum* 1990, **33**:389–393.
A study of 100 patients having follow-up colonoscopy 1 year after removal of an adenoma shows those with multiple polyps initially to be more likely to have a further adenoma at 1 year. Sixty per cent of follow-up adenomas were in the proximal colon, 90% under 1 cm and so thought to be new, although 12/109 (11%) were larger and probably 'missed' initially.

21. LEPPERT M, BURT B, HUGHES JP, SAMOWITZ W, NAKAMURA Y,
•• WOODWARD S, GARDNER E, LALOUEL JM, WHITE R: **Genetic Analysis of an Inherited Predisposition to Colon Cancer in a Family with a Variable Number of Adenomatous Polyps.** *N Engl J Med* 1990, **322**:904–908.
A Utah family of 81 members studied by endoscopy and, genotype characterization and genetic analysis demonstrates the chromosome 5 defect but adenomatous polyposis in only two members with 40 adenomas in eight others — showing that the 'all or none' concept of FAP is wrong.

22. LANSPA SJ, SMYRK TC, LYNCH HT: **The Colonoscopist and the Lynch Syndromes.** *Gastrointest Endosc* 1990, **36**:156–158.
Editorial by Lynch's group suggests that multiple small adenomas (especially if flat) in the proximal colon of patients under 40 should warn of the possibility of a hereditary cancer syndrome.

23. LANSPA SJ, LYNCH HT, SMYRK TC, STRAYHORN P, WATSON P,
• LYNCH JF, JENKINS JX, APPELMAN HD: **Colorectal Adenomas in the Lynch Syndromes. Results of a Colonoscopy Screening Program.** *Gastroenterology* 1990, **98**:1117–1122.
Thirty per cent of 44 colorectal cancer family members (mean age 42 years) submitted to total colonoscopy had adenomas, 20% had more than one adenoma and in 18% adenomas were proximal to the splenic flexure. These results were 3–4 times higher than an age-matched control group and double that of other literature series (but perhaps skewed due to results from one particular multiple-polyp family).

24. SARDELLA W, ROSEN L, SHEETS JA, STASIK JJ, RIETHER RD,
• OLENWINE J, NOLAN P, KHUBCHANDANI IT: **The Value of Colonoscopic Screening in Patients with a Family History of Colon and Rectal Neoplasia.** *Coloproctology* 1990, **5**:265–268.
A retrospective review identified 475 patients (?? asymptomatic) colonoscoped because of a first or second degree relative with polyps or cancer; 16% had neoplasms of which nearly half were malignant, one-third proximal to the splenic flexure.

25. MCCONNELL JC, NIZIN JS, SLADE M: **Colonoscopy in Patients**
• **with a Primary Family History of Colon Cancer.** *Dis Colon Rectum* 1990, **33**:105–107.
One-hundred and twenty-five patients undergoing total colonoscopy because of family history of colorectal cancer (CRC) (no details given) yielded adenomas in 12% of which only 5% were above the reach of the flexible sigmoidoscope — not suggesting colonoscopy as a particularly worthwhile exercise.

26. HOULSTON RS, MURDAY V, HAROCOPOS C, WILLIAMS CB, SLACK J:
• **Screening and Genetic Counselling for Relatives of Patients with Colorectal Cancer in a Family Cancer Clinic.** *Br Med J* 1990, **2**:366–368
Three-hundred and eighty patients with a family history of (CRC) were assessed by geneticists on empiric grounds as having 10% or greater lifetime CRC risk and colonoscoped; two had adenomatous polyposis, five had cancer and 232 had adenomas removed.

27. ORROM WJ, BREZEZINSKI WS, WIENS EW: **Heredity and Colorec-**
• **tal Cancer. A Prospective, Community-based, Endoscopic Study.** *Dis Colon Rectum* 1990, **33**:490–493.
Twenty-three out of 108 asymptomatic patients with family history of colorectal cancer (92% first degree) yielded 21% with neoplasms including two cancers, over 25% in the right colon.

28. KURAMOTO S, IHARA O, SAKAI S, SHUMAZU R, KAMINISHI M,
• OOHARA T: **Depressed Adenoma in the Large Intestine. Endoscopic Features.** *Dis Colon Rectum* 1990, **33**:108–112.
Seven 'depressed adenomas' less than 3 mm diameter were noted in 1000 Japanese colonoscopies, the dysplasia being in the reddened and roughened central area of a tiny mucosal doughnut ring, more easily seen on deflation of the colon.

29. HUNT DR, CHERIAN M: **Endoscopic Diagnosis of Small Flat**
• **Carcinoma of the Colon. Report of Three Cases.** *Dis Colon Rectum* 1990, **33**:143–147.
Three patients with multiple neoplasms also had a 6–8 mm flat cancer without residual adenoma — visible to the endoscopist as small plaques with a reddened and/or depressed central area.

30. OKAMURA S, ASAI T, YAMAGUCHI H, HAMAJIMA E, KATOH T,
• SHIMODAIRA M, ITOH H: **A Clinicopathological Study of IIa + LLc Type Early Colorectal Cancer with Massive Submucosal Invasion.** *Dig Endosc* 1990, **2**:148–155.
Fifty-two 'early' malignancies includes sessile malignant polyps but also details of eight small flat ulcer cancers managed surgically (two with lymph nodes); six were less than 2 cm, three less than 1 cm diameter.

31. SAWADA T, HOJO K, MORIYA Y: **Colonoscopic Management of**
• **Focal and Early Colorectal Carcinoma.** In *Ballieres Clinical Gastroenterology* 1990, 627–645.

A very detailed account of a Japanese experience of 96 'early' invasive carcinomas with focal dysplasia.

32. • WOLFF WL, SHINYA H, CWERN M, HSU M: **Cancerous Colonic Polyps 'hands on' or 'hands off?'** *Am Surg* 1990, **56**:148–152.
Adequate record-keeping, follow-up and histopathological criteria prevent any serious analysis of 104 patients with malignant polyps followed for a mean of 5 years.

33. • PINES A, BAT L, SHEMESH E, RON E, HOROWITZ A, CHETRIT A, BUBIS JJ: **Invasive colorectal Adenomas: Surgery Versus Colonoscopic Polypectomy.** *J Surg Oncol* 1990, **43**:53–55.
Well documented series of 58 patients with 66 malignant polyps (mean 4.4 years follow-up) all pedunculated polyps had uncomplicated follow-up or no residual cancer, whereas nine out of 11 sessile lesions submitted to surgery were Duke's B or C.

34. • WILSON RG, SMITH AN, BIRD CC: **Immunohistochemical Detection of Abnormal Cell Proliferation in Colonic Mucosa of Subjects with Polyps.** *J Clin Pathol* 1990, **43**:744–747.
Simple immunohistochemical technique demonstrates abnormal extension of proliferative cells towards the epithelial surface of affected mucosa of adenoma patients (compared with controls).

35. • BRAVERMAN DZ, STANKIEWICZ H, GOLDSTEIN R, PATZ JK, MORALI GA, JACOBSOHN WZ: **Ornithine Decaryboxylase — An Unreliable Marker for the Identification of Population Groups at Risk for Colonic Neoplasia.** *Am J Gastroenterol* 1990, **85**:723–726.
No difference in levels of ornithine decarboxylase activity of sigmoid colon biopsies taken during total colonoscopy in four patient groups (normals, family history of colorectal cancer, adenomatous polyp subjects and cancer resection patients).

36. • COTHREN RM, RICHARDS-KORTUM R, SIVAK MJ, FITZMAURICE M, RAVA RP, BOYCE GA, DOZTADER M, BLACKMAN R, IVANC TB, HAYES GB, FELD MS, PETRAS RE: **Gastrointestinal Tissue Diagnosis by Laser-induced Fluorescence Spectroscopy at Endoscopy.** *Gastrointes Endosc* 1990, **36**:105–111.
Dye-laser light transmitted down a contact quartz fibre induced sufficient difference in autofluorescence measurements to discriminate between adenomatous and normal (or hyperplastic) tissue with 94% predictive value.

37. •• HILDEBRANDT U, FEIFEL G, ECKER KTW: **Rectal Endosonography.** In *Ballieres Clinical Gastroenterology* 1990, 531–541.
A clear review for the non-initiate of the usefulness of rectal ultrasound in assessing presence or absence of invasion, recurrence or involved lymph nodes (as dark hypoechoic appearances). The authors estimate ultrasound as affecting management in 30% of rectal cancer patients.

38. • ROSCH TH, LOREZ R, SUCHY R, DANCYGIER H, CLASSEN M: **Colonic Endoscopic Ultrasonography: First Results of a New Technique.** *Gastrointest Endosc* 1990, **36**:382–386.
A forward-viewing colonoscope with in-built rotating scanner proves practical for total colonoscopy in spite of the 4 cm rigid tip section and particularly useful for staging of colorectal cancer or assessment of recurrence.

39. • ROSCH T, LORENZ R, CLASSEN M: **Endoscopic Ultrasonography in the Evaluation of Colon and Rectal Disease.** *Gastrointest Endosc* 1990, **36**:S33–S39.
Preliminary experience with the ultrasound colonoscope (seven large sessile adenomas, 25 carcinomas) and a literature review suggest that it should be rather accurate in differentiating benign from malignant lesions and probably more accurate than computed tomography in diagnosing early recurrence.

40. • KIMMEY MB, MARTIN RW, SILVERSTEIN FE: **Endoscopic ultrasound Probes.** *Gastrointest Endosc* 1990, **36**:S40–S46.
Description of a commercial prototype ultrasound probe for use down the channel of standard endoscopes emphasizes that to be small enough the frequency must be high, so penetrates only 7 mm (and will therefore only be useful for superficial lesions).

41. • ARNAUD JP, BERGAMASCHI R, SCHLOEGEL M, OLLIER JC, HAEGELE P, GROB JC, ADLOFF M: **Progress in the Assessment of Lymphatic Spread in Rectal Cancer. Rectal Endoscopic Lymphoscintigraphy.** *Dis Colon Rectum* 1990, **33**:398–401.
Gamma camera scintigraphy after mucosal injection of technetium sulfacolloid has 76% accuracy in predicting presence or absence of lymph node involvement in patients with rectal cancer.

42. •• BRUNETAUD JM, MAUNOURY V, COCHELARD D, ADENIS A, BONIFACE B, CORTOT A, PARIS JC: **Lasers in Rectosigmoid Cancers: Factors Affecting Immediate and Long-term Results.** In *Ballieres Clinical Gastroenterology* 1990, 615–625.
An impressive well-documented summary of a French laser experience, mainly with neodymium-YAG. Palliation of 170 advanced cancer patients with symptom relief in 89% in a mean of 15 days and 2.5 treatments; the effect lasting over 40 months with complications in only 3%.

43. • UNGER SW, STERN JD, ARROYO PJ, RUSSIN DJ: **Endoscopic Nd-YAG Laser Treatment of Colorectal Neoplasms. A Four-year Longitudinal Study.** *Am Surg* 1990, **56**:153–157.
Use of the laser in a heterogenous group of tumour patients, mostly on an out-patient basis, required an average of 2.75 treatments (3 having more than 18) each of 45 min, bringing the calculated long-term cost of therapy to 2/3 that of surgery but sparing poor-risk patients from operation.

44. • PATRICE T, FOULTIER MT, YACTAYO S, ADAM F, GALMICHE JP, DOUET MC, LE BODIC L: **Endoscopic Photodynamic Therapy with Hematoporphyrin Derivatives for Primary Treatment of Gastrointestinal Neoplasms in Inoperable Patients.** *Dig Dis Sci* 1990, **35**:535–552.
Uncontrolled study of photodynamic therapy in 54 gastrointestinal cancers including 16 'inoperable' cancers of the rectosigmoid. Twenty-two per cent major complication rate (mainly stenosis) but promising results in terms of tumour regression, with negative histology in 24 of the 54 cases.

45. • BERRY AR, SOUTER RG, CAMPBELL WB, MORTENSEN NJMC, KETTLEWELL MGW: **Endoscopic Transanal Resection of Rectal Tumours — A Preliminary Report of its Use.** *Br J Surg* 1990, 77:134–137.
Eighty-one patients with benign or malignant tumours managed with aggressive transanal resectoscope technique (under fluid) had 15% major complication rate. The main advantage over laser was cheapness and speed of the procedure, although it requires a general anaesthetic.

46. • MARINI E, FRIGO F, CAVARZERE L, CUTOLO S, PALAZZIN L, ORCALLI F: **Palliative Treatment of Carcinoma of the Rectum by Endoscopic Injection of Polidocanol.** *Endoscopy* 1990, 22:171–173.
Five inoperable rectal cancer patients, three with impending obstruction, were relieved of symptoms by local sclerotherapy (15–20 ml per session every few months according to survival); cheaper than a laser.

47. • PFEIL SA, WEAVER MG, ABUDULKARIM FW, YANG P: **Colonic Lipomas — Outcome of Endoscopic Removal.** *Gastrointest Endosc* 1990, **36**:435–438.
Disastrous experience with major perforation in three broad-based 3–5 cm diameter lipomas of five snared. They conclude surgery is the procedure of choice for lipomas over 2 cm diameter that merit removal.

48. MATSUMOTO T, IIDA M, MATSUI T, HIRAKAWA M, SHIRAISHI A, YAO T, FUJISHIMA M: **Submucosal Tumors of the Terminal Ileum Managed by Endoscopic Polypectomy.** *Gastrointest Endosc* 1990, **36**:505–509.
Case report of a lipoma and a lymphangioma, both pedunculated and prolapsing through the ileo-caecal valve, safely removed by snare polypectomy.

49. CHRISTIE JP: **The Removal of Lipomas.** *Gastrointest Endosc* 1990, **36**:532.
Editorial pointing out that removal of lipomas is rarely indicated and whereas pedunculated lipomas can be snared, over 2 cm broad-based lipomas should usually be managed surgically, if significant bleeding or intussesception indicates it.

50. COLLIN GR, RUSSELL JC: **Endometriosis of the Colon — Its Diagnosis and Management.** *Am Surg* 1990, **56**:275–279.

Clinical review of nine patients with colonic endometriosis causing obstruction; endoscopy in five contributed nothing, surgery was indicated in all.

51. KOTHUR R, MARSH F, POSNER G, DOSIK H: **Endoscopic Leukemic Polyposis.** *Am J Gastroenterol* 1990, **85**:884–886.

Case report of carpeting of the colon with polyps up to 1.5 cm diameter in a patient with disseminated 'lymphosarcoma cell leukaemia' or lymphacytic lymphoma (also involved the upper gastrointestinal tract, generalized lymphadenopathy etc).

52. DUPHARE H, NIJHAWAN S, RANA S, BHARGAVA DK: **Heterotopic**
• **Gastric and Pancreatic Tissue in Large Bowel.** *Am J Gastroenterol* 1990, **85**:68–71.

Case report of bleeding ulcerated polypoid mass at the splenic flexure, in a 30-year-old, surgically resected and shown to be gastric mucosa and pancreatic tissue.

53. NUESSLE WR, MAGILL TR: **Leiomyosarcoma of the Transverse**
• **Colon — Report of a Case with Discussion.** *Dis Colon Rectum* 1990, **33**:323–326.

Case report of a semi-necrotic intussuscepting tumor at the splenic flexure, diagnosed histologically after successful surgical resection (only 45 in the literature).

54. SMITH JA, BHATAL PS, CUTHBERTSON AM: **Angiosarcoma of the**
• **Colon — Report of a Case with Long-term Survival.** *Dis Colon Rectum* 1990, **33**:330–333.

Case report of an ulcerated blue-red dome-like lesion compressing the sigmoid colon of a 16-year-old, (the fourth literature case of angiosarcoma involving the colon).

Colonoscopy and sigmoidoscopy

J.D. Waye

Mount Sinai Medical Center, GI Endoscopy Unit, Mount Sinai Hospital, Lenox Hill Hospital, New York, USA.

This review mentions virtually every article on colonoscopy and sigmoidoscopy (excluding neoplastic disease) in the world's literature during the past year. It demonstrates that knowledge continues to accumulate slowly and that 'new' techniques, devices and descriptions of problems are, in many instances, recycled items that have been known for a long time or previously described and discarded.

Preparation and premedication

Because of problems persuading patients to ingest 4 liters of fluid, in a report by Vilien *et al.* [1•], patients were randomized to drink either 1.5 or 3 liters of an electrolyte preparation, having received bisacodyl on the preceding day. Cleansing was good in 76 and 83% of cases with the smaller and larger volumes, respectively; in half of the remaining patients the result was acceptable and in the other half it was 'poor'. My experience is that one requires at least 3 liters of electrolyte solution; however, these authors currently use 1.5 liters. In a review of the literature, they quote the overall rate of unacceptable cleansing with electrolyte solution as between 3 and 20%. If the rate of poor preparation is as high as 10%, one wonders why electrolyte preparation has received such wide acceptance.

In a comparison of electrolyte preparation and citrate of magnesia with enemas, [2•], elderly patients (over 75 years of age) were randomized to receive an electrolyte solution or an enema preparation. The electrolyte preparation was deemed to be poor in 24% of in-patients compared with 35% of those with the enema preparation. In out-patients, the poor results were seen in 6 and 10%, respectively. A total of 28% receiving the electrolyte solution thought it was difficult or intolerable, compared with 24% of the enema group.

Another hospital in-patient study looked at a small-volume preparation consisting of oral sodium phosphate, a highly osmotic cathartic [3•]. Patients were randomized to receive either the small-volume or a 4-liter preparation of electrolyte. In a patient evaluation questionnaire, 20% of patients were unable to finish the Golytely preparation and another 25% found it to be extremely difficult to finish. Conversely, the majority of patients found the phosphate preparation easy or tolerable. As for effectiveness of cleansing, over 80% of the phosphate-prepared colons were ranked as good or excellent compared with only 33% of those receiving the 4-liter electrolyte preparation, partly because 20% of the patients were unable to tolerate the complete 4-liter preparation (Fig. 1).

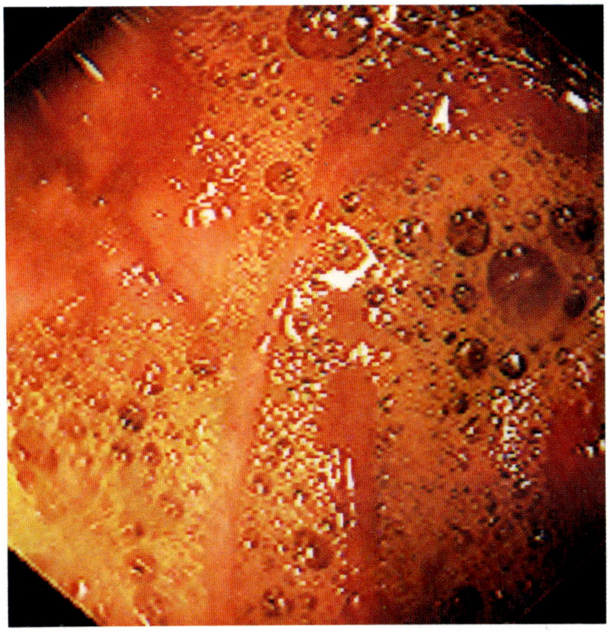

Fig. 1. A 'clean colon' from a 4-liter electrolyte preparation. Unfortunately the quantity of bubbles may interfere with mucosal visualization.

This report may start a trend toward seeking more palatable, smaller-volume preparations for colonoscopy. Until now, the 4-liter electrolyte preparation has been widely embraced, primarily because it obviated the necessity for enemas, although it has been always known that somewhere around 10% of patients would be unprepped with this solution because of its unpalatability. Any other form of preparation must be acceptable and yet totally safe. One of the patients had a syncopal attack with the phosphate preparation and may have had fluid shifts; any patient who receives vigorous cathartics must be instructed to drink copious amounts of fluid to protect against volume depletion.

A randomized clinical trial [4•] compared a Prepacol with 4-liter electrolyte solution. Although the tolerance

© Current Science Ltd ISBN 1-870485-32-7 ISSN 0952-6293

was worse for the electrolyte preparation, the quality of preparation was better [4•]. This group proposed that Prepacol was best suited for patients after previous colorectal resection, in whom both the preparation and tolerance were good.

In an article translated from German [5•], the cardiovascular effects of an electrolyte-polyethylene glycol (PEG) preparation were investigated with no adverse findings.

The group [6•] who introduced the original Golytely preparation has now described a modified lavage solution that has a 'barely perceptible salty taste'. They achieved this by removing some sodium sulfate, increasing the concentration of PEG and making minor adjustments in other salt concentrations. The solution is called Golytely-RSS (reduced sodium sulfate). The authors found that a rate of about 1 liter per hour resulted in a clean colon with somewhat less total volume overall.

Another group [7•] compared this sulfate-free PEG-electrolyte lavage solution with the previous standard PEG-electrolyte preparation. Three-quarters of the patients favored the sulfate-free preparation, but only 82% of all preparations were found to be 'clinically acceptable'. There is no doubt that we have not yet achieved the 'ideal' preparation for colonoscopy. The search goes on.

Difebo *et al.* [8•] compared the reduced-salt PEG-electrolyte solution with a 'standard' preparation consisting of senna tablets, magnesium sulfate and two large-volume water enemas. Eighty-five per cent of the electrolyte group had an adequate preparation compared with 63% who received the 'standard' preparation.

In evaluation of preparations for flexible sigmoidoscopy, a 'mini' study [9•] was performed on 39 consecutive adult out-patients undergoing flexible sigmoidoscopy. Randomization was to enemas containing docusate sodium (Klyx enema) or $1^1/_2$ packets of Picolax by mouth (sodium picosulphate and magnesium citrate dissolved in water; Nordic). Both preparations were given 2–3 hours before the examination. The oral preparation was preferred by the majority of patients but the endoscopist found no significant difference between the effectiveness of the preparations.

An article by Slimak and Fleisher [10•] reminds us that what goes in at the top may come out at the bottom relatively unchanged. A patient whose major problem was hematochezia took cherry-flavored magnesium citrate and had bright red liquid stool, which was mistaken for active bleeding. It is important to advise patients not to take any red substance prior to endoscopy, including red jello and candies.

In an attempt to determine whether enemas caused histological mucosal changes, biopsies were taken through a flexible sigmoidoscope in the unprepared rectum and rebiopsied following a tap-water enema [11•]. The histology and visual appearances were the same in both specimens and it was concluded that a tap-water enema does not give rise to a false diagnosis of mucosal inflammation.

Another group [12•] studied the mucosal effect in normal volunteers of an enema containing 10 mg bisacodyl. Bisacodyl caused injury to the superficial epithelium and upper third of the rectal crypts; pretreatment with topical misoprostol did not prevent epithelial injury. Such changes could be misinterpreted as a mild, acute colitis indistinguishable from idiopathic inflammatory bowel disease.

Two papers [13,14•] considered premedication during endoscopy with 'routine' analgesia. One article [13•], in an anesthesia journal, concluded that both alfentanil and fentanyl combined with midazolam provided satisfactory conditions for out-patient colonoscopy, with no evidence of respiratory depression. However, because of the propensity to induce respiratory depression, although the patient is awake, this combination of medicines will never be used routinely during colonoscopy.

Intravenous droperidol is a potent neuroleptic and may be used as supplementary premedication in selected patients undergoing endoscopy to ensure adequate sedation and co-operation. This drug produces a neuroleptic state characterized by dissociation from the surroundings, decreased motor activity, reduced anxiety and mild sedation. However, the response to painful stimuli and ability to follow verbal commands remains intact. When combined with a narcotic, psychomotor sedation and analgesia (termed neuroleptanalgesia) result. This agent is supposed to be especially useful in patients with active alcohol abuse or withdrawal and in those patients who are difficult to sedate [14•]. Patients received a cocktail of meperidine, diazepam, midazolam and droperidol, and then more medication if necessary. This combination was used in 764 patients during esophagogastroduodenscopy (EGD), endoscopic retrograde cholangiopancreatography (ERCP), and colonoscopy. Hypotension was the most frequent complication, occurring in a little over 1% of patients. In 11 of the patients, the procedure could not be completed because of continued agitation despite droperidol. In a second study [14•], the authors found that the combination of intravenous droperidol with standard pre-medication for endoscopic procedures was highly effective and safe, especially in the actively drinking or withdrawing alcoholic, the drug abuser and the young, active patient. Utilization of such a cocktail of drugs (droperidol, meperidine, diazepam, midazolam) seems rather aggressive when most colonoscopy is performed on ambulatory patients.

In direct opposition to heavy sedation, another article [15•] and subsequent letter [16•] assert that total colonoscopy was successfully performed in 95% of patients in an office setting where 82% of all patients received no analgesia or sedatives.

Monitoring during colonoscopy

Monitoring assumes many forms, the most important of which is the direct observation of the patient by the gastrointestinal assistant during the procedure.

Current monitoring practice [17•] was studied by sending a questionnaire to 509 members of the ASGE members. Excluding sigmoidoscopy, most American patients are routinely sedated for endoscopy, with meperidine being the commonest drug. If a minor tranquilizer was used, midazolam was the agent of choice over diazepam (62% compared with 38%). Pulse oximeters and electrocardiogram (EKG) monitoring were used by 65 and 55% of endoscopists, respectively.

An editorial [18•] questions whether oxygen supplementation, together with monitoring by oximetry when readily available, can reduce the already very low morbidity and mortality of endoscopy. It concludes that endoscopists should recognize the frequency of hypoxemia, however brief, and attempt to prevent it, as it is easy to treat hypoxemia and there is an extra margin of safety by doing so.

Gross and Long [19•] used pusle oximetry during colonoscopy to monitor 59 patients who had been sedated with midazolam or meperidine. Patients were randomized to receive nasal oxygen or air (3 liter/M) via nasal prongs. Those who received oxygen were shown to be less likely to become hypoxic than those who breathed room air. However, the authors concluded that, as hypoxemia may occur even when nasal oxygen is given, continuous monitoring of arterial oxygenation is recommended. No adverse effects were found in any patients, whether breathing room air or oxygen, and one wonders whether this whole business with pulse oximetry monitoring is a 'tempest in a teapot'?

In another series of 39 patients [20•] hypoxia seemed to be related to increased medication given for pain during negotiation of a colonic flexure or during sigmoid looping. Both hypotension and hypoxia were also related to duration of the procedure. Although the authors did not answer the question whether the episodes of hypoxia and hypotension had any clinical relevance, they concluded that mechanical monitoring, and the administration of oxygen when indicated, was worthwhile.

Another study [21•] looked at patients undergoing endoscopy (both upper and lower) with continuous recording of arterial oxygen saturation. Severe arterial oxygen desaturation (less than 85%) was noted in one in three of all patients and in 50% of those having colonoscopy; however, 'no patient... sustained an adverse event related to hypoxia.' In another prospective study [22•], 54% of patients had significant changes in oxygen saturation and in blood pressure, often correlated with medication or painful looping, but without obvious cause in many patients. The authors felt that it 'would seem reasonable to routinely monitor... in an effort to decrease anticipated morbidity.'

Using Holter monitoring in 33 sedated patients having lower gastrointestinal endoscopy, Gupta *et al.* [23•] showed transient EKG abnormalities in 24% of patients, mainly consisting of cardiac arrhythmias, although 4% of patients had ischemic ST-T wave changes. No treatment was necessary but the authors felt that 'it seems advisable to have continuous cardiac monitoring for patients with underlying cardiac or pulmonary disease and patients with baseline electrocardiographic abnormalities when undergoing endoscopic procedures.'

One hundred and three monitored colonoscopies in an office setting [24•] failed to demonstrate any ill effects in spite of a 41% incidence of levels below 90% saturation. A search of the literature found that healthy men may experience desaturation as a physiologic phenomenon during sleep, and passengers travelling on airplanes are also often desaturated because of the reduced oxygen pressure.

Although there is no evidence that oximetry monitoring results in safer endoscopy, almost every paper on this subject concludes that mechanical monitoring is worthwhile. To put the entire situation in context, it is necessary to realize that minor physiologic abnormalities during endoscopy have been reported over many years in various studies. It is now possible to detect these abnormalities as they are occurring, but there is no certainty that they are of any clinical significance.

New findings, new descriptions

Among the new descriptions was a report that approximately 40% of patients who had total colonoscopy with the video endoscope (but not fiberoptic instruments) were found to have a distinctive circinate pattern of 'freckles' near the appendiceal orifice [25•]. Freckle biopsies revealed lymphoid nodules. Their appearance represented an increased aggregation of lymphoid follicles near the appendix, visible as slightly raised spots with pale centers; in the remainder of the colon there was an average of 3.2 lymphoid follicles per cm^3. It should be noted that the same freckles may occasionally be seen in the rectum and sigmoid colon and represent the same lymphoid hyperplasia phenomenon noted by these authors (Fig. 2).

Large lymphoid follicles are relatively uncommon in adults but may occur as smooth-surfaced polypoid nodules throughout the colon, as reported in a 69-year-old man who presented with painless rectal bleeding [26•]. Upper intestinal endoscopy revealed similar findings in the antrum and duodenum. The authors pointed out that, although follicles are relatively commonly reported in the radiologic literature, with a 13% incidence, only a few endoscopic reports exist. In my opinion, this is an extremely rare entity; biopsies should be taken of any such lesions to differentiate them from adenomas.

An interesting colonoscopic sign was described [27•] of areas of bluish discoloration seen throughout the colon which changed in shape and level when the patient's position was altered. On questioning, the patient revealed he had been hospitalized 4 weeks earlier for blunt abdominal trauma. Computed tomography scan confirmed the diagnosis of a splenic injury and the patient was operated on and did well.

Some descriptions purport to be the first report of an entity. A cholecystocolic fistula was found at colonoscopy [28•] for massive bleeding. A polypoid tumor was seen with a fresh clot, which the endoscopist thought was a carcinoma, but at operation proved to be the site of a

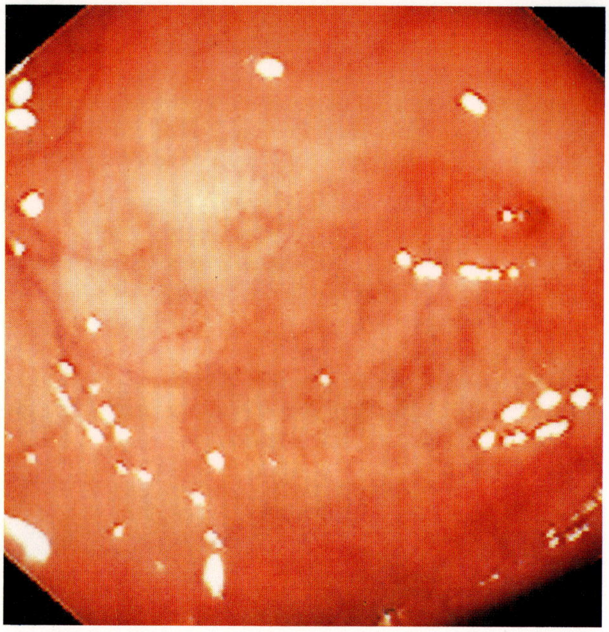

Fig. 2. The 'freckle sign' in the cecum. The circinate red areas with pale centers cluster around the appendiceal orifice.

fistula where the gallbladder stone had eroded into the colon. In another case, colonoscopy was successful in removing an errant gallstone that caused obstruction of the sigmoid colon [29•].

Finding gastric mucosa in the colon is also a rare event. In a 30-year-old man with massive rectal bleeding, barium enema confirmed an ulcerated mass at the splenic flexure [30•]. Colonoscopy revealed a polypoid ulcerated lesion about 4 cm in diameter at the splenic flexure from which blood was oozing. After surgery the resected mass was shown to consist of heterotopic gastric mucosa and pancreatic tissue.

Occult gastrointestinal bleeding is a common feature of Henoch–Schonlein purpura but little information has been reported about colonic lesions associated with bleeding. Cappell and Gupta [31•] report on two patients with the condition, both of whom had multiple 2–3 mm erythematous lesions throughout the colon. These were similar to the vasculitic lesions seen on the skin of the lower extremities.

The gastrointestinal group from Pittsburgh [32•] performed colonoscopy and upper endoscopy in 412 patients who were evaluated for possible liver transplantation. Of 57 subjects with primary sclerosing cholangitis, 30 had ulcerative colitis and eight had Crohn's disease. Overall, 20% of patients had 'non-specific colon edema' and 11% had 'inflammatory changes in the colon'. Unfortunately, there was no control group and the degree of edema was not correlated with Child's classification of liver disease. However, this paper bears witness to the fact that if you do many procedures in many patients you will eventually collect enough data to write a paper and have it published (perhaps even in *Gastroenterology*).

Little has been written on 'top-and-tail' endoscopy, also called single-session panendoscopy [33•]. This is most often performed to investigate a positive fecal occult blood test, anemia or iron deficiency. Colonoscopy is suggested as the first procedure, followed immediately by upper-intestinal endoscopy if the large bowel is normal. The EGD portion adds little to the overall time of the procedure, but circumvents the necessity for the patient to return at a future date or to go elsewhere for an upper gastrointestinal barium radiograph.

New devices

Similar papers from two different groups [34,35•] on autofluorescence appeared in 1990. An interesting autofluorescent technique has been developed which can discriminate between adenomas and normal tissues [34•]. Hyperplastic polyps show the same autofluorescent spectrum as normal tissue. In this study, a helium-cadmium laser fiber directly contacted the tissue surface. Both light and reflected autofluorescence could be measured through the same single fiber without tissue damage.

Cothren *et al.* [35•] reported that laser autofluorescence spectra of mucosal abnormalities differentiated adenomas from both normal mucosa and hyperplastic polyps in 97% of the specimens studied. This is a marked increase in sensitivity compared with the 75% accuracy of endoscopic observation in distinguishing hyperplastic polyps from adenomas. The technique could possibly be developed in the future so that spectral information from a lesion would be instantly available to guide an endoscopist to take biopsies from areas most likely to yield positive results, minimizing sampling error for instance. This technology would be extremely important in looking for dysplasia of the colon in inflammatory bowel disease as well as in differentiating adenomas from hyperplastic polyps. Although this work is preliminary, the future may allow laser scanning of an entire visual field in real time to provide instantaneous feedback to the endoscopist. Unfortunately, at present direct fiber contact with the tissue surface is required in order to induce the necessary fluorescence spectrum.

A 'prototype' stiffening device [36•] has been described which can be passed through the channel of a standard colonoscope. By cranking the handle, a variable amount of stiffening will occur. With this 'wonderful' device the authors performed colonoscopy to the cecum in 22 out of 25 patients. Being 'the old man' in colonoscopy, I am amused by this since in the early 1970s ACMI had a similar 'variable stiffening device' which was thought to be 'the answer' to the performance of colonoscopy but which fell into disuse because it proved not to be helpful. The identical tool is unlikely to prove to be any more valuable in the 1990s than it was in the 1970s.

Techniques new and old

Under the heading of 'controversies', two sides of the question whether fluoroscopy should or should not be used during colonoscopy were once again debated. Rogers [37•] suggested that there are a number of 'failed colonoscopies that result from a lack of fluoroscopic control'; if colonoscopy fails with fluoroscopy, it simply cannot be done, and therefore it is not worthwhile to refer the case to another colonoscopist. Waye [38•] responded that fluoroscopy is not necessary in passage of the colonoscope to the cecum and that techniques of non-fluoroscopic intubation and loop removal can be learned readily. He cautioned that the instrument should only be advanced with the lumen in view and the fluoroscope should not be used to blindly point the instrument in the direction of the lumen and then push. Old attitudes die hard. However, it is a truism that most colonoscopists no longer use fluoroscopy, even for difficult cases. The next generation of colonoscopists will probably never use fluoroscopy, even during training.

The standard Starck 'crank'-type dilator was described in 1924 for dilatation of achalasia. The 50 cm long dilator can be placed through a rigid proctosigmoidoscope under general anesthesia and opened under direct vision. This technique was used in four patients with low anastomotic strictures [39•], but modern-day endoscopists would prefer to use a TTS balloon for proximal colonic strictures or a Savary dilator (over an endoscopically placed guidewire using fluoroscopic control) for distal strictures.

A case report [40•] of successful use of Savary dilators in a radiation stricture in a single session shows radiographic pictures of a 50 French (F) Savary dilator assuming a pretzel-shape in the sigmoid colon, enough to make even the strongest endoscopist somewhat weak-kneed. It would be my practice to dilate at a slower rate, taking more than one session to do the job. Pietropaola *et al.* [41•] report an overall failure rate of 2.4% in a series of balloon dilatations of postoperative colon strictures. The balloon was successful in one application in 77% of patients, compared with a single bougeinage in 52% of patients.

A 40 mm balloon was used for dilatation of rectal strictures [42•] and passed over a fluoroscopically placed guidewire initially introduced via colonoscopy. Only one patient had a restenosis which was successfully re-dilated. Be careful! A 4 cm balloon is a big dilator, and would wreck havoc higher up in the colon.

In a brief but pointed reply to a letter to the editor, Herman [16•] asserted that the trick in colonoscoping patients without sedation is to avoid any painful loop while advancing the scope. The author wrote: 'most endoscopists I have watched tend to do the opposite. They progressively advance the scope while pushing and attempt to straighten loops only after they have formed. Furthermore, many doctors are afraid to withdraw the instrument for fear they are losing ground in their attempt to reach the cecum. Actually, the opposite seems to be true. Basically this technique involves constantly advancing and withdrawing the instrument while rotating the colonoscope clockwise. The premise is that this motion not only avoids loops but telescopes the colon over the instrument concurrently. Most lateral (right/left) motion and some vertical (up/down) motion of the colonoscope tip is achieved by torqueing the instrument and not predominantly by the dial controls. External abdominal pressure by the nurse is most helpful as well. The cecum can be reached in under 90 cm most of the time with this technique.' This is a succinct and worthwhile description to bring to the attention of all endoscopists. However, it may not be possible to avoid formation of a loop at all times, and occasionally it is necessary to advance the instrument shaft and 'push through a loop', knowing that it will cause some degree of patient discomfort. It is for this reason that I prefer to give medication for most colonoscopies. The trick to performing total colonoscopy is not how much one pushes; rather, the magic occurs by frequent withdrawal of the shaft (and removal of loops) during intubation.

The prize for the longest colonoscopy (8 hours) must go to Langdon [43•]. An indwelling scope was left behind in patients with intermittent gastrointestinal bleeding when no bleeding site was found on total colonoscopy, and scans were negative. The colonoscope was taped to the buttocks and when bleeding occurred the light was turned on and air insufflated; upon seeing blood flow from the ileocecal valve, diagnosis was made of a bleeding site proximal to the colon. The only complaint from the patients was of limited mobility. Of all the new techniques of 1990, this one seems the least likely to be accepted by endoscopists and patients alike.

Nakagawa *et al.* [44•] describe a small-caliber choledochoscope (BR3-type, external diameter 6.5 mm; Olympus, Tokyo) used to inspect fistulas. Foreign bodies could be seen, sutures could be removed, and biopsies could be performed through this technique. Only two out of 15 cases required dilation (every other day) of too-narrow fistulas, and patients tolerated fistuloscopy quite well.

Sigmoidoscopy

Three articles were published during this past year on sigmoidoscopy, only one of which was relevant to sigmoidoscopy in its comparison with colonoscopy (discussed below under 'Lower gastrointestinal bleeding'). The American Medical Association has gathered a large panel to assess diagnostic and therapeutic technology [45•]. They have concluded that rigid sigmoidoscopy is safe regardless of the availability of flexible sigmoidoscopy, and it is effective if flexible sigmoidoscopy is not readily available. A literature review in the accompanying article pointed out that flexible sigmoidoscopy was considerably more comfortable, took longer, but reached further and so had a diagnostic yield two to three times greater than with the rigid sigmoidoscope. The perforation rate in rigid sigmoidoscopy ranges from 1 in 10 000 to 1 in 20 000, whereas in flexible sigmoidoscopy the rate is estimated to be 1 in 5000. Although a 35 cm and a 60 cm flexible sigmoidoscope are currently available, 95% of instruments sold to family practitioners have been the 60 cm model. Historically, the 30 cm scope has been a fiasco, introduced by insecure colonoscopists who were concerned that non-experts would be tempted to 'go all the way' if they became adept with a 60 cm scope.

Rex *et al.* [46•] reported on the use of a standard colonoscope to perform screening 'sigmoidoscopy' in 500 asymptomatic, unsedated patients. Only five patients had polyps detected above 60 cm. The average depth of penetration was 66 cm with this long instrument, with a mean time of 9.3 min. The authors concluded that the use of instruments longer than 60 cm gives very little additional yield, but ignored the fact that a 60 cm scope does not actually reach 60 cm into the colon in the vast majority of patients. The paper by Rex *et al.* at least leaves no doubt that one can perform flexible sigmoidoscopy with a long colonoscope and do it easily and relatively quickly. This reviewer notes that one could use outmoded flexible upper endoscopes for sigmoidoscopy as well. Older gastroscopes that are 'hanging around gathering dust' could easily be used for flexible sigmoidoscopies and should be pressed into service rather than allowed to deteriorate in the closet.

Many physicians are concerned that an air (or double) contrast barium enema (ACBE/DCBE) will not be accurate if performed immediately after flexible sigmoidoscopy. Some have advocated carbon dioxide insufflation during flexible sigmoidoscopy to ensure that air does not interfere with the ACBE. A randomized clinical trial [47•] showed that although there is more air after a routine flexible sigmoidoscopy than when carbon dioxide is used, the quality of an ACBE is not affected (and is also not significantly different from examinations performed on separate days).

Old problems revisited

Diversion colitis is an inflammatory process that develops in the bypassed segment of the large bowel after diversion of the fecal stream. Among the endoscopic findings are erythema with a granular friable mucosa and aphthous ulcers. Histologically the biopsies may mimic idiopathic inflammatory bowel disease. Various causes have been proposed for diversion colitis, including bacterial overgrowth, prolonged contact with toxic products, disturbance of the symbiotic bacterial-mucosal relationships and deprivation of essential nutrients, specifically short-chain fatty acids. The most effective way to treat diversion colitis is to re-establish colonic continuity, as the endoscopic and histologic abnormalities in all cases returned to normal after re-establishment of colon continuity. This condition can respond to medical treatment when indicated by symptoms, six patients improving after being given short-chain fatty acids into the bypassed segment [48•].

Eighty-five patients having a colostomy with a distal loop of excluded bowel were evaluated over a 9-year period [49•]. About one-half of the patients had no symptoms, but the endoscopy revealed mucus plugs and scybala in the excluded colon. There was a relatively high incidence of diversion colitis in the non-functioning colonic segments of 86% of patients following diverticulitis, and in 25% of patients following operations for carcinoma. The authors assert that even asymptomatic patients should be examined annually using endoscopy, but this seem, to be an unnecessary exercise for the endoscopist, with no discernible benefit for the patient.

Two sisters who presented with the apparent diagnosis of multiple polyposis had the correct diagnosis made by puncture deflation of cysts of pneumatosis coli [50•] using a sclerotherapy-type needle.

Air cysts in pneumatosis coli can be deflated with multiple, progressively deeper biopsies, but the method of puncture deflation is easier and quicker. The important factor in making the diagnosis, however, is not their deflation, but first suspecting the diagnosis on visual grounds.

Pneumatosis cystoides intestinalis has been reported after organ transplantation, although most cases resolve spontaneously with consecutive management (even if pneumoperitoneum is present). Andorsky [51•] reports on a case with mild gastrointestinal symptoms 4 months after cardiac transplantation. Colonoscopy revealed the changes of pneumatosis.

Foreign bodies should always be considered as a cause of colon abnormalities, but only one article [52•] was written on this during 1990. A 61-year-old patient presented with diffuse abdominal discomfort and rectal bleeding. Flexible sigmoidoscopy demonstrated a firm object transverse in the lumen and penetrating the opposing walls of the sigmoid colon.This was grasped, withdrawn and found to be a 6 cm toothpick. Blood culture showed *Erysipelothrix rhusiopathiae*, an unusual bacterium found worldwide as a normal inhabitant in a number of domestic animals, wild rodents and fowl. The patient was started on appropriate antibiotics and did well.

Transplant patients seem to be particularly vulnerable to gastrointestinal insults. One report [53•] described 13 cases of Ogilvie's syndrome (pseudoobstruction) 1–13 days following renal transplantation. Five of the six patients with and two of the seven without colonoscopy had resolution. In this series, a total of seven patients had perforation of the colon. Early surgery is suggested to salvage these acutely ill patients.

A retrospective study of patients with endometriosis [54•] revealed that endoscopy was performed in five patients, in each of whom the finding was of an extramucosal mass compressing the lumen but with normal results from biopsies. This simply demonstrates the known inability of the colonoscope to detect submucosal pathology.

Teaching colonoscopy

There was a paucity of articles concerning teaching. A group with roots in the UK [55•] has developed a computer simulation model that may be a cheap and harmless method to teach trainees control of the endoscope. An endoscope head and partial shaft are fitted with appropriate sensors to detect torque, up/down, in/out, and right/left control movement, air insufflation and use of the suction button. Computer graphics produce a schematic image as the physician manipulates the instrument control head. Pushing the shaft forward causes the concentric rings on the screen to expand, giving the illusion of forward movement, which can be reversed by withdrawing the shaft. Similarly, up/down controls create screen movement to simulate the 'real thing'. Although the development is brilliant, the computer score is derived by the number of times that one 'bangs into the wall', over-inflates, or pushes too hard.The technique shows great promise and could allow an attempt at eye–hand co-ordination without the necessity of actually putting the instrument into a patient. However, this author tried the model and came out with the highest score of errors ever recorded. I guess this means I will never perform colonoscopy successfully and should never try it in a patient?

In a more patient-oriented teaching article [56•], trainees in diagnostic radiology performed a total of 1578 consecutive colonoscopic examinations over a 10-year interval. The endoscopic examination was completed to the cecum in 66% of cases, but in some a limited examination was adequate to solve the problem posed on a previous barium enema examination. In patients who underwent both radiography and endoscopy, the barium enema failed to diagnose 23% of the neoplastic lesions subsequently found during colonoscopy (including nine cancers). Half of the falsely negative enemas were performed by consultant staff and half by trainees. The performance of colonoscopy by radiologists was demonstrated to improve the liaison between radiologists and gastroenterologists, and to make the radiologist aware of the value of colonoscopy as both a diagnostic and a therapeutic tool.

It may not be practical or necessary to have the radiologist actually handle the instrument but certainly there is a great deal of practical information that can be gained from the correlation of radiographic with gross anatomical demonstrations of pathology through flexible endoscopes. Every gastrointestinal radiologist should, during the training period, be obliged to spend some time on a regular basis observing endoscopies of the upper and lower gastrointestinal tract.

Lower gastrointestinal bleeding

On evaluation of 1000 consecutive patients [57•] referred for colonoscopy, the endoscopist was requested to make a judgment immediately before colonoscopy about the most likely endoscopic findings. Concurrence between pre-endoscopic predictions and colonoscopic findings was only 61%. The level of accuracy was not improved by having a previous barium enema examination.

An important message from this study is that rectal bleeding should alert the clinician. In patients referred because of bleeding, the diagnosis was malignancy in 12%, polyps in 18% and inflammatory bowel disease in 13%, whereas in patients with abdominal pain and/or constipation the yield was relatively low. The authors considered the prime reasons for colonoscopy to be visible rectal bleeding, occult fecal blood, an abnormality on a previous barium enema (or endoscopy), and the detection of synchronous/metachronous tumors either before or shortly after an operation for colorectal carcinoma.

Dent *et al.* [58•] studied how long people delay before presenting to their doctor with rectal bleeding. The period between onset of symptoms and presenting for medical attention ranged from 0 to 249 days, but with a median of only 7 days. Fifty per cent of patients stated that this episode was not the first occurrence and they were more likely to have delayed seeking attention than those in whom bleeding occurred for the first time. The 46% of patients who always looked at either the toilet paper or their feces were less likely to have delayed seeking medical care than other patients. It is remarkable that these authors found a median of only 7 days from rectal bleeding to seeking medical attention, whereas studies a decade ago demonstrated that for colon cancer in an American population the median delay was 11 weeks before diagnosis, and in a British series the delay was 22 weeks. It is possible that the message is getting through to patients that rectal bleeding is an important presenting symptom of colorectal cancer.

A randomized, controlled clinical trial [59••] comparing colonoscopy with flexible sigmoidoscopy and ACBE was performed to evaluate which of these procedures seemed to have the best diagnostic yield for patients with suspected lower gastrointestinal bleeding. Over 300 patients were enrolled. Total colonoscopy was possible in 92% of 151 patients; obstructing cancers accounted for lack of total intubation. Thirty-two per cent of patients initially randomized to flexible sigmoidoscopy and ACBE had subsequent colonoscopy, whereas only 8% of patients initially randomized to colonoscopy had subsequent ACBE because of inability to advance the colonoscope to the cecum. The diagnostic yield for either of the approaches was similar. Procedural charges were:

Flexible sigmoidoscopy -	$154
ACBE -	$255
Diagnostic colonoscopy -	$543
Polypectomy -	$137

The mean total charge for all investigations of the flexible sigmoidoscopy-and-ACBE group was $609.64 (including any colonoscopies needed) and for the colonoscopy-first group was $603.11.

One of the conclusions in this paper was that initial colonoscopy may be preferable in populations with poor compliance because a diagnostic examination could be coupled with biopsy or polypectomy in one procedure. The authors suggested that in patients over 55 years of age with suspected lower gastrointestinal bleeding, colonoscopy as the initial study is more cost-effective for the detection of significant neoplasms than flexible sigmoidoscopy and ACBE (because polyps can be removed at colonoscopy) whereas, because of lower yields in people aged less than 55 years, the latter approach seems to be the most cost-effective.

Another study, of debatable cost-effectiveness, used colonoscopy to study the cause of lower gastrointestinal bleeding in marathon runners [60•]. Seven out of nine runners who developed stool occult blood after a marathon had EGD and colonoscopy; two out of three who had endoscopic examinations within 48 hours of the event had antral erosions and the other had patchy areas of erythema and erosions at the splenic flexure. No pathology was found when endoscopy was delayed beyond 48 hours after running. It is postulated that the injuries were secondary to relative gut ischemia which normalized rapidly.

A 66-year-old patient had undergone placement of a right aorto-iliac Dacron graft 12 years earlier [61•]. Colonoscopy demonstrated the prosthesis extruding into the lumen of the ascending colon. Another patient had a graft placed 4 years before endoscopy and, because of gastrointestinal hemorrhage 1 year later, underwent a right axillo-femoral graft with a cross-over graft. Colonoscopy performed for evaluation of non-bloody diarrhea revealed both limbs of the aorto-iliac graft in the sigmoid colon. Aorto-enteric fistulas result from low-grade infection of the proximal graft suture line, causing a pseudo-aneurysm with subsequent fistula formation between the graft, lumen and bowel. On the other hand, paraprosthetic-enteric fistula are believed to originate as a result of pressure necrosis of the bowel from constant pulsation of the graft, resulting in eventual erosion of the graft into the bowel lumen itself. Bleeding is rarely massive, although the patient may present with hemorrhage, sepsis or abdominal and back pain. Endoscopy should be performed with caution in these patients since dislodgement of a clot from the fistula may result in fatal gastrointestinal hemorrhage.

Emergency colonoscopy is taking its place in the diagnosis of acute colorectal bleeding. In one patient, emergency colonoscopy was performed without preparation [62•], using 6 liters of water flushed through the scope to obtain bowel cleansing. When a 1 cm diverticulum with pulsating arterial hemorrhage was seen, the neck of the diverticulum was injected with 16 ml 1/10 000 adrenaline solution; immediate hemostasis averted surgery. Injection therapy for gastrointestinal bleeding is becoming a commonly used modality in the colon as well as in the upper gastrointestinal tract. I find this to be so useful for immediate hemostasis (such as after polypectomy) that a 20 cm injector/sclerotherapy needle is the only piece of equipment that I carry by hand when travelling to demonstrate colonoscopy in a foreign land.

Inflammatory bowel disease

A few interesting papers were written, most of which re-enforced the overall feeling that endoscopy is not the best way to follow patients with inflammatory bowel disease. An overview [63•] on the role of colonoscopy in inflammatory bowel disease discussed the indications for endoscopy and its problems, providing a balanced look at the current state of knowledge on this subject.

When assessing drug therapy in the upper intestinal tract endoscopy is the 'gold standard' against which response of healing is measured. However, in the area of inflammatory bowel disease the response has always been measured by clinico-biologic parameters and not by any fixed endoscopic criteria. Twenty-eight different parameters were collected during endoscopic and clinical evaluation of 142 patients with active colonic or ileocolonic Crohn's disease treated with oral steroids in a multicenter prospective study [64•]. One hundred and thirty-one patients went into clinical remission but only 38 developed a true endoscopic remission. Using a complex, but manageable, index for evaluating the percentage of colon segments involved by disease taking into account nine separate items (pseudopolyp, healed ulceration, frank erythema, frankly swollen mucosa, aphthoid ulceration, superficial or shallow ulceration, deep ulceration, non-ulcerated stenosis, and ulcerated stenosis), the study shows no correlation between any of the clinical activity indices of Crohn's disease and any of the endoscopic data. Thus, the clinical severity of an attack of Crohn's disease is not related to the nature, extent or severity of endoscopic lesions. For instance, it is surprising that erythema and aphthoid ulcers, usually considered as early and relatively minor lesions in Crohn's disease, were not at all influenced by steroid therapy. This elegant study demonstrates a fact that many of us have stated for several years: one cannot and should not use repeated interval colonoscopies to assess the results of therapy in inflammatory bowel disease. Indeed, this paper lends great support to the ongoing need for clinical evaluation in these patients instead of trying to assess the results of therapy by the endoscopic appearance.

Along these same lines, in a group of patients with ulcerative colitis or with Crohn's disease, a significant discrepancy was seen between the degree of clinical disease activity and the extent and degree of mucosal inflammation at endoscopy and on histologic assessment [65•]. Patients often had no (or minimal) clinically apparent disease activity, despite mucosal inflammatory activity of a moderate or severe degree at endoscopy and/or histology. The authors suggest that the commonly used classifications of clinical inflammatory bowel disease activity do not reflect mucosal inflammation satisfactorily and that total colonoscopy is necessary to establish the extent and degree of mucosal inflammation. One wonders why that is necessary, as the important parameters as far as therapy are concerned rest with the clinical status of patients.

A prospective colonoscopic evaluation [66•] of the anastomotic area was conducted in 89 patients who had an ileo-colonic anastomosis for active Crohn's disease. In 73% of patients, endoscopy within 1 year of surgery revealed recurrent lesions in the neoterminal ileum, although only 20% of these patients had symptoms. Three years after surgery, the endoscopic recurrence rate had increased to 85%, although only 34% had symptoms of recurrence. The authors postulate that early lesions in the neoterminal ileum after Crohn's resection do not originate from foci of microscopic inflammation in this bowel segment at the time of surgery, but are actually new areas of involvement. They also suggest that the postoperative clinical course of Crohn's disease is best predicted by the severity of endoscopic lesions during the first year following resection. Control of recurrence in the small-bowel near the anastomosis is a good model for studying the value of various new therapeutic modalities.

Olaison *et al.* [67•] report on the clinical-endoscopic disparity in eight patients with Crohn's disease who had ileo-ascending colon anastomosis (six patients) or ileorectal anastomosis (two patients). The patients all had some degree of small bowel involvement and were treated with prednisolone. Good subjective improvement was seen in all eight, but post-therapy endoscopy demonstrated improvement of the ileum in only two patients.

In the presence of gastrointestinal tract involvement with Crohn's disease, barium radiography may not demonstrate any abnormalities. This point was made in a survey [68•] of 528 children with the clinical diagnosis of Crohn's disease. Thirty-seven of them did not fulfill the minimal radiographic criteria for gut involvement, but endoscopic biopsies were positive for granulomas. Some had repeat radiographs 3 years later, and in 14 patients evidence of disease was shown. In a third of the children, the original biopsies showing epithelioid granulomas were taken from macroscopically normal mucosa, and granulomas were found in a surprisingly high proportion (57%) of initial rectal biopsies. It is my experience in adult practice that granulomas are only demonstrated in about 5% of endoscopic biopsies in Crohn's disease and that the endoscopic diagnosis is a more important parameter than the histologic, unless granulomas are reported.

In an overview, authors from the Cleveland Clinic [69•] asserted that they currently rely primarily on colonoscopy to evaluate the patient with suspected colonic inflammatory bowel disease because it permits visualization of the mucosa, provides biopsies and appears to be more sensitive for the detection of subtle mucosal changes and for judging the extent of disease than is barium radiography, (sensitivity of 85% for colonoscopy in the diagnosis of colonic Crohn's disease versus 48% for barium enema).

All endoscopists, radiologists and gastrointestinal clinicians agree that looking at the mucosa with a colonoscope will allow the detection of ulcers and inflammation in a fashion superior to that provided by radiology. The broader question is whether the extra information gained is meaningful as regards disease prognosis or therapeutic decisions. Rutgeerts *et al.* [66•] pointed out that prognosis is related to severity of disease and it is the impression of both gastroenterologists and radiologists that the more serious areas of involvement will be detected by barium studies. Modigliani *et al.* [64•] also suggest that most therapeutic decisions in inflammatory bowel disease are based on the patient's symptoms and not on endoscopic findings.

Endoscopic evaluation was performed in the evaluation of an oral agent, olsalazine (composed of two 5-amino salicylate molecules linked by an azo bond). When administered orally it is split by colonic bacteria to liberate 5-ASA. This drug lacks the sulfapyridine moiety found in sulfasalazine. A randomized double blind placebo-controlled trial was conducted [70•] with endoscopic evaluation. The olsalazine group showed an improvement in the colonoscopic score whereas the placebo group showed a worsening in the score. However, there are problems with the conculsions of this paper because of the withdrawals and failures to perform follow-up colonoscopies. These data could have make a vast difference in the overall colonoscopic scores. One cannot rely on studies such as this to make endoscopic comparisons with drug treatment. Indeed, in view of the preceding papers, should endoscopy be the parameter by which improvement is judged?

Forty-seven patients who had colectomy with mucosal proctectomy and ileal pouch-anal anastomosis were followed for an average of 1½ years [71•]. Forty-one patients (87%) had no pouchitis symptoms and quality of life was judged good by 85% of all patients. The other six patients (all with ulcerative colitis) developed recurrent 'pouchitis', the main endoscopic feature being that of an acute non-specific inflammation involving all of the mucosa of the neorectum and, in one case, extension into the ileum. Granularity, edema, mucosal hemorrhages, contact bleeding, mucus hypersecretion and multiple superficial ulcers were present to some degree in all cases of pouchitis. Occasionally, features of a pseudomembranous enteritis were encountered with small punctate white-yellow pseudomembranes covering the surface of the mucosa. In all patients, Crohn's disease was excluded on reassessing the colonic surgical specimens. A review of the literature revealed the frequency of pouchitis to vary from 7 to 44% of patients but apparently the true frequency is somewhere between 10 and 15% of patients. Although the pathogenesis of pouchitis is unknown, the hypothesis is of abnormal bacterial growth, favored by stasis of intestinal contents within the pouch.

Colitis, ischemia and colon ulcers

Boley [72•] reminisces over a life-time of work in the field of bowel ischemia. He asserts that the vast majority of patients with colonic ischemia have no identifiable cause, no iatrogenic injury, no preceding problem and no precipitating event. The ischemic episode is usually spontaneous and may involve any part of the colon, although the transverse and splenic flexures are the most commonly affected sites. He suggests that when a patient with colonic ischemic injury remains symptomatic for more than 2–3 weeks surgery is to be recommended because of the high probability of perforation. In summarizing the lessons learned over the past 25 years, he states that the diagnosis of ischemia can be made either by barium enema or by colonoscopy, but there is no role for angiography as most cases are non-occlusive in nature.

Approximately 3% of a large group [73•] of renal transplant recipients developed colitis. Previous literature reviews have pointed out that approximately 9% of renal transplant patients have gastrointestinal complications of which one in 10 are colonic, including acute colitis, colonic perforation and diverticulitis.

Collagenous or microscopic colitis is a rare condition characterized clinically by chronic diarrhea and histologically by a thickened subepithelial collagenous band on colonic biopsies in an endoscopically normal colon. Another case of collagenous colitis has been added to the more than 200 cases so far described [74•]. This patient presented with chronic watery diarrhea of 6 months' duration and was found to have collagenous colitis on biopsies from a normal-appearing colon. An upper intestinal endoscopy also appeared grossly normal, but biopsy in the duodenal bulb revealed a deposition of collagen fibers which mimicked that in the colon. With the increasing frequency of collagenous colitis, it is important that endoscopists are aware of the need to biopsy normal colonic mucosa in patients being examined for colonic diarrheal symptoms. Perhaps gastroduodenal involvement is not so rare, as most patients with the diagnosis of collagenous colitis do not have upper intestinal endoscopy and biopsies.

Although most patients with collagenous colitis are women, two men have been reported [75•] in whom the onset of colitis was related to non-steroidal anti-inflammatory drugs. One patient had a completely normal colonoscopic appearance and the other had pseudomembranes on the surface of the colon. Both had typical findings of collagenous colitis and responded to sulfasalazine or prednisone.

Familial occurrence had never previously been described but two families have now been reported [76•] in whom first-degree relatives had collagenous colitis. In one family, two sisters were affected by chronic diarrhea and a number of autoimmune disorders, including thyroid disease, rheumatoid arthritis and pernicious anemia. One sister had collagenous colitis and the other had microscopic colitis but in a review of biopsies from the latter colon (11 years previously) the colon showed histologic features consistent with collagenous colitis. In the other family, both a father and son with diarrhea for several years had a diagnosis of collagenous colitis from endoscopic biopsies.

Microscopic colitis was diagnosed in five children (mean age 5–7 years) who underwent rectosigmoidoscopy with multiple biopsies [77•]. Their mean age was 5.7 years. They presented with chronic diarrhea with or without vomiting, abdominal pain or anorexia. In all patients the mucosa was endoscopically normal but biopsies met the usual pathologic criteria for microscopic colitis. It is suggested that, in the evaluation of children with chronic undiagnosed diarrhea, biopsies be taken to search specifically for microscopic colitis.

Okada *et al.* [78•] reported on a patient with solitary rectal ulcer syndrome in whom the lesion was found to change dramatically over a course of $2^1/_2$ years. The biopsy findings were typical, with fibromuscular obliteration of the lamina propria and goblet cell depletion. As opposed to most patients with solitary rectal ulcer whose prolapsing folds are internal, this patient had external rectal prolapse and over the course of observation developed large edematous rectal folds with multiple broad-based polypoid lesions having ulcerated surfaces. These lesions were localized to the rectum and extended between 3 and 15 cm from the anal margin. This report is interesting, as most solitary rectal ulcers tend not to change much over several years of observation.

In a large series of cases, 22 patients with solitary rectal ulcer and typical histological features were described from India [79•]. In 15 a single rectal ulcer was found, whereas in seven two ulcers were present. Of the 29 ulcers, 19 were on the anterior or anterolateral wall of the rectum and 10 were on the posterior or posterolateral wall.

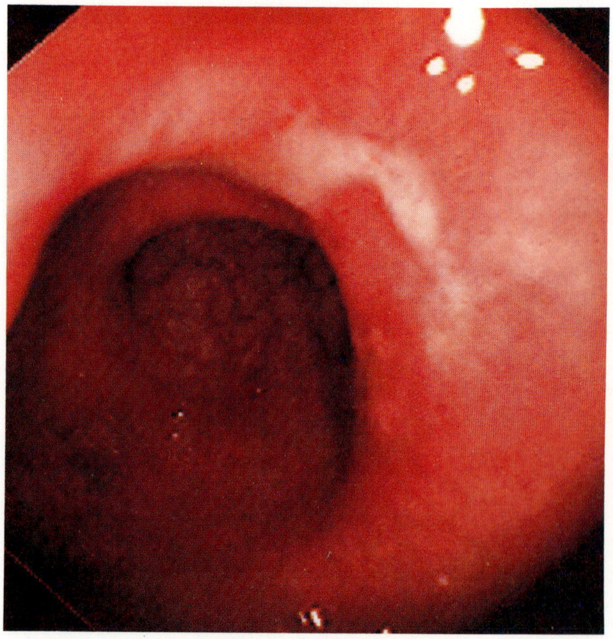

Fig. 3. Stellate ulcer in rectum ('solitary rectal ulcer').

Rectal ulcers can also be secondary to certain medications [80•]. Apparently, suppositories containing non-steroidal anti-inflammatory drugs may induce ulcerative, hemorrhagic proctitis giving rise to symptoms of urgency, tenesmus, and rectal bleeding. The proctitis regresses after discontinuation of therapy but one of the three cases presented had progressed to rectal stenosis, presumably secondary to the ulcerative proctitis caused by these medication-suppositories (Fig. 3).

The diffuse intestinal ulcerations due to enteric graft-versus-host disease in general are erosive or ulcerative lesions which in most cases are segmental and irreversible. Severe hemorrhage from the lower intestinal tract occurred in a 29-year-old patient who had received a bone marrow transplantation for leukemia [81•]. On colonoscopy, multiple erosions, ulcers and diffuse bleeding were seen in the colon.

An unusual cause of multiple colonic ulcerations has been described by Japanese authors [82•]. They saw multiple irregular shallow ulcers throughout the entire length of the large bowel in a patient with abdominal pain, nausea, diarrhea, and purpura on both legs. The ulcers had the features of necrotizing vasculitis and the diagnosis was made of allergic granulomatous angiitis or Churg–Strauss syndrome (CSS), a variant of periarteritis nodosa. The Churg–Strauss syndrome is characterized by asthma, hypereosinophilia, necrotizing vasculitis, and extravascular granulomas. Perforating gastrointestinal ulcerations may occur in both the large and small bowel. The authors considered the ulcers to be a complication of the vasculitis, as they were similar to ulcerations seen in Behcet's disease, systemic lupus erythematosis and Henoch–Schonlein purpura. The patient responded to steroid therapy.

Infectious colon diseases

In a colonoscopic *tour de force* [83•] 25 patients with acute colitis caused by *Shigella dysenteriae* were studied with a total of 115 colonoscopic examinations, most patients having weekly colonoscopy until no disease remained. Mucosal edema was the predominant finding in the first week of disease, but all patients developed star-shaped mucosal ulcers and friability in the second and third weeks. Punctate hemorrhagic spots with normal intervening mucosa in the absence of any persisting symptoms were evidence of healing, seen from the fourth week onward. Involvement of the colon was total in only five patients. The average duration of mucosal disease was approximately 39 days. The rectosigmoid and left colon were the area of greatest disease, which was continuous in distribution, in contrast to amebiasis, which is usually discontinuous and frequently spares the rectum, showing small, discrete ulcers with strikingly normal intervening mucosa. The paper offers an excellent description of the serial changes in shigellosis, starting with mucosal edema in the first week of disease, development of star-shaped mucosal ulcers and friability in the 2nd and 3rd weeks with punctate hemorrhagic spots but normal intervening mucosa in the healing phase.

The terminal ileum was affected in all of eight patients with *Yersinia enterocolitica* infection, with involvement of the ileocecal region in some [84•]. The terminal ileum showed round or oval elevations with or without ulcers and small ulcers were seen on the ileocecal valve and in the cecum for up to 5 weeks after the onset of symptoms. The right-sided distribution described is not always found and previous reports have demonstrated that aphthoid ulcers and edematous, erythematous mucosa may be seen in the left side of the colon in some cases.

Whenever *Streptococcus bovis* is isolated from the blood, cerebrospinal fluid or an abscess, a thorough investigation should be made to exclude occult neoplasm of the gastrointestinal tract. Patients with carcinoma of the colon have a carriage rate of *Streptococcus bovis* that is four to five times greater than that of the general population, possibly because of exposure of underlying blood vessels to the fecal flora. In seeking a cause for a patient's brain abscess a colonoscopy was performed (in spite of the absence of any gastrointestinal symptoms) and revealed a 3 cm villous adenoma on a short stalk near the splenic flexure [85•]. Infection with toxin-producing *Escherichia coli* 0157:H7 caused hemorrhagic colitis with endoscopic findings including edema, erythema and superficial ulceration, usually in a patchy and right-sided distribution. Clinical differential diagnosis includes other infectious colitidies, *Clostridium difficile*-associated colitis, idiopathic inflammatory bowel disease and ischemic colitis. If a patient has hemorrhagic colitis, stools should be specifically screened for *E. coli* 0257:H7, as routine culture media will not distinguish it from other strains of *E. coli* normally present in the stool.

Herpes simplex virus type 1 (HSV-1) usually affects the oropharynx whereas herpes simplex virus type 2 (HSV-2) affects the genital area. The internal organ most commonly involved in this viral infection is the esophagus and only rarely is herpetic involvement of the colon identified. A 76-year-old woman with bloody stools was described [87•] in whom colonoscopy showed erythema and friability of the cecal mucosa, aphthous ulcers and inflammatory pseudopolypoid lesions in the transverse and descending colon and necrotic ulcerative lesions in the rectosigmoid area. HSV-1 was isolated from the colonic biopsies and stool specimens, although intranuclear inclusions were not identified histologically. Three other cases have been reported in the literature.

Cytomegalovirus (CMV) gastroenteritis was reported in three cases [88•] in which isolated CMV ileitis was found during colonoscopy in immunocompromised patients with diarrhea after bone marrow transplantation. The colonic mucosa was normal but ileal findings ranged from extensive ulceration of to confluent exudate. Biopsies showed the CMV inclusions.

CMV anal lesions have not often been reported although rectal biopsies show CMV in about 25% of patients with the aquired immunodeficiency syndrome who have diarrhea. In a report by Puymontbrun *et al.* [89•], all of the six affected patients complained of severe or intense rectal pain and had single or multiple anal ulcers with raised edges. The taking of biopsy specimens may require general anesthesia because of the intense anal pain.

Colonic tuberculosis may be difficult to diagnose at colonoscopy. In a 71-year-old woman with diarrhea, barium enema revealed a long narrowed segment in the descending colon which, on colonoscopy, had superficial ulcerations with a prominent crater [90•]. Biopsies demonstrated only necrotic and inflammatory material with granulation tissue, but culture was positive for *Mycobacterium tuberculosis*. The authors state in their discussion that colonic tuberculosis tends to be segmental and may affect any region of the colon including the rectum and that the affected segment is usually short (5–7 cm).

Reports such as these last three are disturbing, as endoscopists do not often request bacterial or viral cultures from biopsy material. This should be thought of in any group at high–risk for a specific infection or on finding a peculiar lesion or diffuse ulcers that are obviously not malignant.

In an evaluation of 58 human immunodeficiency virus-infected patients with diarrhea [91•], neither ACBE or colonoscopy added to the diagnostic information provided by sigmoidoscopy and biopsy. This confirms the existing previous opinion of most colonoscopists.

Pinworm (threadworm) infestation is seen frequently by endoscopists (Fig. 4) but has, amazingly, never been reported. Goldenberg and Marignani [92•] demonstrate the typical thread-like undulating worms and give a brief account of the life cycle of *Enterobius vermicularis.*

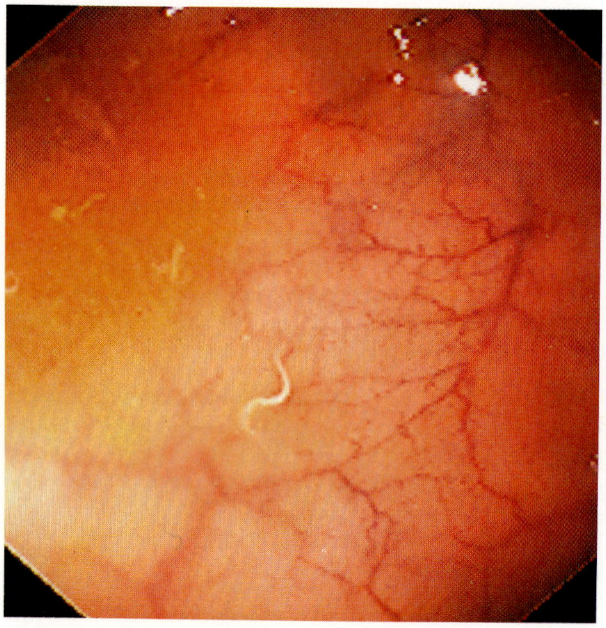

Fig. 4. Filamentous pinworm, which wriggles furiously when illuminated.

A report from Saudi Arabia [93•] details the colonoscopic appearance of schistosomiasis (*Schistosoma mansoni*) in 216 patients with colonic disease, nearly half of whom had neoplastic polyps or colorectal cancer. The endoscopic appearance was one of patchy mucosal congestion with petechia or erosions/ulcerations or both. Rectal or colonic biopsies are examined for Schistosoma ova using the 'squash' technique of crushing a fresh biopsy specimen, which is simple and rapid, and more effective than histological examination by paraffin section. Biopsies were frequently positive, even when the colonic mucosa looked normal.

The small intestine

The small intestine may be observed with a 'push' enteroscope, a Sonde-small bowel enteroscope, or endoscopy of surgically fashioned small bowel pouches or stomas. In a series of patients with Peutz–Jeghers syndrome, intraoperative colonoscopy was used to treat polyps in the small bowel [94•]. The authors used a Kocher maneuver to mobilize the duoendum surgically and to facilitate transit through the small bowel after the colonoscope was passed transorally, telescoping the small bowel on to the scope and examining the lumen as the instrument was withdrawn. We find it unnecessary to 'Kocherize' the duodenum and, although the described technique is satisfactory when looking for polyps, pleating of the small bowel tightly over the colonoscope causes so many traumatic 'crush artifacts' that inspection of each 6–10 cm segment before pleating is necessary when exploring for the site of small bowel bleeding. If an arteriovenous malformation is visualized, a serosal marking suture is placed at the site to facilitate subsequent eradication.

Complications

A review of the literature [95•] on complications of endoscopy included one short paragraph on complications of colonoscopy. With the most recent reference in 1986 and most of the data from complications referring to an article published in 1976, this review may be the latest, but it is not the greatest.

For anyone still worried about intracolonic explosions an article appeared in which the potential risk of colonic explosions was evaluated by sampling gas during colonoscopy [96•]. The authors found no case in which the gas concentration was more than 1/6 of combustible levels (4% for hydrogen, 6% for methane). They calculated, tongue-in-cheek, that if every person on earth were colonoscoped 200 million times, one explosion might be expected. However, if a polyp is found in the rectum or sigmoid colon, and its removal is attempted before total bowel preparation for total colonoscopy, the dilutional effect of air insufflation may not yet have occurred and there is a risk that explosive gases could still be present and ignite during electrocautery.

Three more cases were reported this year of splenic injury. One patient was operated for a ruptured spleen which had become symptomatic with abdominal pain 3 days following an uneventful diagnostic colonoscopy [97•]. Two others were reported [98•] who developed symptoms of pain and hypotension some hours after 'uneventful' colonoscopy. Both had the diagnosis of splenic injury confirmed by computed tomography scan and were managed non-operatively.

The endoscopic appearance of shifting blue areas due to extracolonic blood has been described above [27•].

This year, many common problems have been published for the first time. Colonoscope insertion was impeded [99•] after entering a left inguinal hernia. Any attempts

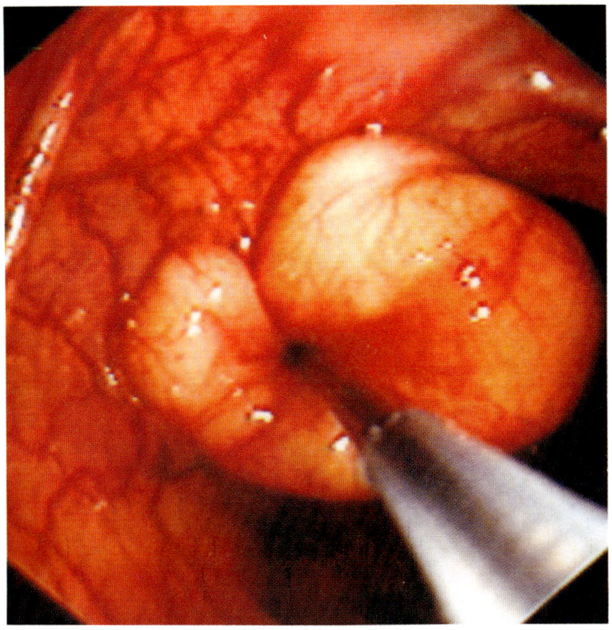

Fig. 5. Lipoma with forceps indentation (the 'pillow sign').

to withdraw increased the patient's pain; external pressure resulted in the release of the endoscope and its safe removal. During insertion the looped shaft becomes tighter and tighter in the hernial sac and then, on withdrawal of the instrument, a tight 'alpha' loop forms which 'locks' the instrument in position until external pressure is applied. My patient with this occurernce suffered no ill-effect and apparently neither did the one reported. In another case [100•] it was impossible to advance the colonoscope beyond the sigmoid colon in spite of fluoroscopic assistance. A subsequent barium enema revealed the inguinal hernia. Perforation is a sobering event but can occur in the best of hands.

The overall frequency of perforation during colonoscopy ranges from 0.06 to 0.6%. Seven perforations were reported [101•] out of 1832 colonoscopic examinations over a $2^1/_2$-year interval with an incidence of 0.38%. Perforations varied from 0.5 to 4 cm in length at surgery. Despite a 'prepared' bowel, endoscopic colonoscopic perforation invariably leads to bacterial spillage and establishment of infection over time. The authors suggest an aggressive approach with early surgical intervention when the diagnosis is made. Patients who complain of persistent pain or distention after colonoscopy deserve a careful clinical examination because radiological evidence of free gas in the peritoneal cavity is not always evident. The vast majority of the perforations occur in the rectosigmoid and mid-sigmoid regions. A primary repair or resection can be performed with safety if the interval from perforation to surgery is less than 5 hours but when fecal contamination is considerable, repair of the injured bowel with a proximal diverting colostomy should be performed.

A 'benign pneumoperitoneum' may occur following an uneventful (or eventful) colonoscopy but, in the absence of any symptoms, surgery may be withheld, although antibiotics should be instituted. Such patients should remain under careful observation in the hospital with frequent re-evaluation to assess signs of developing peritonism, in which event surgery should be considered. Any patient with a large amount of free air under the diaphragm or complaint of abdominal pain, or in whom the peritoneal cavity is visualized during colonoscopy, should have immediate surgery.

Ileus is reported after a polypectomy, the patient presenting with vomiting and abdominal pain and the radiograph showing no free air [102•]. Although the authors felt that the ileus could be related to administration of opiates it would be my impression this may be a burn response to diathermy current, a variation of the 'colon coagulation syndrome' when a full-thickness wall burn occurs. The patient may present with signs and symptoms of peritoneal irritation. Ileus could occur under this circumstance. As with this patient, most patients with colon coagulation syndrome improve spontaneously.

A rather dramatic occurrence of pneumatosis cystoides coli with palpable subcutaneous emphysema occured 7 hours following resection of two small sessile polyps from the sigmoid colon [103•]. There was a small amount of intra-abdominal air, but the patient remained afebrile and responded to 5 days of parenteral antibiotics with complete resolution of all of the air.

The danger of removing large lipomas is described in a series of seven lipomas removed over a 5-year period with three perforations. It is well known that there is a substantial risk of perforation when lipomas are removed colonoscopically and that their removal is rarely indicated if the lesions are correctly identified at endoscopy (Fig. 5). In an accompanying editorial, Christie [105•] asserts that pedunculated lipomas which are producing symptoms can and should be removed endoscopically. However, sessile lipomas larger than 2 cm are technically difficult to remove and perforation may ensue. Christie feels strongly that endoscopic excision of large sessile lipomatous lesions is inappropriate and places the patient at great risk for perforation.

A letter [106•] concerned a patient who had undergone an uneventful 'hot biopsy' diminutive polypectomy and 1 week later had massive bleeding with hypotension treated with angiography; upon recurrence colonoscopy demonstrated acutely inflamed mucosa with areas of necrosis in the cecum. The caution is issued that power settings should be diminished when working in the cecum.

Informed consent is still the vaguest area in the entire field of colonoscopy. There has been an attempt at some sort of understanding of this aspect of the examination [107•] but most physicians remain reluctant to be 'upfront' with this difficult part of the patient interface.

References and recommended reading

Papers of special interest, published within the annual period of review, have been highlighted as:

- • Of interest
- •• Of outstanding interest

1. • VILJEN M, RYTKONEN M: **Golytely Preparation for Colonoscopy — 1.5 Liters is Enough for Outpatients.** *Endoscopy* 1990, 22:168–170.

A smaller volume of electrolyte solution is sufficient for out-patient colonoscopy.

2. • LASHNER BA, WINANS CS, BLACKSTONE MO: **Randomized Clinical Trial of Two Colonoscopy Preparation Methods for Elderly Patients.** *J Clin Gastroenterol* 1990, 12:405–408.

Electrolyte lavage solution was about as effective as citrate of magnesia and enemas.

3. • VANNER SJ, MACDONALD PH, PATERSON WG, PRENTICE RS, DA COSTA LR, BECK IT: **A Randomized Prospective Trial Comparing Oral Sodium Phosphate with Standard Polyethylene Glycol-based Lavage Solution (Golytely) in the Preparation of Patients for Colonoscopy.** *Am J Gastroenterol* 1990, 85:422–427.

Fleet phospho-soda may be as effective as the electrolyte preparation.

4. • KOHLER L, VESTWEBER KH, MENNIGEN R, SOMMER H, TROIDL H: **Whole Gut Irrigation and Prepacol Laxative Preparation for Colonoscopy: a Comparison.** *Br J Surg* 1990, 77:527–529.

The electrolyte solution resulted in a better preparation.

5. • GROSSMANN R, KITTNER I, BERGBAUER M, BORSCH G, RICKEN D: **Cardiovascular Effects of Electrolyte and Polyethlene Glycol Lavage as a Method of Bowel Preparation for Colonoscopy.** *Med Welt* 1990, 41:365–370.

Electrolyte lavage is well tolerated cardiovascularly.

6. • FORDTRAN JS, SANTA-ANA CA, CLEVELAND MB: **A Low-sodium Solution for Gastrointestinal Lavage.** *Gastroenterology* 1990, **98**:11–16.

A reduced sodium sulfate electrolyte preparation is effective.

7. • DIPALMA JA, MARSHALL JB: **Comparison of a New Sulfate-free Polyethylene Glycol Electrolyte Lavage Solution Versus a Standard Solution for Colonoscopy Cleansing.** *Gastrointest Endosc* 1990, 36:285–289.

Sulfate-free electrolyte solution is safe and effective, and the taste is preferred.

8. • DIFEBO G, GIZZI G, CALO G, SIRINGO S, BRUNETTI G: **Comparison of a New Colon Lavage Solution (ISO-Giuliani) with a Standard Preparation for Colonoscopy — a Randomized Study.** *Endoscopy* 1990, 22:214–217.

An electrolyte preparation is compared with standard laxatives.

9. • HICKSON DE, COX JG, TAYLOR RG, BENNETT JR: **Enema or Picolax as Preparation for Flexible Sigmoidoscopy.** *Postgrad Med J* 1990, 66:210–211.

There was no difference between two preparations for flexible sigmoidoscopy.

10. • SLIMAK G, FLEISCHER D: **Blood-red Residual After Cherry-flavored Magnesium Citrate [letter].** *Gastrointest Endosc* 1990, 36:79–80.

Red magnesium citrate may cause effluent that looks like blood.

11. • NIV Y: **Enema Preparation for Proctosigmoidoscopy Does Not Cause Mucosal Changes.** *Endoscopy* 1990, 22:199–200.

Tap water enemas do not cause mucosal changes histologically.

12. • SAUNDERS DR, HAGGITT RC, KIMMEY MB, SILVERSTEIN FE: **Morphological Consequences of Bisacodyl on Normal Human Rectal Mucosa: Effect of a Prostaglandin E1 Analog on Mucosal Injury.** *Gastrointest Endosc* 1990, 36:101–104.

Histological effects of a Fleet enema on rectal mucosa are not prevented by a preceding prostaglandin enema.

13. • HOLLOWAY AM, LOGAN DA: **Pain Relief for Outpatient Colonoscopy: a Comparison of Alfentanil with Fentanyl.** *Anaesth Intensive Care* 1990, **18**:210–213.

An anesthesiologist's preference for colonoscopic sedation.

14. • WILCOX CM, FORSMARK CE, CELLO JP: **Utility of Droperidol for Conscious Sedation in Gastrointestinal Endoscopic Procedures.** *Gastrointest Endosc* 1990, **36**:112–115.

A method to sedate the agitated patient.

15. • HERMAN FN: **Avoidance of Sedation During Total Colonoscopy.** *Dis Colon Rectum* 1990, **33**:70–72.

Good results without drugs.

16. • HERMAN FN: **Avoidance of Sedation During?** *Dis Colon Rectum* 1990, 33:540–541.

A description of the technique for painless colonoscopy; frequent withdrawal is the secret.

17. • KEEFFE EB, OCONNOR KW: **1989 A/S/G/E Survey of Endoscopic Sedation and Monitoring Practices.** *Gastrointest Endosc* 1990, **36**(Suppl):S13–S18.

Result of a nationwide survey on sedation and monitoring during endoscopy.

18. • FINE JM: **Is Brief Arterial Oxygen Desaturation During Endoscopy Dangerous.** *Am J Gastroenterol* 1990, **85**:1314.

Suggests that hypoxia, no matter how brief, should be treated whenever it is diagnosed.

19. • GROSS JB, LONG WB: **Nasal Oxygen Alleviates Hypoxemia in Colonoscopy Patients Sedated with Midazolam and Meperidine.** *Gastrointest Endosc* 1990, **36**:26–29.

Patients receiving oxygen during colonoscopy were less likely to become hypoxic than those who did not.

20. • LANCASTER JF, GOTLEY D, BARTOLO DC, LEAPER DJ: **Hypoxia and Hypotension During Endoscopy and Colonoscopy.** *Aust NZ J Surg* 1990, **60**:271–273.

Hypoxia during colonoscopy was related to duration of the procedure.

21. • DARK DS, CAMPBELL DR, WESSELIUS LJ: **Arterial Oxygen Desaturation During Gastrointestinal Endoscopy.** *Am J Gastroenterol* 1990, **85**:1317.

Patients may desaturate during colonoscopy.

22. • FENNERTY MB, EARNEST DL, HUDSON PB, SAMPLINER RE: **Physiologic Changes During Colonoscopy.** *Gastrointest Endosc* 1990, **36**:22–25.

In many patients there is no known cause for changes in monitored events during colonoscopy.

23. • GUPTA SC, GOPALSWAMY N, SARKAR A, SURYAPRASAD AG, MARKERT RJ: **Cardiac Arrhythmias and Electrocardiographic Changes During Upper and Lower Gastrointestinal Endoscopy.** *Milit Med* 1990, **155**:9–11.

Holter monitoring during colonoscopy reveals 25% of patients with arrhythmias and 4% with transient ischemic changes.

24. • BILOTTA JJ, FLOYD JL, WAYE JD: **Arterial Oxygen Desaturation During Ambulatory Colonoscopy: Predictability, Incidence, and Clinical Insignificance.** *Gastrointest Endosc* 1990, **36**:S5–S8.

Pulse oximetry monitoring may not be worthwhile after all.

25. • FLESHNER PR, ACKROYD FW, SHELLITO PC: **The Freckle Sign — an Endoscopic Feature of the Cecum.** *Dis Col Rectum* 1990, 33:836–839.

Lymphoid nodules in the cecum produce a 'freckle' appearance with the video endoscope.

26. • COLARIAN J, CALZADA R, JASZEWSKI R: **Nodular Lymphoid Hyperplasia of the Colon in Adults — is it Common?.** *Gastrointest Endosc* 1990, 36:421–422.

Large lymphoid follicles may occur throughout the entire colon in adults.

27. PARITHIVEL VS, ROSARIO PG, SUBBARAO M: **Shifting Blue Hue**
• **Sign.** *Gastrointest Endosc* 1990, 36:422–422.
Splenic rupture may be associated with blood free in the abdominal cavity causing an interesting colonoscopic appearance.

28. SAKURAI Y, ITOH M, TSUCHIYA H, *ET AL.*: **Acute Cholecysto-**
• **colic Fistula Detected by Colonoscopy [letter].** *Gastrointest Endosc* 1990, 36:163–164.
A gallstone eroding into the colon causes an odd polypoid appearance.

29. ROBERTS SR, CHANG C, CHAPMAN T, KOONTZ PG JR, EARLY GL:
• **Colonoscopic Removal of a Gallstone Obstructing the Sigmoid Colon.** *J Tenn Med Assoc* 1990, 83:18–19.
A technique for removal of a gallstone causing colonic obstruction.

30. DUPHARE H, NIJHAWAN S, RANA S, BHARGAVA DK: **Heterotopic**
• **Gastric and Pancreatic Tissue in Large Bowel.** *Am J Gastroenterol* 1990, 85:68–71.
Gastric and pancreatic mucosa may be encountered in the colon — in this case the endoscopist thought it was a cancer.

31. CAPPELL MS, GUPTA AM: **Colonic Lesions Associated with**
• **Henoch-Schonlein Purpura.** *Am J Gastroenterol* 1990, 85:1186–1188.
Vasculitis caused ulceration resulting in occult gastrointestinal bleeding in this disease.

32. RABINOVITZ M, SCHADE RR, DINDZANS VJ, BELLE SH, VAN THIEL
• DH, GAVALER JS: **Colonic Disease in Cirrhosis. An Endoscopic Evaluation in 412 Patients.** *Gastroenterology* 1990, 99:195–199.
A description of colonoscopic findings in liver transplant candidates.

33. UNGER SW, SARANTO JR, FURLONG RJ, SCOTT JS: **Single Session**
• **Panendoscopy. Indications and Expectations for Yield.** *Am Surg* 1990, 56:144–147.
In the search for a cause of occult blood loss, perform colonoscopy first.

34. KAPADIA CR, CUTRUZZOLA FW, O'BRIEN KM, STETZ ML, ENRIQUEZ
• R, DECKELBAUM LI: **Laser-induced Fluorescence Spectroscopy of Human Colonic Mucosa. Detection of Adenomatous Transformation.** *Gastroenterology* 1990, 99:150–157.
A new contact modality which may in the future be useful to differentiate adenomas from other tissue.

35. COTHREN RM, RICHARDS KORTUM R, SIVAK MV JR, *ET AL.*: **Gas-**
• **trointestinal Tissue Diagnosis by Laser-induced Fluorescence Spectroscopy at Endoscopy.** *Gastrointest Endosc* 1990, 36:105–111.
A contact probe may distinguish adenomas from normal mucosa and hyperplastic polyps.

36. SULLIVAN MJ: **Variable Stiffening Device for Colonoscopy.**
• *Gastrointest Endosc* 1990, 36:642–643.
Description of a colonoscope stiffening device accessory.

37. ROGERS BH: **Colonoscopy with Fluoroscopy [editorial].** *Gas-*
• *trointest Endosc* 1990, 36:71–72.
Colonoscopy is better with fluoroscopy. One side of the story.

38. WAYE JD: **Colonoscopy Without Fluoroscopy [editorial].** *Gas-*
• *trointest Endosc* 1990, 36:72–73.
Fluoroscopy is not necessary for colonoscopy. One side of the story.

39. DUCE AM, BADIA-DE-YEBENES A, GARCES G: **Instrument for Di-**
• **lation of Stenotic Colorectal Anastomosis.** *Dis Col Rectum* 1990, 33:160–161.
A novel use of an old rigid dilator for dilatation of anastomotic rectal strictures.

40. TRIADAFILOPOULOS G, SARKISIAN M: **Dilatation of Radiation-in-**
• **duced Sigmoid Stricture Using Sequential Savary-guilliard Dilators — a Combined Radiologic-Endoscopic Approach.** *Dis Col Rectum* 1990, 33:1065–1067.
Use of Savary dilators in a radiation stricture.

41. PIETROPAOLO V, MASONI L, FERRARA M, MONTORI A: **Endoscopic**
• **Dilation of Colonic Postoperative Strictures.** *Surg Endosc* 1990, 4:26–30.
Postoperative anastomotic strictures may be treated with either balloon or bougies.

42. FREGONESE D, DIFALCO G, DITOMA F: **Balloon Dilatation of**
• **Anastomotic Intestinal Stenoses: Long-term Results.** *Endoscopy* 1990, 22:249–253.
Anastomotic strictures respond to balloon dilation.

43. LANGDON DE: **Extended Colonoscopy.** *Gastrointest Endosc*
• 1990, 36:637.
The longest colonoscopic examination in the world (8 hours).

44. NAKAGAWA K, MOMONO S, SASAKI Y, FURUSAWA A, UJIIE K: **Endo-**
• **scopic Examination for Fistula.** *Endoscopy* 1990, 22:208–211.
Fistulas can be dilated and entered with a tiny endoscope.

45. : **Diagnostic and Therapeutic Technology Assessment. Rigid**
• **and Flexible Sigmoidoscopies.** *JAMA* 1990, 264:89–92.
The rigid sigmoidoscope is still acceptable.

46. REX DK, LEHMAN GA, HAWES RH, O'CONNOR KW, SMITH JJ: **Per-**
• **forming Screening Flexible Sigmoidoscopy Using Colonoscopies: Experience in 500 Subjects.** *Gastrointest Endosc* 1990, 36:486–488.
Flexible sigmoidoscopy was performed with standard-length colonoscopes and the mean depth of penetration was 66 cm.

47. MARSHALL JB, HOYT TS, SEGER RM, REID JC, BEYER KL, BUTT
• JH: **Air-contrast Barium Enema Studies After Flexible Proctosigmoidoscopy: Randomized Controlled Clinical Trial.** *Radiology* 1990, 176:549–551.
ACBE can be accurately performed after flexible sigmoidscopy using room air.

48. KOMOROWSKI RA: **Histologic Spectrum of Diversion Colitis.**
• *Am J Surg Pathol* 1990, 14:548–554.
Treatment of diversion colitis with short-chain fatty acid enemas.

49. HAAS PA, FOX TA JR, SZILAGY EJ: **Endoscopic Examination**
• **of the Colon and Rectum Distal to a Colostomy.** *Am J Gastroenterol* 1990, 85:850–854.
A description of endoscopic findings in diverted colon segments.

50. SPIGELMAN AD, WILLIAMS CB, ANSELL JK, RUTTER KR, PHILLIPS
• RK: ***Pneumatosis coli*: a Source of Diagnostic Confusion.** *Br J Surg* 1990, 77:155.
A report of two sisters with pneumatosis, the previous diagnosis of polyposis disproved by needle deflation of the cysts.

51. ANDORSKY RI: **Pneumatosis Cystoides Intestinalis After Organ**
• **Transplantation.** *Am J Gastroenterol* 1990, 85:189–194.
Pneumatosis can occur in the post-transplant patient and the etiology is unknown.

52. CALLON RA JR, BRADY PG: **Toothpick Perforation of**
• **the Sigmoid Colon: an Unusual Case Associated with Erysipelothrix rhusiopathiae Septicemia.** *Gastrointest Endosc* 1990, 36:141–143.
A toothpick impacted in the colon was removed endoscopically.

53. KONERU B, SELBY R, O'HAIR DP, TZAKIS AG, HAKALA TR, STARZL
• TE: **Nonobstructing Colonic Dilatation and Colon Perforations Following Renal Transplantation.** *Arch Surg* 1990, 125:610–613.
Renal transplant recipients may develop Ogilvie's syndrome.

54. COLLIN GR, RUSSELL JC: **Endometriosis of the Colon — its**
• **Diagnosis and Management.** *Am Surg* 1990, 56:275–279.
Colonoscopy is not helpful in obstructing at colonic endometriosis.

55. WILLIAMS CB, BAILLIE J, GILLIES DF, BORISLOW D, COTTON PB:
• **Teaching Gastrointestinal Endoscopy by Computer Simulation: a Prototype for Colonoscopy and ERCP.** *Gastrointest Endosc* 1990, 36:49–54.
Computers may help to teach eye–hand coordination required in endoscopy.

56. RAWLINSON J, TATE JJ, SHEPHERD DF, ROYLE GT, BRUNTON FJ:
• **Through the Colonoscope — a Radiologist's View.** *Clin Radiol* 1990, 41:253–257.

Radiology registrars performed colonoscopy and learned from the appreciation of instant correlation with barium radiographs.

57. BRENNA E, SKREDEN K, WALDUM HL, *ET AL.*: **The Benefit of**
• **Colonoscopy.** *Scand J Gastroenterol* 1990, **25**:81–88.
Colonoscopy is worthwhile in investigation of lower gastrointestinal bleeding.

58. DENT OF, GOULSTON KJ, TENNANT CC, *ET AL.*: **Rectal Bleed-**
• **ing — Patient Delay in Presentation.** *Dis Col Rectum* 1990, 33:851.
A study of the reason why patients with rectal bleeding delayed seeking medical attention.

59. REX DK, WEDDLE RA, LEHMAN GA, *ET AL.*: **Flexible Sig-**
•• **moidoscopy Plus Air Contrast Barium Enema Versus Colonoscopy for Suspected Lower Gastrointestinal Bleeding.** *Gastroenterology* 1990, **98**:855–861.
A scientific look at the yield and indications for colonoscopy versus flexible sigmoidoscopy and ACBE. The conclusions are interesting.

60. SCHWARTZ AE, VANAGUNAS A, KAMEL PL: **Endoscopy to Evaluate**
• **Gastrointestinal Bleeding in Marathon Runners.** *Ann Intern Med* 1990, **113**:632–633.
Bleeding in runners may be ischemic.

61. WILCOX CM, OSTROFF JW: **Colonoscopic Diagnosis of**
• **Paraprosthetic-Enteric Fistula [letter].** *Gastrointest Endosc* 1990, **36**:166–167.
Intra-abdominal grafts may erode into the bowel; don't disturb any clot seen or massive bleeding may result.

62. BERTONI G, CONIGLIARO R, RICCI E, MORTILLA MG, BEDOGNI G,
• FORNACIARI G. **Endoscopic Injection Hemostasis of Colonic Diverticular Bleeding — a Case Report.** *Endoscopy* 1990, 22:154–155.
A bleeding diverticulum treated with epinephrine injection.

63. WAYE JD: **Endoscopy in Inflammatory Bowel Disease: Indi-**
• **cations and Differential Diagnosis.** *Med Clin North Am* 1990, 74:51-65.
An overview on the role of colonoscopy in inflammatory bowel disease.

64. MODIGLIANI R, MARY JY, SIMON JF, *ET AL.*: **Clinical, Biological,**
• **and Endoscopic Picture of Attacks of Crohn's Disease. Evolution on Prednisolone. Groupe d'Etude Therapeutique des Affections Inflammatoires Digestives.** *Gastroenterology* 1990, **98**:811–818.
A multicenter study took into account nine separate variables in the colon and showed a lack of correlation between clinical activity and endoscopic findings in inflammatory bowel disease.

65. HOLMQUIST L, AHREN C, FALLSTROM SP: **Clinical Disease Activ-**
• **ity and Inflammatory Activity in the Rectum in Relation to Mucosal Inflammation Assessed by Colonoscopy. A Study of Children and Adolescents with Chronic Inflammatory Bowel Disease.** *Acta Paediatr Scand* 1990, 79:527–534.
In inflammatory bowel disease there is a poor correlation between clinic disease activity and the amount of inflammation seen on endoscopy.

66. RUTGEERTS P, GEBOES K, VANTRAPPEN G, BEYLS J, KERREMANS
• R, HIELE M: **Predictability of the Postoperative Course of Crohn's Disease.** *Gastroenterology* 1990, 99:956–963.
There is a high endoscopically identified recurrence rate following ileocolonic anastomosis for Crohn's disease.

67. OLAISON G, SJODAHL R, TAGESSON C: **Glucocorticoid Treat-**
• **ment in Ileal Crohn's Disease: Relief of Symptoms but not of Endoscopically Viewed Information.** *Gut* 1990, 31:325–328.
There is a lack of correlation between endoscopic findings and patient's symptoms in inflammatory bowel disease.

68. KELLER KM, BENDER SW, KIRCHMANN H, *ET AL.*: **Diagnostic**
• **Significance of Epithelioid Granulomas in Crohn's Disease in Children. Multicenter Paediatric Crohn's Disease Study Group.** *J Pediatr Gastroenterol Nutr* 1990, **10**:27–32.
Granulomas were found in 57% of rectal biopsies in patients with Crohn's disease.

69. BOZDECH JM, FARMER RG: **Diagnosis of Crohn's Disease.**
• *Hepato-gastroenterol* 1990, **37**:8–17.
Colonoscopy has a role in the diagnosis of Crohn's disease.

70. ZINBERG J, MOLINAS S, DAS KM: **Double-blind Placebo-con-**
• **trolled Study of Olsalazine in the Treatment of Ulcerative Colitis.** *Am J Gastroenterol* 1990, **85**:562.
A drug evaluation in ulcerative colitis using the colonoscope.

71. DIFEBO G, MIGLIOLI M, LAURI A, *ET AL.*: **Endoscopic Assess-**
• **ment of Acute Inflammation of the Ileal Reservoir after Restorative Ileo-anal Anastomosis.** *Gastrointest Endosc* 1990, 36:6–9.
A description of pouchitis within ileal reservoirs.

72. BOLEY SJ: **Colonic Ischemia — 25 Years Later.** *Am J Gas-*
• *troenterol* 1990, **84**:931–934.
'State-of-the-art' review lecture on this favorite topic.

73. INDUDHARA R, KOCHHAR R, MEHTA SK, CHUGH KS, YADVA RVS:
• **Acute Colitis in Renal Transplant Recipients.** *Am J Gastroenterol* 1990, **85**:964–968.
Severe progressive colitis may occur in renal transplant recipients.

74. STOLTE M, RITTER M, BORCHARD F, KOCHSCHERRER G: **Collage-**
• **nous Gastroduodenitis on Collagenous Colitis.** *Endoscopy* 1990, 22:186–187.
Similar to collagenous colitis can also affect the duodenum — normal appearance, abnormal histology.

75. GIARDIELLO FM, HANSEN FC III, LAZENBY AJ, *ET AL.*: **Collagenous**
• **Colitis in Setting of Nonsteroidal Antiinflammatory Drugs and Antibiotics.** *Dig Dis Sci* 1990, **35**:257–260.
Men can also get collagenous colitis although it is commoner in women.

76. VAN TILBURG AJ, LAM HG, SELDENRIJK CA, *ET AL.*: **Familial Oc-**
• **currence of Collagenous Colitis. A Report of Two Families.** *J Clin Gastroenterol* 1990, **12**:279–285.
Collagenous colitis can occur in families.

77. MASHAKO MN, SONSINO E, NAVARRO J, *ET AL.*: **Microscopic Coli-**
• **tis: a New Cause of Chronic Diarrhea in Children.** *J Pediatr Gastroenterol Nutr* 1990, **10**:21–26.
Microscopic colitis can occur in children.

78. OKADA M, IMAMURA K, YAO T, SAKURAI T, IWASHITA A, MURAYAMA
• H: **The Evolution of the Lesion in the Solitary Rectal Ulcer Syndrome.** *Gastrointest Endosc* 1990, 36:621–623.
A chronicle of solitary rectal ulcer evolving into multiple raised rectal lesions.

79. TANDON RK, ATMAKURI SP, MEHRA NK, MALAVIYA AN, TANDON
• HD, CHOPRA P: **Is Solitary Rectal Ulcer a Manifestation of a Systemic Disease?** *J Clin Gastroenterol* 1990, 12:286–290.
An unconvincing attempt to involve systemic disease with solitary rectal ulcers.

80. GIZZI G, VILLANI V, BRANDT G, PAGANELLI GM, DIFEBO G, BIASCO
• G. **Ano-rectal Lesions in Patients Taking Suppositories Containing Non-Steroidal Anti-inflammatory Drugs (NSAID).** *Endoscopy* 1990, 22:146–148.
Severe progressive rectal lesions may occur from non-steroidal anti-inflammatory drug suppositories.

81. SAITO H, OSHIMI K, NAGASAKO K, *ET AL.*: **Endoscopic Appear-**
• **ance of the Colon and Small Intestine of a Patient with Hemorrhagic Enteric Graft-vs-host Disease.** *Dis Col Rectum* 1990, 33:695.
Transplant recipients may develop diffuse intestinal ulcerations.

82. SHIMAMOTO C, HIRATA I, OHSHIBA S, FUJIWARA S, NISHIO M:
• **Churg-Strauss Syndrome (Allergic Granulomatous Angiitis) with Peculiar Multiple Colonic Ulcers.** *Am J Gastroenterol* 1990, **85**:316–319.
A systemic syndrome with vasculitis causing multiple ulcers.

83. KHUROO MS, MAHAJAN R, ZARGAR SA, *ET AL.*: **The Colon**
• **in Shigellosis: Serial Colonoscopic Appearances in Shigella Dysenteriae I.** *Endoscopy* 1990, 22:35–38.
Frequently repeated colonoscopies document the edema-ulceration-resolution sequence.

84. MATSUMOTO T, IIDA M, MATSUI T, *ET AL.*: **Endoscopic Findings**
• **in Yersinia-enterocolitica Enterocolitis.** *Gastrointest Endosc* 1990, 36:583–587.
Description of ileo-colonic ulceration in eight cases.

85. EMILIANI VJ, CHODOS JE, COMER GM, HOLNESS LG, SCHWARTZ
• AJ: **Streptococcus bovis Brain Abscess Associated with an Occult Colonic Villous Adenoma.** *Am J Gastroenterol* 1990, 85:78–80.
When *Streptococcus bovis* is in the blood one should look in the colon too — a villous adenoma was found.

86. GRIFFIN PM, OLMSTEAD LC, PETRAS RE: ***Escherichia coli*** **0157-**
• **H7-associated Colitis — a Clinical and Histological Study of 11 Cases.** *Gastroenterology* 1990, 99:142–149.
Ask the laboratory to look specifically for this organism in hemorrhagic colitis (they won't find it routinely).

87. COLEMONT LJ, PEN JH, PELCKMANS PA, DEGRYSE HR, PATTYN
• SR, VAN MAERCKE YM: **Herpes Simplex Virus Type 1 Colitis: an Unusual Cause of Diarrhea.** *Am J Gastroenterol* 1990, 85:1182–1185.
Colitis following viral infection.

88. LEPINSKI SM, HAMILTON JW: **Isolated Cytomegalovirus**
• **Ileitis Detected by Colonoscopy.** *Gastroenterology* 1990, 98:1704–1706.
CMV can selectively affect the small bowel in immunosuppressed patients.

89. PUYMONTBRUN T, GANANSIA R, LEMARCHAND N, DELECHENAULT
• P, DENIS J: **Anal Ulcerations Due to Cytomegalovirus in Patients with AIDS — Report of 6 Cases.** *Dis Colon Rectum* 1990, 33:1041–1043.
CMV may cause severe ulcers and rectal pain associated with anal ulcerations.

90. MEDINA E, ORTI E, TOME A, QUILES F, CANELLES P, MERTINEZ
• A: **Segmental Tuberculosis of the Colon Diagnosed by Colonoscopy.** *Endoscopy* 1990, 22:188–190.
Another description of colonic tuberculosis, a case with descending colon stricture.

91. CONNOLLY GM, FORBES A, GLEESON JA, GAZZARD BG: **The Value**
• **of Barium Enema and Colonoscopy in Patients Infected with HIV.** *AIDS* 1990, 4:687–689.
It is not worthwhile to colonoscope patients with human immunodeficiency virsus presenting with diarrhea.

92. GOLDENBERG SP, MARIGNANI P: **The Endoscopic Diagnosis of**
• **Colonic Enterobiasis.** *Gastrointest Endosc* 1990, 36:309–310.
The first endoscopic description of pinworms in the colon.

93. MOHAMED AR, AL KARAWI M, YASAWY MI: **Schistosomal Colonic**
• **Disease.** *Gut* 1990, 31:439–442.
A description of the endoscopic appearance of schistosomal disease in 216 patients.

94. PANOS RG, POELKA FG, NOGUERAS JJ: **Peutz-Jeghers Syndrome**
• **— a Call for Intraoperative Enteroscopy.** *Am Surg* 1990, 56:331–333.
Intraoperative enteroscopy is useful for small bowel location of polyps.

95. HART R, CLASSEN M: **Complications of Diagnostic Gastroin-**
• **testinal Endoscopy.** *Endoscopy* 1990, 22:229.
An overview of endoscopic complications (with outdated colonic references).

96. STROCCHI A, BOND JH, ELLIS C, LEVITT MD: **Colonic Concen-**
• **trations of Hydrogen and Methane Following Colonoscopic Preparation with an Oral Lavage Solution.** *Gastrointest Endosc* 1990, 36:580–582.
Colonic explosions are unlikely.

97. MERCHANT AA, CHENG EH: **Delayed Splenic Rupture After**
• **Colonoscopy [letter].** *Am J Gastroenterol* 1990, 85:906–907.
A post-colonoscopic ruptured spleen, symptomatic 3 days later.

98. ROCKEY DC, WEBER JR, WRIGHT TL, WALL SD: **Splenic**
• **Injury Following Colonoscopy.** *Gastrointest Endosc* 1990, 36:306–309.
Two cases with splenic rupture following colonoscopy.

99. LEISSER A, DELPRE G, KADISH U: **Colonoscope Incarceration**
• **— an Avoidable Event.** *Gastrointest Endosc* 1990, 36:637–638.
Take care not to let the colonoscope stick in an inguinal hernia; resolve it by pushing externally.

100. FULP SR, GILLIAM JH III. **Beware of the Incarcerated Hernia**
• **[letter].** *Gastrointest Endosc* 1990, 36:318–319.
A hernia resulted in difficulty passing the colonoscope.

101. SOON JC, SHANG NS, GOH PM, RAUFF A: **Perforation of the**
• **Large Bowel During Colonoscopy in Singapore.** *Am Surg* 1990, 56:285–288.
Early surgical exploration after colonoscopic perforation is advised.

102. STERMER E, LEVY N: **Ileus as a Complication of Colonoscopy**
• **[letter].** *Am J Gastroenterol* 1990, 85:333–334.
Ileus followed polypectomy.

103. MCCOLLISTER DL, HAMMERMAN HJ. **Air, Air, Everywhere: Pneu-**
• **matosis Cystoides Coli after Colonoscopy [letter].** *Gastrointest Endosc* 1990, 36:75–76.
Pneumatosis following polypectomy.

104. PFEIL SA, WEAVER MG, ABDUL-KARIM FW, YANG P: **Colonic Lipo-**
• **mas: Outcome of Endoscopic Removal.** *Gastrointest Endosc* 1990, 36:435–438.
Three out of four patients who had large lipomas resected endoscopically resulted in perforation.

105. CHRISTIE JP: **The Removal of Lipomas.** *Gastrointest Endosc*
• 1990, 36:532–533.
A plea for leaving these benign tumors alone as most do not require removal.

106. NELSON AM: **Delayed Hemorrhage Following 'Hot Biopsy'**
• **of a Diminutive Colonic Polyp.** *Gastrointest Endosc* 1990, 36:418.
Be careful using the hot biopsy forceps.

107. MARK JS, SPIRO H: **Informed Consent for Colonoscopy. A**
• **Prospective Study.** *Arch Intern Med* 1990, 150:777–780.
Physicians are paternalistic in their attitude toward informed consent.

Bibliography of the current world literature

This bibliography is compiled by gastrointestinal endoscopists from the journals listed at the end of this publication. It is based on literature entered into our database between 1st January 1990 and 31st December 1990 (articles are generally added to the database about two and a half months after publication). In addition, the bibliography contains every paper annotated by reviewers; these references were obtained from a variety of bibliographic databases and published between the beginning of the review period and the time of going to press. The bibliography has been grouped into topics that relate to the reviews in this issue.

● Papers considered by the reviewers to be of interest.
●● Papers considered by the reviewers tq be of outstanding interest.

The number in square brackets following a selected paper, e.g. [7], refers to its number in the annotated references of the corresponding review.

Contents

Endoscopy of the oesophagus

Aguado JM, Napal J, Alsar MJ: **Pneumococcal Bacteraemia - a Late Complication Following Endoscopic Variceal Sclerotherapy [letter].** *Postgrad Med J* 1990, **66**:790–791.

● Anderson JR: **Oesophageal Injury. Part 1. The Changing Face of the Management of Instrumental Perforations.** *Gullet* 1990, **1**:10–15. **[30].**

Bailey AD, Goldner F: **Can Clinicians Accurately Assess Esophageal Dilation Without Fluoroscopy.** *Gastrointest Endosc* 1990, **36**:373–375.

Bancewicz J: **Cancer of the Oesophagus [editorial].** *Br Med J [Clin Res]* 1990, **300**:3.

● Barcena R, Erdozain JC, Lopez-San Roman A, Perez Hernandez F, Ledo L, Boixeda D: **Tuberculous Mediastinal Adenopathy Mimicking Esophageal Leiomyoma.** *Endoscopy* 1990, **22**:57–58. **[33].**

● Barkin JS, Guelrud M, Reiner DK, Goldberg RI, Phillips RS: **Forceful Balloon Dilation: an Outpatient Procedure for Achalasia.** *Gastrointest Endosc* 1990, **36**:123–126. **[25].**

●● Barr H, Krasner N, Raouf A, Walker RJ: **Prospective Randomized Trial of Laser Therapy Only and Laser Therapy Followed by Endoscopic Intubation for Palliation of Malignant Dysphagia.** *Gut* 1990, **31**:252–257. **[39].**

● Bartelsman JFWM, Lange JMA, Van Leeuwen R, Van Der Tweel JG, Tytgat GNJ: **Acute Primary HIV-Esophagitis.** *Endoscopy* 1990, **22**:184–187. **[6].**

● Bhutiawi RP, Warrington AJ: **Not a Way to do Esophageal Bougienage.** *Endoscopy* 1990, **22**:239. **[31].**

● Bonacini M, Laine L, Gal AA, Lee MH, Martin SE, Strigle S: **Prospective Evaluation of Blind Brushing of the Esophagus for Candida Esophagitis in Patients with Human Immuno-Deficiency Virus Infection.** *Am J Gastroenterol* 1990, **85**, **4**:385–389. **[5].**

●● Boyce WH Jr: **Drug-induced Esophageal and Gastric Damage.** *Current Topics in Gastroenterology and Hepatology, Edited by Tytgat GNJ, Van Blankenstein M. New York, Stuttgart: Thiem* 1990, :pp 170–195. **[11].**

●● Buset M, Des Marez B, Cremer M: **Endoscopic Palliative Intubation of the Esophagus Invaded by Lung Cancer.** *Gastrointest Endosc* 1990, **36**:357–359. **[43].**

Buset M, Marez BD, Cremer M: **Endoscopic Palliative Intubation of the Esophagus Invaded by Lung Cancer.** *Gastrointest Endosc* 1990, **36**:357–359.

Buto SK, Tsang TK, Sielaff GW, Gutstein LL, Meiselman MS: **Bay Leaf Impaction in the Esophagus and Hypopharynx.** *Ann Intern Med* 1990, **113**:82–83.

Carrlocke DL: **Acute Gallstone Pancreatitis and Endoscopic Therapy [Review].** *Endoscopy* 1990, **22**:180–183.

● Chowhan NM: **Injurous Effects of Radiation on the Esophagus.** *Am J Gastroenterol* 1990, **85**:115–120. **[13].**

Claudel-Bonvoisin S, Descos L, Chatelard P, Souquet JC, Pasquier J: **Carcinoma of the Esophagus and Sclerotherapy for Esophageal Varices (in French) [letter].** *Gastroenterol Clin Biol* 1990, **14**:189.

Desmorat H, Cales P, Vinel JP, Maquin P, Caucanas JP, Combis JM, Pascal JP: **Obstructive Intramural Hematoma of the Esophagus - an Unusual Complication of Endoscopic Variceal Sclerotherapy [in French].** *Gastroenterol Clin Biol* 1990, **14**:581–585.

Domingo JJ, Lorenzo AD, Castro LS, Franco DC, Menchen P: **Endoscopic Management of Foreign Bodies in the Gastrointestinal Tract [in Spanish].** *Rev Esp Enferm Dig* 1990, **77**:259–262.

Domingo JJS, Castro LS, Lorenzo AD, Franco DC, Deayala VP, Senent C: **Endoscopy in Corrosive Oesophagitis and Gastritis [in Spanish].** *Rev Esp Enferm Dig* 1990, **77**:176–178.

● Domschke W, Foerster ECh, Matek W, Rödl W: **Self-expanding Mesh Stent for Esophageal Cancer Stenosis.** *Endoscopy* 1990, **22**:134–136. **[45].**

Donnelly PK, Lavelle J, Carrlocke D: **Massive Haemorrhage Following Endoscopic Transgastric Drainage of Pancreatic Pseudocyst.** *Br J Surg* 1990, **77**:758–759.

Dumas O, Barthelemy C, Billard F, Dumollard JM, Boucheron S, Calmard P, Rousset H, Audigier JC: **Isolated Melanosis of the Esophagus — Systematic Endoscopic Diagnosis [letter].** *Endoscopy* 1990, **22**:94–95.

● Eda Y, Asaki S, Yamagata L, *et al.*: **Endoscopic Treatment for Submucosal Tumors of the Esophagus: Studies in 25 Patients.** *Gastroenterol JPN* 1990, **25**, **4**:411–416. **[34].**

● Fennerty B, Sampliner R, Garewal H: **Esophageal Ulceration Assocaited with 13-*cis*-Retinoic Acid Therapy in Patients with Barrett's Esophagus.** *Gastrointest Endosc* 1989, **35**, **5**:442–443. **[3].**

● Ferguson MK, Migliore M, Staszak VM, Little AG: **Early Evaluation and Therapy for Caustic Esophageal Injury.** *Am J Surg* 1989, **157**:116–120. **[10].**

Fernandez CM, Ledo L, Cunqueiro R, Naranjo A, Rodriguez D, Pereira S, Pallares A: **Early Esophageal Crohn's Disease — an Endoscopic View.** *Gastrointest Endosc* 1990, **36**:303–304.

● Fleischer D: **Non-laser Techniques for Palliative Cancer Treatment.** *In Current Topics in Gastroenterology and Hepatology Edited by Tytgat GNJ, Van Blankenstein M. New York, Stuttgart: Geo* 1990, :pp 330–335. **[38].**

● Fregonese D, Di Falco G, Di Toma F: **Balloon Dilatation of Anastomotic Intestinal Stenoses: Long-term Results.** *Endoscopy* 1990, **22**:153–249. **[24].**

● Függer R, Niederle B, Jantsch H, Schiessel R, Schultz F: **Endoscopic Tube Implantation for the Palliation of Malignant Esophageal Stenosis.** *Endoscopy* 1990, **22**:101–104. **[42].**

●● Goldschmid S, Boyce Jr HW, Brown JI, Brady PG, Nord HJ, Lyman GH: **A New Objective Measurement of Esophageal Lumen Patency.** *Am J Gastroenterol* 1989, **84**:12545–1258. **[20].**

Graham JR: **Upper Esophageal Sphincter Spasm as a Marker of Monilial Esophagitis.** *Gastrointest Endosc* 1990, **36**:77.

Gubbins GP, Nensey YM, Schubert TT, Batra SK: **Barogenic Perforation of the Esophagus Distal to a Stricture after Endoscopy.** *J Clin Gastroenterol* 1990, **12**:310–312.

Hashizume M, Kitano S, Yamaga H, Wada H, Sugimachi K: **Eradication of Oesophageal Varices Recurring after Portal Non- Decompressive Surgery by Injection Sclerotherapy.** *Br J Surg* 1990, **77**:940–943.

● Hayashi R, Nakayama J, Inoue A, Komatsu O, Katsuyama T, Inoue K: **Squamous Cell Papilloma of the Esophagus — a Report of Two Cases and a Review of the Literature.** *Dig Endosc* 1990, **2**:377–382. **[32].**

HORDIJK ML, DEES J, VAN BLANKENSTEIN M: **The Management of Malignant Esophago-**
● **Respiratory Fistulas with a Cuffed Prosthesis.** *Endoscopy* 1990, **22**:241–244. **[44].**

HORNTRICH J, HINKEL M: **The Exstirpation of Strictures by Cauterization of the Oesophagus — an Alternative of the Bougienage Treatment.** *Z Klin Med* 1990, **45**:1665–1708.

INK O, LASCAR G, PELLETIER G, SCHOUX JB, ETIENNE JP: **Hepatocellular Carcinoma and Variceal Sclerotherapy [in French].** *Gastroenterol Clin Biol* 1990, **14**:524–528.

ISAACS PET, MARTINS JCR, EDWARDS S, FAGG NLK, MAISEY MN, SLADEN GE: **Assessment of Gastro-esophageal Reflux Disease — Comparison of Reflux Scintigraphy with Endoscopy Biopsy and Esophageal PH Monitoring.** *Hepatogastroenterology* 1990, **37**:198–200.

ISOLAURI OF, AIRO I: **Benign Mucous Membrane Pemphigoid Involving the**
● **Esophagus: a Report of Two Cases Treated with Dilation.** *Gastrointest Endosc* 1989, **35, 6**:569–571. **[18].**

KA L, WU W-X: **A New Retrograde Dilation Method for Esophageal Cicatrical**
● **Stenosis: Gulp and Pull Dilator with Cushion.** *Dig Surg* 1990, **7**:175–178. **[22].**

KIM OD, CANTAVE I, SCHLESINGER PK: **Esophageal Involvement by Cutaneous T-cell Lymphoma, Mycosis Fungoides Type: Diagnosis by Endoscopic Biopsy.** *J Clin Gastroenterol* 1990, **12**:178–182.

KLEIN I: **Resourceful Management of Esophageal Food Impaction.** *Gastrointest*
● *Endosc* , :3680. **[28].**

LAM TS, LACK E, BENJAMIN SB: **Compact Parakeratosis of Esophageal Mucosa: a Non-**
● **specific Lesion Mimicking 'Leukoplakia'.** *Gastrointest Endosc* 1990, **36**:397–399. **[15].**

LIGHTDALE CJ, BOTET JF: **Esophageal Carcinoma: Pre-operative Staging and Evaluation of Anastomotic Recurrence.** *Gastrointest Endosc* 1990, **36 (suppl)**:S11–S16.

MAI H, SANOWSKI RA: **Endoscopic Diagnosis of the Panje Prosthesis in a Patient with Upper Esophageal Stricture.** *Gastrointest Endosc* 1990, **36**:404–406.

MASCLEE AAM, DE BEST ACAM, DE GRAAF R, CLUYSENAER OJJ, JANSEN JBMJ: **Ambulatory 24-hour PH-metry in the Diagnosis of Gastroesophageal Reflux Disease. Determination of Criteria and Relation to Endoscopy.** *Scand J Gastroenterol* 1990, **25**:225–230.

MATHUR SK, SHIRHATTI RGP, DALVI AN, GONDHALEKAR RA, SABNIS SB: **Endoscopic Esophageal Intubation for Treatment of Chronic Esophago-cutaneous Fistula.** *Gastrointest Endosc* 1990, **36**:67–68.

MAXTON DG: **Guide Wire Distance Marks for Oesophageal Dilatation.** *Gut* 1990, **31**:564.

MCCLAVE SA, WRIGHT RA, BRADY PG: **Prospective Randomized Study of Maloney**
●● **Esophageal Dilation —Blinded Versus Fluoroscopic Guidance.** *Gastrointest Endosc* 1990, **36**:272–275. **[23].**

MCCORD GS, CLOUSE RE: **Pill-induced Esophageal Strictures: Clinical Features and**
● **Risk Factors for Development.** *Am J Med* 1990, **88**:512–517. **[12].**

MISUMI A, HARADA K, MURAKAMI A, ARIMA K, KONDO H, AKAGI M, YAGI Y, IKEDA T, BABA K,
● KABORI Y, MATSUKANE H: **Role of Lugol Dye Endoscopy in the Diagnosis of Early Esophageal Cancer.** *Endoscopy* 1990, **22**:12–16. **[36].**

MISUMI A, HARADA K, MURAKAMI A, ARIMA K, KONDO H, AKAGI M, YAGI Y, IKEDA T, KABORI Y,
● MATSUKANE H, BABA K: **Early Diagnosis of Esophageal Cancer: Analysis of 11 Cases of Esophageal Cancer.** *Ann Surg* 1989, **210**:732–739. **[35].**

MORETO M, ZABALLA M, IBANEZ S: **Endoscopic Incision as an Alternative to**
● **Bougienage in the Treatment of Peptic Esophageal Stricture.** *Endoscopy* 1990, **22**:105–109. **[21].**

PALAZZO L, GAYET B, VILGRAIN V, MOLAS G, AMOUYAL P, ROSEAU G, PONSOT P, AMOUYAL G, FEKETE F, PAOLAGGI JA: **Endoscopic Ultrasound and Esophageal Carcinoma — Results of a Prospective Study [in French].** *Gastroenterol Clin Biol* 1990, **14**:428–436.

PATERLINI A, BUFFOLI F, CESARI P, GRAFFEO M: **£alliative Treatment with the Bicap of Recurrent Neoplastic Stenosis of the Colon-rectum Anastomosis [letter].** *Endoscopy* 1990, **22**:96.

PAYNE-JAMES JJ, SPILLER RC, MISIEWICZ JJ, SILK DBA: **Use of Ethanol-induced Tumor**
● **Necrosis to Palliate Dysphagia in Patients with Esophagogastric Cancer.** *Gastrointest Endosc* 1990, **36**:43–46. **[40].**

PEDRO-BOTET J, MIRALLES R, SAULEDA J, RUBIÉS-PRAT J: **Idiopathic Ulcer of the**
● **Esophagus in the AIDS Syndrome: a Potential Life-threatening Complication.** *Gastrointest Endoscopy* 1989, **35, 5**:470476. **[7].**

PREMACHANDRA DJ, MCRAE D, PRINSLEY P: **Biopsy of Neck Lumps in Adults Should be Preceded by Examination of the Upper Aerodigestive Tract.** *Postgrad Med J* 1990, **66**:113–115.

RABINOVICI R, KATZ E, GOLDIN E, AYALON A: **The Danger of High Compliance Balloons**
● **for Esophageal Dilatation in Achalasia.** *Endoscopy* 1990, 22:63–64. **[26].**

RENÉ E, VERDON R, AIDS GIT GROUP: **Upper Gastrointestinal Tract Infections in**
● **AIDS.** *Clin Gastroenterol Bailieres* 1990, **4**:339–359. **[9].**

SAEED ZA, MICHALETZ PA, FEINER SD, WOODS KL, GRAHAM DY: **A New Endoscopic**
● **Method for Managing Food Impaction in the Esophagus.** *Endoscopy* 1990, **22**:226–228. **[27].**

SALA T, PONCE J, PERTEJO V, LINARES M, GARRIGUES V, BERENGUER J: **Early Complications of Pneumatic Dilatation in the Treatment of Motor Disorders of the Esophagus [in Spanish].** *Rev Esp Enferm Dig* 1990, **77**:255–258.

SARTORI S, MIELSEN I, TREVISANI L, PAZZI P, MALACARNE P: **Barrett's Esophagus after**
● **Antineoplastic Chemotherapy.** *Endoscopy* 1990, **22**:152. **[2].**

SASAJIMA K, WATANABE M, TAKUBO K, TAKAI A, YAMASHITA K, ONDA M: **Mucoepidermoid Carcinoma of the Esophagus — Report of Two Cases and Review of the Literature.** *Endoscopy* 1990, **22**:140–143.

SHERLOCK S: **Esophageal Varices.** *Am J Surg* 1990, **160**:9–13.

STARITZ M, RAMBOW A: **Measurement of Hydrostatic Pressure in Oesophageal Varices (in German).** *Dtsch Med Wochenschr* 1990, **115**:382–385.

STOOPACK PM, DE SILVA R, RAUFMAN J-P: **Inflammatory Double-barrelled Esophagus**
● **in Two Patients with AIDS.** *Gastrointest Endoscopy* 1990, **36**:394–396. **[8].**

TADA S, *ET AL.*: **Endoscopic and Biopsy Findings of Upper Digestive Tract in**
● **Patients with Amyloidosis.** *Gastrointest Endosc* 1990, **36**:10–14. **[14].**

TYTGAT GNJ: **Dilatation Therapy of Benign Esophageal Stenoses.** *World J Surg* 1989, **13**:142–148. **[19].**

TYTGAT GNJ: **Esophageal Perforation: Diagnosis, Prevention and Therapy.** *Eur J*
●● *Gastroenterol Hepatol* 1990, **2**:193–202. **[29].**

TYTGAT GNJ: **Endoscopic Therapy of Esophageal Cancer: Possibilities and**
● **Limitations.** *Endoscopy* 1990, **22**:263–267. **[37].**

TYTGAT GNJ, NICOLAI JJ, REMAN FC: **Efficacy of Different Doses of Cimetidine in the**
● **Treatment of Reflux Esophagitis. A Review of Three Large, Double-Blind Controlled Trials.** *Gastroenterology* 1990, **99**:629–634. **[1].**

WANG WM, CHEN CY, JAN CM, CHEN LT, WU DC: **Central Nervous System Infection after Endoscopic Injection Sclerotherapy.** *Am J Gastroenterol* 1990, **85**:865–867.

WESTABY D, WILLIAMS R: **Status of Sclerotherapy for Variceal Bleeding in 1990.** *Am J Surg* 1990, **160**:32–36.

WITTE JT, ICKEN JN, LLOYD ML: **Induction of Esophageal Bullae by Endoscopy in**
● **Benign Mucous Membrane Pemphigoid.** *Gastrointest Endosc* 1989, **35**:566–568. **[17].**

WRIGHT RA, O'CONNOR KW: **A Pilot Study of Endoscopic Injection**
● **Chemo/Sclerotherapy of Esophageal Carcinoma.** *Gastrointest Endosc* 1990, **36**:47–48. **[41].**

Endoscopy of the stomach

AABAKKEN L, LARSSEN S, OSNES M: **Visual Analogue Scales for Endoscopic Evaluation**
● **of Nonsteroidal Anti-Inflammatory Drug-induced Mucosal Damage in the Stomach and Duodenum.** *Scand J Gastroenterol* 1990, **25**:443–448. **[9].**

AMANO Y, ISHIHARA S, TAKATORI Y, IMAOKA T, WATANABE M, FUKUMOTO S: **Endoscopic**
● **Retrospective Study on Gastric Malignant Lymphoma — with Special Reference to the Appearance of the Initial Lesion.** *Dig Endosc* 1990, **2**:396–401. **[36].**

ANAI H, OKADA Y, OKUBO K, *ET AL.*: **Gastric Syphilis Simulating Linitis Plastica Type**
● **of Gastric Cancer.** *Gastrointest Endosc* 1990, **36**:624–626. **[13].**

ANDRUS CH, DEAN PA, PONSKY JL: **Evaluation of Safe, Effective Intravenous Sedation**
● **for Utilization in Endoscopic Procedures.** *Surg Endosc* 1990, **4**:179–183. **[2].**

AWAD JA, LEE EY, WANG TC, DESCHRYVER-KECSKEMETI K, CLOUSE RE: **Effect of Mucosal Thickening Near Gastric Carcinoma on the Endoscopic Diagnosis of Malignancy.** *Dig Dis Sci* 1990, **35**:317–320. **[33].**

BERMAN IR: **Monitoring and Patient Safety [letter].** *Gastrointest Endosc* 1990, **36**:160. **[6].**

BHASIN DK, NAGI B, KOCHHAR R, SINGH L, GUPTA NM, MEHTA SK: **Endoscopic Manage-**
● **ment of Chronic Organo-**
Axonial Volvulus of the Stomach. *Am J Gastroenterol* 1990, **85**:1486–1488. **[51].**

BINMOELLER KF, KATON RM: **Bipolar Electrocoagulation for Watermelon Stomach.**
● *Gastrointest Endosc* 1990, **36**:399–402. **[12].**

CASTEEL HB, FIEDOREK SC, KIEL EA: **Arterial Blood Oxygen Desaturation in Infants**
● **and Children During Upper Gastrointestinal Endoscopy.** *Gastrointest Endosc* 1990, **36**:489–493. **[4].**

CHAMBON J, GAUDRIC M, AMOUYAL P, CHAUSSADE S, CHAPUIS Y, LOUVEL A, GUERRE J: **Achalasia Associated with Gastric Leiomyoma - Value of Endoscopic Sonography [in French] [letter].** *Gastroenterol Clin Biol* 1990, **14**:605–607.

CHAWLA SK, RAMANI K, PRESTI PL: **The Honeycomb Stomach: Coalesced Gastric**
● **Angiodysplasia.** *Gastrointest Endosc* 1990, **36**:516–518. **[41].**

CHINITZ MA, BERTRAND G: **Endoscopic Removal of Toothbrushes.** *Gastrointest Endosc* 1990, **36**:527–530. **[44].**

CHUNG RS, SCHERTZER M: **Pathogenesis of Complications of Percutaneous**
● **Endoscopic Gastrostomy. A Lesson in Surgical Principles.** *Am Surg* 1990, **56**:134–137. **[22].**

CULLADO MJ, SLEZAK FA, PORTER JA: **Repeat Percutaneous Endoscopic Gastrostomy (PEG): an Outpatient Procedure.** *Surg Endosc* 1990, **4**:173–174. **[21].**

DAVIS JB JR, BOWDEN TA JR, RIVES DA: **Percutaneous Endoscopic Gastrostomy. do**
● **Surgeons and Gastroenterologists Get the Same Results?** *Am Surg* 1990, **56**:47–51. **[16].**

DEMIRCI S, GOHCHI A: **A Comparative Study for Fiberoptic and Video Endoscope**
● **Determination of the Extent in Minimal Changes of Gastric Mucosa Using Indigo Dye Spraying.** *Surg Endosc* 1990, **4**:80–82. **[30].**

DOMINGO JJ, LORENZO AD, CASTRO LS, FRANCO DC, MENCHEN P: **Endoscopic Management of Foreign Bodies in the Gastrointestinal Tract [in Spanish].** *Rev Esp Enferm Dig* 1990, **77**:259–262.

DONAHUE PE, CARVALHO PJPC, DAVIS PE, SHEN Y-JE, MIIDLA I, BOMBECK T, NYHUS LM:
● **Endoscopic Sclerosis of the Gastric Cardia for Prevention of Experimental Gastroesophageal Reflux.** *Gastrointest Endosc* 1990, **36**:253–256. **[50].**

ESCOURROU J, DELVAUX M, BUSCAIL L, DARMANA R, FREXINOS J, MORUCCI JP, RIBET A: **First**
● **Clinical Evaluation and Experimental Study of a New Mechanical Suture Device for Endoscopic Hemostasis.** *Gastrointest Endosc* 1990, **36**:494–497. **[49].**

ESKER AH, HALL CH JR: **Replacement of the Damaged Percutaneous Endoscopic Gastrostomy Feeding Tube in the Immature Tract.** *Gastrointest Endosc* 1990, **36**:380–391. **[27].**

FAY DE, LUTHER R, GRUBER M: **A Single Procedure Endoscopic Technique for Replacing Partially Extruded Percutaneous Endoscopic Gastrostomy Tubes.** *Gastrointest Endosc* 1990, **36**:298–300. **[24].**

FRUHMORGEN P, PFAHLER A: **Komplikationen Bei 39397 Endoskopischen**
● **Untersuchungen — Eine 7-jährige Prospektive Dokumentation Uber Art Und Haufigkeit.** *Leber Magen Darm* 1990, **1**:20–32. **[7].**

FUKUMOTO S, ADACHI K, OHTSU K, *ET AL.*: **Pedunculated Submucosal Ectopic Mucosa of the Stomach Treated by Endoscopic Polypectomy: Report of Two Cases.** *Dig Endosc* 1990, **2**:434–438. **[39].**

FULP SR, GILLIAM JH: **Beware of the Incarcerated Hernia [letter].** *Gastrointest Endosc* 1990, **36**:318–319.

GLASER D, MASON AT, DETARNOWKSY GO: **Tube Migration in PEG [letter].** *Gastrointest Endosc* 1990, **36**:161.

GOLDENBERG SP, DELUCA VA JR, MARIGNANI P: **Endoscopic Treatment of Dieulafoy's Lesion of the Duodenum.** *Am J Gastroenterol* 1990, **85**:452–454.

HARUMA K, SUMII K, INOUE K, TESHIMA H, KAJIYAMA G: **Endoscopic Therapy in Patients**
● **with Inoperable Early Gastric Cancer.** *Am J Gastroenterol* 1990, **85**:522–526. **[31].**

HASHIZUME M, KITANO S, YAMAGA H, KOYANAGI N, SUGIMACHI K: **Endoscopic**
• **Classification of Gastric Varices.** *Gastrointest Endosc* 1990, **36**:276–280. **[52].**

HEDENBRO JL, HÄGERSTAND I, RYCHTEROVA V: **Parietal Cell Carcinoma — a New Differential Diagnosis for Submucosal Gastric Tumours.** *Endoscopy* 1990, **22**:47–48. **[34].**

KADOTA T, HIRAIDE H, IMAI J, TAMAKUMA S: **An Easy and Safe Modified Method of**
• **Endoscopic Balloon Dilation for Postgastrectomy Anastomotic Stricture.** *Surgery Gyn Obstet* 1990, **170**:445–447. **[46].**

KANG JY, CHAN-WILDE C, WEE A, CHEW R, TI TK: **Role of Computed Tomography and Endoscopy in the Management of Alimentary Tract Lipomas.** *Gut* 1990, **31**:550–553.

KERRIGAN DD, BROWN SR, HUTCHINSON GH: **Open Access Gastroscopy: Too Much to**
• **Swallow?** *Br Med J* 1990, **300**:374–376. **[1].**

KLEIN S, HEARE BR, SOLOWAY RD: **The 'Buried Bumper Syndrome': a Complication of Percutaneous Endoscopic Gastrostomy.** *Am J Gastroenterol* 1990, **85**:448–451. **[23].**

KOZAREK RA, BOTOMAN VA, PATTERSON DJ: **Long-term Follow-up in Patients Who have**
• **Undergone Balloon Dilatation for Gastric Outlet Obstruction.** *Gastrointest Endosc* 1990, **36**:558–561. **[45].**

LAU WY: **Intraoperative Enteroscopy —Indications and Limitations.** *Gastrointest Endosc* 1990, **36**:268–271.

MANSBERGER JA, KAVOUKLIS JH: **Combined Endoscopic and Surgical Gastrostomy**
• **when Percutaneous Endoscopic Gastrostomy is Contraindicated.** *Am Surg* 1990, **56**:138–140. **[20].**

MAŘATKA Z: **Early Gastric Stump Cancer: Macroscopic and Microscopic Appearance.** *Gastrointest Endosc* 1990, **36**:88.

MCGOVERN R, BARKIN JS, GOLDBERG RI, PHILLIPS RS: **Duo-**
• **Denal Obstruction: a Complication of Percutaneous Endoscopic Gastrostomy Tube Migration.** *Am J Gastroenterol* 1990, **85**:1037–1038. **[28].**

MELATO M, LAURINO L: **Gastric Stump — a Malignancy Promoter [letter].** *Am J Surg Pathol* 1990, **14**:596–597.

MISRA SP, DWIVEDI M, MISRA V, AGARWAL SK, GUPTA R, GUPTA SC, MITAL VP: **Endoscopic**
• **and Histologic Appearance of the Gastric Mucosa in Patients with Portal Hypertension.** *Gastrointest Endosc* 1990, **36**:575–579. **[11].**

MORAN BJ, TAYLOR MB, JOHNSON CD: **Percutaneous Endoscopic Gastrostomy.** *Br J*
• *Surg* 1990, **77**:858–862. **[15].**

MOUSSA SE, TUNUGUNTLA K, CHAN CH, SEDARAT A, RYBNICEK K: **Endoscopic Removal of an Intact Anti-reflux Prosthesis 6 Years after Implantation.** *Gastrointest Endosc* 1990, **36**:525–527. **[43].**

NAKANO H, PERSSON B, SLEZAK P: **Study of the Gastric Mucosal Background in**
• **Patients with Gastric Polyps.** *Gastrointest Endosc* 1990, **36**:39–42. **[37].**

OBATA S, TSUKAMOTO A, KIMURA K, MAEDA K, KAWAMURA R: **Adult T-cell Leukemia Presenting a IIa + 11c-like Lesions in the Stomach on Endoscopic Examination.** *Endoscopy* 1990, **22**:81–82. **[35].**

PFEIL S, BLADES E, YANG P: **Complications of Percutaneous Endoscopic**
• **Gastrostomy Removal.** *Gastrointest Endosc* 1990, **36**:316. **[25].**

SAINI S, MUELLER PR, GAA J, *ET AL*: **Percutaneous Gastrostomy with Gastropexy:**
•• **Experience in 125 Patients.** *AJR* 1990, **154**:1003–1006. **[18].**

SATALOFF DM, LIEBER CP, SEINIGE UL: **Strictures Following Gastric Stapling for**
• **Morbid Obesity. Results of Endoscopic Dilatation.** *Am Surg* 1990, **56**:167–174. **[47].**

SAVALGI RS, CORBISHLEY CM, CAYGILKL C, HILL M, COOK MG, KIRKHAM JS, NORTHFIELD TC:
• **Relation Between Severity and Extent of Precancerous Lesions in the Postoperative Stomach.** *Lancet* 1990, **336**:413–416. **[29].**

SCHWARTZ AE, VANAGUNAS A, KAMEL PL: **Endoscopy to Evaluate Gastrointestinal**
• **Bleeding in Marathon Runners.** *Ann Intern Med* 1990, **113**:632–633. **[53].**

SHERMAN A, ZINGLER BM: **Successful Endoscopic Retrieval of a Cocaine Packet from**
• **the Stomach.** *Gastrointest Endosc* 1990, **36**:152–154. **[42].**

SPANDRE M, CAVALLERO M, PENNAZIO M, *ET AL*: **Needle Biopsy of Submucosal Lesions**
• **of the Gastrointestinal Tract.** *Surg Endosc* 1990, **4**:161–163. **[38].**

STEFFES CP, SUGAWA C, WILSON RF, HAYWARD SR: **Oxygen Saturation Monitoring**
• **During Endoscopy.** *Surg Endosc* 1990, **4**:175–178. **[3].**

STIEGMANN GV, GOFF JS, SILAS D, PEARLMAN N, SUN J, NORTON L: **Endoscopic Versus**
•• **Operative Gastrostomy: Final Results of a Prospective Randomized Trial.** *Gastrointest Endosc* 1991, **36**:1–5. **[17].**

STOLTE M, RITTER M, BORCHARD F, KOCH-SCHERRER G: **Collagenous Gastroduodenitis on Collagenous Colitis.** *Endoscopy* 1990, **22**:186–187. **[14].**

SWETECH J, HASAN S: **Combined Endoscopic and Surgical Modalities for Percutaneous Endoscopic Gastrostomy Placement in the Setting of Subtotal Gastrectomy with a Gastric Pull Up [letter].** *Gastrointest Endosc* 1990, **36**:316–317.

WALDRON R, KERIN M, ALI A, MCANENA OJ, MCGUIRE M, MCCARTHY CH, GIVEN HF:
• **Evaluation of the Role of Endoscopic Biopsies and Cytology in the Detection of Gastric Malignancy.** *Br J Surg* 1990, **77**:62–63. **[32].**

WARRINGTON SJ, DEBBAS NMG, FARTHING M, *ET AL*: **Lornoxicam, Indomethacin and**
• **Placebo: Comparison of Effects of Faecal Blood Loss and Healthy Upper Gastrointestinal Endoscopic Appearances in Healthy Men.** *Postgrad Med J* 1990, **66**:622–626. **[10].**

WOLFSEN HC, KOZAREK RA, BALL TJ, PATTERSON DJ, BOTOMAN VA, RYAN JA: **Value of**
• **Diagnostic Upper Endoscopy Preceding Percutaneous Gastrostomy.** *Am J Gastroenterol* 1990, **85**:249–251. **[19].**

YAKSHE PN, ALBERT F, RAGSDALE B, TRAVERS R, BENJAMIN S: **An Unusual Vascular Lesion in a Patient with Hereditary Hemorrhagic Teleangiectasia.** *Gastrointest Endosc* 1990, **36**:513–516. **[40].**

Endoscopy of the small bowel and duodenum

AABAKKEN L, LARSEN S, OSNES M: **Visual Analogue Scales for Endoscopic Evaluation**
• **of Nonsteroidal Anti-inflammatory Drug-induced Mucosal Damage in the Stomach and Duodenum.** *Scand J Gastroenterol* 1990, **25**:443–448. **[28].**

BEMELMAN WA, BRUMMELKAMP WH, BARTELSMAN JFWM: **Endoscopic Balloon Dilation of the Pylorus after Esophagogastrostomy Without a Drainage Procedure.** *Surg Gynecol Obstet* 1990, **170**:424–426.

BILOTTA JJ, WAYE JD: **Hydrogen Peroxide Enteritis: the 'Snow White' Sign.**
• *Gastrointest Endosc* 1989, **35**:428–430. **[33].**

BOZDECH JM, FARMER RG: **Diagnosis of Crohn's Disease.** *Hepatogastroenterology* 1990, **37**:8–17. **[20].**

CADONI S, OTTONELLO R, MAXIA G, GEMINI S, COCCO P: **Endoscopic Treatment of a Duodeno-Cutaneous Fistula with Fibrin Tissue Sealant (Tissucol) [letter].** *Endoscopy* 1990, **22**:194–195.

CHEN LT, CHEN CY, JAN CM, WANG WM, LAN TS, HSIEH MY, LIU GC: **Gastrointestinal Tract Involvement in Hepatocellular Carcinoma — Clinical, Radiological and Endoscopic Studies.** *Endoscopy* 1990, **22**:118–123.

DAURIA DA, NAIDORF T, HASHMI MA, LEVINE SM: **Endoscopic Excision of a Foreign Body in the Pyloric Channel.** *Gastrointest Endosc* 1990, **36**:406–408.

DI FEBO G, MIGLIOLI M, LAURI A, *ET AL*: **Endoscopic Assessment of Acute Inflammation of the Ileal Reservoir after Restorative Ileo-anal Anastomosis.** *Gastrointest Endosc* 1990, **36**:6–9. **[22].**

DISARIO JA, FOUTCH PG, SANOWSKI RA: **Poor Results with Percutaneous Endoscopic**
• **Jejunostomy.** *Gastrointest Endosc* 1990, **36**:257–260. **[25].**

ETIENNE PL, RAOUL JL, BRETAGNE JF, RAMEE MP, MALIER F, GOSSELIN M: **Gastroduodenal Intussusception - a Radioendoscopic Description [in French].** *Gastroenterol Clin Biol* 1990, **14**:589–592.

FERNANDEZ-MELONE JH, TRIADAFILOPOULOS G, CHANDLER JG: **Nodular Duodenitis and Single Duodenal Nodules.** *Am Surg* 1990, **56**:175–177. **[32].**

FOUTCH PG, SAWYER R, SANOWSKI RA: **Push-enteroscopy for Diagnosis of Patients**
• **with Gastrointestinal Bleeding of Obscure Origin.** *Gastrointest Endosc* 1990, **36**:337–341. **[2].**

FRUCHT H, NORTON JA, LONDON JF, *ET AL*: **Detection of Duodenal Gastrinomas by**
• **Operative Endoscopic Transillumination.** *Gastroenterology* 1990, **99**:1622–1627. **[13].**

FUJITA S *ET AL*: **Preoperative Endoscopy in Peutz-Jeghers Syndrome [letter].** *Lancet* 1990, **335**:415.

GEBOES K, ECTORS N, HEIDBUCHEL H, RUTGEERTS P, DESMET V, VANTRAPPEN G: **Whipple's**
• **Disease: Endoscopic Aspects Before and after Therapy.** *Gastrointest Endosc* 1990, **36**:247–251. **[29].**

GROUP D'ETUDES THERAPEUTIQUES DES AFFECTIONS INFLAMMA-
• TOIRES DU TUBE DIGESTIF (GETAID) PRESENTED BY MARY JY, MODIGLIANI R: **Development and Validation of an Endoscopic Index of the Severity for Crohn's Disease: a Prospective Multicentre Study.** *Gut* 1989, **30**:983–989. **[18].**

KANG JY, CHAN-WILDE C, WEE A, CHEW R, TI TK: **Role of Computed Tomography and Endoscopy in the Management of Alimentary Tract Lipomas.** *Gut* 1990, **31**:550–553. **[15].**

KIMMEL ME, BOYLAN JJ: **Use Suction Catheters to Dilate Ostomy Site [letter].** *Gastrointest Endosc* 1990, **36**:161.

LAU WY: **Intraoperative Enteroscopy —Indications and Limitations.** *Gastrointest*
• *Endosc* 1990, **36**:268–271. **[6].**

LEWIS BS: **Perform PEJ, not PED [editorial].** *Gastrointest Endosc* 1990, **36**:311–312.
• **[24].**

LEWIS BS: **The Rapid Placement of Jejunal Feeding Tubes: the Seldinger**
• **Technique Applied to the Gut.** *Gastrointest Endosc* 1990, **36**:139–141. **[26].**

LIPSON A, BARTRAM CI, WILLIAMS CB, SLAVIN G, WALKER-SMITH J: **Barium Studies and Ileoscopy Compared in Children with Suspected Crohn's Disease.** *Clin Radiol* 1990, **41**:5–8. **[19].**

MADDEN MV, FARTHING MJG, NICHOLLS RJ: **Inflammation in Ileal Reservoirs:**
• **'Pouchitis'.** *Gut* 1990, **31**:247–249. **[21].**

MATSUMOTO T, LIDA M, MATSUI T, *ET AL*: **Submucosal Tumours of the Terminal Ileum Managed by Endoscopic Polypectomy.** *Gastrointest Endosc* 1990, **36**:505–508. **[16].**

MINOLI G: **Development and Validation of an Endoscopic Severity Index for Crohn's Disease [letter].** *Gastrointest Endosc* 1990, **36**:168.

ODDSSON E, GUDJONSSON H, THJODLEIFSSON B: **Endoscopic Findings in the Stomach and Duodenum after Treatment with Enteric-coated and Plain Naproxen Tablets in Healthy Subjects.** *Scand J Gastroenterol* 1990, **25**:231–234.

OLAISON G, SJODHL R, TAGESSON C: **Glucocorticoid Treatment in Ileal Crohn's**
• **Disease: Relief of Symptoms But not of Endoscopically Viewed Inflammation.** *Gut* 1990, **31**:325–328. **[17].**

PANOS RG, OPELKA FG, NOGUERAS JJ: **Peutz-Jeghers Syndrome: a Call for**
• **Intraoperative Enteroscopy.** *Am Surg* 1990, **56**:331–333. **[3].**

PATEL AS, DERIDDER PH: **Endoscopic Appearance and Significance of Functional Lymphangiectasia of the Duodenal Mucosa.** *Gastrointest Endosc* 1990, **36**:376–378. **[31].**

ROLNY P, EKMAN R, SJOLUND K, WICKBOM G, OHRN PG: **Endoscopic Diagnosis and Treatment of Duodenal Gastrinoma.** *Gastrointest Endosc* 1990, **36**:511–513. **[14].**

SHIKE M, WALLACH C, BLOCH A, BRENNAN MF: **Combined Gastric Drainage and Jejunal Feeding Through a Percutaneous Endoscopic Stoma.** *Gastrointest Endosc* 1990, **36**:290–292.

SPIGELMAN AD, THOMSON JP, PHILLIPS RK: **Towards Decreasing the Relaparotomy**
•• **Rate in the Peutz–Jeghers Syndrome: the Role of Peroperative Small Bowel Endoscopy.** *Br J Surg* 1990, **77**:301–302. **[12].**

STOLTE M, RITTER M, BORCHARD F, KOCHSCHERRER G: **Collagenous Gastroduodenitis on Collagenous Colitis.** *Endoscopy* 1990, **22**:186–187.

TADA S, LIDA M, IWASHITA A, *ET AL*: **Endoscopic and Biopsy Findings of the Upper**
• **Digestive Tract in Patients with Amyloidosis.** *Gastrointest Endosc* 1990, **36**:10–14. **[30].**

WARRINGTON SJ, DEBBAS NMG, FARTHING M, HORTON M, JOHNSTON A, THILLAINAYAGAM A, TURNER P, FERBER H: **Lornoxicam, Indomethacin and Placebo - Comparison of Effects on Faecal Blood Loss and Upper Gastrointestinal Endoscopic Appearances in Healthy Men.** *Postgrad Med J* 1990, **66**:622–626.

WESTFALL SH, ANDRUS CH, NAUNHEIM KS: **A Reproducible, Safe Jejunostomy Replacement Technique by a percutaneous Endoscopic Method.** *Am Surg* 1990, **56**:141–143.

WILLIAMS CB, BAILLIE J, GILLIES DG, BORISLOW D, COTTON PB: **Teaching Gastrointestinal Endoscopy by Computer Simulation: a Prototype for Colonoscopy and ERCP.** *Gastrointest Endosc* 1990, **36**:49–54.

WOLFSEN HC, KOZAREK RA, BALL TJ, PATTERSON DJ, BOTOMAN VA: **Tube Dysfunction Following Percutaneous Endoscopic Gastrostomy and Jejunostomy.** *Gastrointest Endosc* 1990, **36**:261–263.

Endoscopy of upper gastrointestinal bleeding

AGUADO J, NAPAL J, ALSAR MJ: **Pneumococcal Bacteremia: a Late Complication Following Endoscopic Variceal Sclero-Therapy.** *Postgrad Med J* 1990, **66**:790–791. **[28].**
●

BALANZO J, VILLANUEVA C, SAINZ S, ESPINOS JC, MENDEZ C, GUARNER C, VILLARDELL F: **Injection Therapy of Bleeding Peptic Ulcer. A Prospective, Randomized Trial Using Epinephrine and Thrombin.** *Endoscopy* 1990, **22**:157–159. **[64].**
●

BELLARY SV, ISAACS P: **Disseminated Intravascular Coagulation (DIC) after Endoscopic Injection Sclerotherapy with Ethanolamine Oleate [letter].** *Endoscopy* 1990, **22**:151.

BENDTSEN F, SKOVGAARD LT, SORENSEN TIA, MATZEN P: **Agreement Among Multiple Observers on Endoscopic Diagnosis of Esophageal Varices Before Bleeding.** *Hepatology* 1990, **11**:341–347. **[6].**
●

BERTONI G, FORNACIARI G, BELTRAMI M, CONIGLIARO R, MORTILLA MG, RICCI E, CASTAGNETTI E, BEDOGNI G, PLANCHER AC: **Nadolol for Prevention of Variceal Rebleeding During the Course of Endoscopic Injection Sclerotherapy: a Randomized Pilot Study.** *J Clin Gastroenterol* 1990, **12**:364–365. **[18].**
●

BOURBON P, ZARSKI JP, KITMACHER P, BOURLARD P, MACHECOURT J, DENIS B, RACHAIL M: **Esophageal Varice Sclerotherapy: Influence on Portal Pressure and Azygos Blood Flow (in French).** *Gastroenterol Clin Biol* 1990, **14**:244–247.

BRANICKI FJ, COLEMAN SY, FOK PJ, PRITCHETT CJ, FAN ST, LAI ECS, MOK FPT, CHEUNG WL, LAU PWK, TUEN HH, LAM SK, HUI WM, NG MMT, LAM DKH, TSE MCK, TANG APK, WONG J: **Bleeding Peptic Ulcer: a Prospective Evaluation of Risk Factors for Rebleeding and Mortality.** *World J Surg* 1990, **14**:262–270. **[60].**
●●

CALES P, ZABOTTO B, MESKENS C, CAUCANAS JP, VINEL JP, DESMORAT H, FERMANIAN J, PASCAL JP: **Gastro-esophageal Endoscopic Features in Cirrhosis. Observer Variability, Interassociations, and Relationship to Hepatic Dysfunction.** *Gastroenterology* 1990, **98**:156–162. **[4].**
●

CALETTI GC, BROCCHI E, LABRIOLA E, GASBARRINI G, BARBAR L: **Pericarditis: a Probably Overlooked Complication of Endoscopic Variceal Sclerotherapy** *Endoscopy* 1990, **22**:144–145. **[30].**
●

CARVALHO PJPC, DONAHUE PE, MIIDLA I, DAVIS PE, SHEN Y-J, BOMBECK CT, NYHUS LM: **Fibrosis of Gastric Cardia after Endoscopic Sclerosis: Mechanism for Control of Experimental Reflux?** *Am Surg* 1990, **56**:163–166.

CHAWLA YK, DILAWARI JB, RAMESH GN, KAUR U, MITRA SK, WALIA BNS: **Sclerotherapy and Extrahepatic Portal Venous Obstruction.** *Gut* 1990, **31**:213–216. **[47].**
●●

CLAUDEL-BONVOISIN S, DESCOS L, CHATELARD P, SOUQUET JC, PASQUIER J: **Carcinoma of the Esophagus and Sclerotherapy for Esophageal Varices (in French) [letter].** *Gastroenterol Clin Biol* 1990, **14**:189.

COTTER J: **Endoscopic Treatment of Bleeding Peptic Ulcers - Good in Every Situation [letter].** *Endoscopy* 1990, **22**:201.

DESMORAT H, CALES P, VINEL JP, MAQUIN P, CAUCANAS JP, COMBIS JM, PASCAL JP: **Obstructive Intramural Hematoma of the Esophagus - an Unusual Complication of Endoscopic Variceal Sclerotherapy [in French].** *Gastroenterol Clin Biol* 1990, **14**:581–585.

FAVRE O, GENIN G, SOUQUET JC: **Obstructive Hematoma of Esophagus: an Unusual Complication of Sclerotherapy of Esophageal Varices (in French) [letter].** *Gastroenterol Clin Biol* 1990, **14**:100.

FLICK JA: **Antibody Prophylaxis During Sclerotherapy for Esophageal Varices.** *J Paediatrics* 1990, **116**:156–157. **[29].**
●

FULLARTON GM, BIRNIE GG, MACDONALD A, MURRAY WR: **The Effect of Introducing Endoscopic Therapy on Surgery and Mortality Rates for Peptic Ulcer Hemorrhage. A Single Centre Analysis of 1125 Cases.** *Endoscopy* 1990, **22**:110–113. **[67].**
●

FULLARTON GM, MURRAY WR: **Prediction of Rebleeding in Peptic Ulcers by Visual Stigmata and Endoscopic Doppler Ultrasound Criteria.** *Endoscopy* 1990, **22**:68–71. **[72].**
●

GRACE ND: **A Hepatologists View of Variceal Bleeding.** *Am J Surg* 1990, **160**:26–31. **[2].**
●

GRACE ND: **Prevention of Recurrent Variceal Bleeding — is Surgical Rescue the Answer?** *Ann Intern Med* 1990, **112**:242–244. **[58].**
●

GRACE ND: **A Hepatologists View of Variceal Bleeding.** *Am J Surg* 1990, **160**:26–31.

HASHIZUME M, KITANO S, YAMAGA H, KOYANAGI I, SUGIMACHI K: **Endoscopic Classification of Gastric Varices.** *Gastrointest Endosc* 1990, **36**:276–280. **[45].**
●

HENDERSON JM, KUTNER M, MILLIKAN WJ, GALAMBOS JT, RIEPE SP, BROOKS WS, BRYAN FC, WARREN WD: **Endoscopic Variceal Sclerosis Compared with Distal Splenorenal Shunt to Prevent Recurrent Variceal Bleeding in Cirrhosis.** *Ann Intern Med* 1990, **112**:262–269. **[52].**
●●

HESELTINE D, BRAMBLE M, COLE A, CLARKE D, CASTLE W: **Weber-Christian Disease Producing Splenic Vein Occlusion and Bleeding Gastric Varices: Successful Treatment with Sclero-Therapy.** *Postgrad Med J* 1990, **66**:321–325. **[46].**
●

IDEZUKI Y, SANJO K, BANDAI Y, KAWASAKI S, OHASHI K: **Current Strategy for Esophageal Varices in Japan.** *Am J Surg* 1990, **160**:98–104.

JENSEN LS, KRARUP N: **Propranolol May Prevent Recurrence of Esophageal Varices after Obliteration by Endoscopic Sclero-Therapy.** *Scand J Gastroenterol* 1990, **25**:352–356. **[20].**
●

KOCHHAR R, GOENKA MK, MEHTA S, MEHTA SK: **A Comparative Evaluation of Sclerosants for Esophageal Varices: a Prospective Randomized Controlled Study.** *Gastrointest Endosc* 1990, **36**:127–130. **[10].**
●

KOKUDO N, SANJO K, UMEKITA N, HARIHARA Y, TADA Y, IDEZUKI Y: **Squamous Cell Carcinoma after Endoscopic Injection Sclerotherapy for Esophageal Varices.** *J Gastroenterol* 1990, **85**:861–864. **[41].**
●

KOVACS TO, JENSEN DM: **Electrothermal Modalities in the Treatment of Non-variceal Upper Gastrointestinal Bleeding.** *Eur J Gastroenterol Hepatol* 1990, **2**:87–93. **[59].**
●●

LAVY A: **A Technique for Preventing Iatrogenic Bleeding During Sclerotherapy.** *Gastrointest Endosc* 1990, **36**:79.

LI V, ZARSKI JP, BOULARD JC, FRICAMPS-PIRONI C, RACHAIL M: **Intramural Pharyngo-esophageal Hematoma: an Unusual Complication of Endoscopic Injection Sclerotherapy (in French) [letter].** *Gastroenterol Clin Biol* 1990, **14**:101.

LIN HJ, LEE FY, CHAN CY, HUANG ZC, KANG WM, LEE CH, LEE SD, TSAI YT: **Heat Probe Thermocoagulation as a Substitute for Surgical Intervention to Arrest Massive Peptic Ulcer Hemorrhage - an Experience in 153 Cases.** *Surgery* 1990, **108**:18–21.

LIN HJ, LEE FY, KANG WM, TSAI YT, LEE SD, LEE CH: **Heat Probe Thermocoagulation and Pure Alcohol Injection in Massive Peptic Ulcer Hemorrhage: a Prospective Randomized Controlled Trial.** *Gut* 1990, **31**:753–757. **[65].**
●

LIN HJ, LEE FY, KANG WM, TSAI YT, LEE SD, LEE CH: **Heat Probe Thermocoagulation and Pure Alcohol Injection in Massive Peptic Ulcer Haemorrhage: a Prospective, Randomised Controlled Trial.** *Gut* 1990, **31**:753–757.

LIN HJ, LEE FY, KANG WM, YANG TT, LEE SD, LEE CH: **A Controlled Study of Therapeutic Endoscopy for Peptic Ulcer with Non-Bleeding Visible Vessel.** *Gastrointest Endosc* 1990, **36**:241–246. **[68].**
●

LIN HJ, LEE FY, TSAI YT, LEE SD, LEE CH: **What Kind of Non-Bleeding Visible Vessel in a Peptic Ulcer Needs Aggressive Therapy.** *Endoscopy* 1990, **22**:8–11. **[61].**
●

LIN HJ, LEE FY, TSAI YT, LEE SD, LEE CH: **What Kind of Non-bleeding Visible Vessel in a Peptic Ulcer Needs Aggressive Therapy — Long-term Clinical Observation.** *Endoscopy* 1990, **22**:8–11.

MADONIA S, TRAINA M, MONTALBANO L, D'AMICO G: **Variceal Ulceration Following Sclerotherapy: Normal Consequence or Complication.** *Gastrointest Endosc* 1990, **36**:76–77. **[36].**
●

MATHUR SK, DALVI AN, SOMESHWAR V, SUPE AN, RAMAKANTAN R: **Endoscopic and Radiological Appraisal of Gastric Varices.** *Br J Surg* 1990, **77**:432–435. **[44].**
●

MICHALETZ PA, GRAHAM DY: **The Effect of Endoscopic Hemostasis with Alcohol on the Mortality Rate of Non-variceal Upper Gastrointestinal Hemorrhage.** *Gastrointest Endosc* 1990, **36**:87.

OKANO H, TSUJI H, KODAMA T, TAKINO T, MURAKAMI M: **Effect of Endoscopic Sclerotherapy and Propranolol on the Blood Flow of Esophageal Varices.** *Am J Gastroenterol* 1990, **85**:30–33. **[21].**
●

PANES J, FORNE M, BAGENA F, VIVER J: **Endoscopic Sclerosis in the Treatment of Bleeding Peptic Ulcers with a Visible Vessel.** *Am J Gastroenterol* 1990, **85**:252–254. **[63].**
●

PAQUET KJ, MERCADO MA: **Surgical Procedures for Bleeding Oesophagogastric Varices when Sclerotherapy Fails: a Prospective Study.** *Am J Surg* 1990, **160**:43–47. **[57].**
●

PEILLON C, DUHAMEL C, LEREBOURS E, COLIN R, TESTART J, BONMARCHAND G, LEROY J: **Dissecting Duodenal Hematoma: a Complication of Endoscopic Hemostasis in Duodenal Ulcer Bleeding (in French) [letter].** *Gastroenterol Clin Biol* 1990, **14**:289–290.

RABINOVITZ M, YOO YK, SCHADE RR, DINDZANS VJ, VAN THIEL DH, GAVALER JS: **Prevalence of Endoscopic Findings in 510 Consecutive Individuals with Cirrhosis Evaluated Prospectively.** *Dig Dis Sci* 1990, **35**:705–710. **[3].**
●

ROGGO A, FILIPPINI L: **Endoscopic Injection Treatment of Acute Non-Varicose Upper Gastrointestinal Bleeding [in German].** *Dtsch Med Wochenschr* 1990, **115**:1227–1231.

SAKAI P, BOAVENTRUA S, ISHIOKA S, MIES S, SETTE H, PINOTTI HW: **Sclerotherapy of Bleeding Esophageal Varices in Schistosomiasis.** *Endoscopy* 1990, **22**:5–7. **[49].**
●

SAKAI P, BOAVENTURA S, ISHIOKA S, MIES S, SETTE H, PINOTTI HW: **Sclerotherapy of Bleeding Esophageal Varices in Schistosomiasis — Comparative Study in Patients with and Without Previous Surgery for Portal Hypertension.** *Endoscopy* 1990, **22**:5–7.

SALENA BJ, SIVAK MV: **Injection Therapy in the Treatment of Upper Gastrointestinal Hemorrhage.** *Eur J Gastroenterol Hepatol* 1990, **2**:79–86. **[1].**
●

SARIN SK, KUMAR A: **Sclerosants for Variceal Sclerotherapy: a Critical Appraisal.** *Am J Gastroenterol* 1990, **85**:641–649. **[9].**
●●

SAUERBRUCH T: **Treatment and Prevention of Bleeding from Oesophageal Varices [in German].** *Dtsch Med Wochenschr* 1990, **115**:940–943.

SHEMESH E, CZERNIAK A, KLEIN E, PINES A, BAT L: **A Comparison Between Emergency and Delayed Endoscopic Injection Sclerotherapy of Bleeding Esophageal Varices in Nonalcoholic Portal Hypertension.** *J Clin Gastroenterol* 1990, **12**:5–9. **[15].**
●

SINGAL A, SARIN SK, SOOD GK, BROOR SL: **Ulcers after Intravariceal Sclerotherapy: Correlation of Symptoms and Factors Affecting Healing.** *J Clin Gastroenterol* 1990, **12**:250–254. **[35].**
●

SPINA GP, SANTAMBROGIO R, OPOCHER E, COSENTINO F, ZAMBELLI A, PASSONI GR, CUCCHIARO G, MACRI M, MORANDI E, BRUNO S, PEZZUOLI G: **Distal Splenorenal Shunt Versus Endoscopic Sclerotherapy in the Prevention of Variceal Rebleeding.** *Ann Surg* 1990, **211**:178–186. **[53].**
●

STIEGMANN GV, GOFF JS, SUN JH, HRUZA D, REVEILLE RM: **Endoscopic Ligation of Esophageal Varices.** *Am J Surg* 1990, **159**:21–26. **[50].**
●●

TAKASE Y, SHIBUYA S, CHIKAMORI F, ORII K, IWASAKI Y: **Recurrence Factors Studied by Percutaneous Transhepatic Portography Before and after Endoscopic Sclerotherapy for Esophageal Varices.** *Hepatology* 1990, **11**:348–352. **[51].**
●

TAM F, CHOW H, PRINDIVILLE T, CORNISH D, HAULK T, TRUDEAU W, HOEPRICH P: **Bacterial Peritonitis Following Esophageal Injection Sclerotherapy for Variceal Hemorrhage.** *Gastrointest Endosc* 1990, **36**:131–133. **[26].**
●

TERADA T, NAKANUMA Y, YONEJIMA M, YOKOYAMA H, KOIKE N: **Portal, Mesenteric and Splenic Venous Thrombosis after Endoscopic Injection Sclerotherapy.** *J Clin Gastroenterol* 1990, **12**:238–239. **[34].**
●

TERBLANCHE J: **Has Sclerotherapy Altered the Management of Patients with Variceal Bleeding?** *Am J Surg* 1990, **160**:37–42. **[8].**
●

THAPA BR, MEHTA S: **Endoscopic Sclerotherapy of Esophageal Varices in Infants and Children.** *J Pediatr Gastroenterol Nutr* 1990, **10**:430–434.

TRINCHET JC: **Is Endoscopic Sclerotherapy of Esophageal Varices Responsible for an Increase in Portal Hypertension? [editorial] (in French).** *Gastroenterol Clin Biol* 1990, **14**:241–243.

VAIRA D, HOLTON J, OSBORN J, DANNA L, ROMANOS A, FALZON M, MCNEIL I: **Endoscopy in Dyspeptic Patients — is Gastric Mucosal Biopsy Useful.** *Am J Gastroenterol* 1990, **85**:701–704.

VAN ZAANEN HCT, SCHOTBORGH RH, CHAMULEAU RAFM: **Meningococcus Septicemia: a Complication of Endoscopic Injection Sclerotherapy.** *Am J Gastroenterol* 1990, **85**:631–632. **[27].**
●

VANSTIEGMANN G, GOFF JS, SUN JH, HRUZA D, REVEILLE RM: **Endoscopic Ligation of Esophageal Varices.** *Am J Surg* 1990, **159**:21–26.

VANZAANEN HCT, SCHOTBORGH RH, CHAMULEAU RAFM: **Meningococcus Septicemia — a Complication of Endoscopic Injection Sclerotherapy [letter].** *Am J Gastroenterol* 1990, **85**:631–632.

WESTABY D, POLSON RJ, GIMSON AES, HAYES PC, HAYLLAR K, WILLIAMS R: **A Controlled ●● Trial of Oral Propranolol Compared with Injection Sclerotherapy for the Long-Term Management of Variceal Bleeding.** *Hepatology* 1990, **11**:353–359. **[16].**

WESTABY D, WILLIAMS R: **Status of Sclerotherapy for Variceal Bleeding in 1990.** *Am J* ●● *Surg* 1990, **160**:32–35. **[7].**

WINKELTAU G, ARLT G, TREUTNER KH, SCHUBERT T, SCHUMPELICK V: **Endoscopic Therapy ● and Early Elective Operation as a Therapeutic Regimen in Ulcer Bleeding.** *Hepatogastroenterol* 1990, **37**:121–123. **[69].**

WINKELTAU G, ARLT G, TREUTNER KH, SCHUBERT T, SCHUMPELICK V: **Endoscopic Therapy and Early Elective Operation as a Therapeutic Regimen in Ulcer Bleeding.** *Hepatogastroenterology* 1990, **37**:121–123.

Lasers and tumor probes

BARR H, KRASNER N, RAOUF A, WALKER RJ: **Prospective Randomized Trial of Laser ●● Therapy Only and Laser Therapy Followed by Endoscopic Intubation for the Palliation of Malignant Dysphagia.** *Gut* 1990, **31**:252–258. **[13].**

BROWN PE, WRIGHT RA: **The Water Jet-guided Nd:YAG Laser in the Treatment of Gastroduodenal Ulcer with a Visible Vessel [letter].** *Gastrointest Endosc* 1990, **36**:171.

CAVE DR: **Photodynamic Therapy for Esophageal Tumors.** *Gastrointest Endosc* 1990, **36**:85.

CHOI PM, SCHNEIDER L: **Endoscopic Nd:YAG Laser Treatment of Granular Cell Tumor of the Esophagus.** *Gastrointest Endosc* 1990, **36**:144–145.

COHEN MA, SANCHEZ MJG, MONROY E, RUIZ JM, NOGUERAS FM: **Electrocoagulation of Rectal Cancer [in Spanish].** *Rev Esp Enferm Dig* 1990, **78**:23–26.

COTHREN RM, RICHARDS-KORTUM R, SIVAK MV, *ET AL.*: **Gastrointestinal Tissue Diagnosis ●● by Laser-induced Fluorescence Spectroscopy at Endoscopy.** *Gastrointest Endosc* 1990, **36**:105–111. **[24].**

DOWLATSHAHI K, BANGERT JD, HAKLIN MF, RHODES CK, WEINSTEIN RS, ECONOMOU SG: ●● **Protection of Fiber Function by Para-axial Fluid Flow in Interstitial Laser Therapy of Malignant Tumors.** *Lasers Surg Med* 1990, **10**:322–327. **[28].**

ECKHAUSER ML: **Palliative Therapy of Upper Gastrointestinal Malignancies Using the Nd-YAG Laser.** *Am Surg* 1990, **56**:158–162.

FLOWERS BF, SASLAWSKY MJ, MATHES GL, TONKIN AK: **Use of the Pulsed Dye Laser and ● Ultrasonic Lithotriptor for Removal of Multiple Intrahepatic Gallstones.** *Surg Gyn Obstet* 1990, **170**:443–444. **[17].**

GANA TJ, SOENEN GM, KOO J: **A Controlled Study of Human Resting Gastric ● Mucosal Blood Flow by Endoscopic Laser-Doppler Flowmetry.** *Gastrointest Endosc* 1990, **36**:264–267. **[23].**

GOLDENBERG SP, DELUCA VA JR, MARIGNANI P: **Endoscopic Treatment of Dieulafoy's Lesion of the Duodenum.** *Am J Gastroenterol* 1990, **85**:452–454.

GOSTOUT CJ: **Gastrointestinal Laser Endoscopy: Future Horizons.** *Mayo Clin Proc* ● 1990, **65**:509–517. **[4].**

HAHL J, HAPPIAINEN R, OVASKA J, PUOLAKKAINEN P, SCHRODER T: **Laser-induced ● Hyperthermia in the Treatment of Liver Tumors.** *Lasers Surg Med* 1990, **10**:319–321. **[26].**

HARUMA K, SUMII K, INOUE K, TASHIMA H, KAJIYAMA G: **Endoscopic Therapy in Patients ● with Inoperable Early Gastric Cancer.** *Am J Gastro* 1990, **85**:522–526. **[5].**

HARUMA K, SUMII K, INOUE K, TESHIMA H, KAJIYAMA G: **Endoscopic Therapy in Patients with Inoperable Early Gastric Cancer.** *Am J Gastroenterol* 1990, **85**:522–526.

KREVSKY B, PUSATERI JP: **Laser Lysis of an Esophageal Web.** *Gastrointest Endosc* 1989, ● **35**:451–453. **[20].**

LABENZ J, BORSCH G: **Endoscopic Laser Therapy of Coloproctological Diseases.** ● *Colo-proctology* 1989, **12**:132–136. **[3].**

LEUNG JWC, SUNG JY, BANEZ VP, WU ZM, AGAS FV, LING TKW, CHUNG SCS: **Endoscopic Cholangiopancreatography in Hepatic Clonorchiasis - a Follow-Up Study.** *Gastrointest Endosc* 1990, **36**:360–363.

LOIZOU LA, GRIGG D, BOULOS PB, BOWN SG: **Endoscopic Nd : YAG Laser Treatment of ● Rectosigmoid Cancer.** *Gut* 1990, **31**:812–816. [2].

MANG TS: **Combination Studies of Hyperthermia Induced by the Neodymium- ● Yttrium-Aluminium-Garnet (Nd : YAG) Laser as an Adjuvant to Photodynamic Therapy.** *Lasers Surg Med* 1990, **10**:173–179. **[25].**

MARCON NE: **Lasers in Gastrointestinal Haemorrhage.** *Euro J Gastro Hepat* 1990, ● 2:94–98. **[9].**

MATHUS-VLIEGEN EMH, TYTGAT GNJ: **Analysis of Failures and Complications of ● Neodymium-YAG Laser Photocoagulation in Gastrointestinal Tract Tumors: a Retrospective Survey of 8 Years.** *Endoscopy* 1990, **22**:17–23. **[7].**

MATHUSVLIEGEN EMH, TYTGAT GNJ: **Analysis of Failures and Complications of Neodymium — YAG Laser Photocoagulation in Gastrointestinal Tract Tumors — a Retrospective Survey of 8 Years Experience.** *Endoscopy* 1990, **22**:17–23.

MAUNOURY V, TURCK D, BRUNETAUD JM, MARTI R, CORTOT A, FARRIAUX JP, PARIS JC: **Blue ● Rubber Bleb Nevus Syndrome.** *Gastroenterol Clin Biol* 1990, **14**:593–595. **[21].**

MCCAUGHAN JS, NIMS TA, GUY GT, *ET AL.*: **Photodynamic Therapy for Esophageal ● Tumors.** *Gastrointest Endosc* 1990, **36**:85–86. **[18].**

NAVEAU S, AUBERT A, POYNARD T, CHAPUT JC: **Long-term Results of Treatment of ● Vascular Malformations of the Gastrointestinal Tract by Neodymium-YAG Laser Photocoagulation.** *Dig Dis Sci* 1990, **35**:821–826. **[11].**

NAVEAU S, CHIESA A, POYNARD T, CHAPUT JC: **Endoscopic Nd : YAG Laser Therapy ●● as Palliative Treatments for Esophageal and Cardial Cancer: Parameters Affecting Long-term Outcome.** *Dig Dis Sci* 1990, **35**:294–301. **[6].**

NEUHAUS H: **Endoscopic Tumor Therapy.** *Endoscopy* 1989, ● **21**:357–360. **[16].**

PANJEHPOUR M, OVERHOLT BF, MILLIGAN AJ, SWAGGERTY MW, WILKINSON JE, KLEBANOW ER: ● **Nd : YAG Laser-induced Interstitial Hyperthermia Using a Long Frosted Contact Probe.** *Lasers Surg Med* 1990,**10**:16–24. **[27].**

PATRICE T, FOULTIER MT, YACTAYO S, ADAM F, GALMICHE JP, DOUET MC, LEBODIC L: ●● **Endoscopic Photodynamic Therapy with Hematoporphyrin Derivative for Primary Treatment of Gastrointestinal Neoplasms in Inoperable Patients.** *Dig Dis Sci* 1990, **35**:545–552. **[19].**

PFEFFER R, REINUS JF, BRANDT LJ: **Endoscopic Laser Treatment for Rectosigmoid Villous Adenoma [letter].** *Gastrointest Endosc* 1990, **36**:170.

RADFORD CM, AHLQUIST DA, GOSTOUT CJ, VIGGIANO TR, BALM RK, ZINSMEISTER AR: ● **Prospective Comparisons of Contact with Non-contact Nd : YAG Laser Therapy for Palliation of Esophageal Carcinoma.** *Gastrointest Endosc* 1989, **35**:394–397. **[12].**

RADFORD CM, AHLQUIST DA, SARR MG, WOLD LE, ZINSMEISTER AR, GOSTOUT CJ: **Endoscopic ● Gastric Vagotomy: a Feasibility Study Using Laser in Dogs.** *Gastrointest Endosc* 1989, **35**:419–424. **[15].**

RIARD P, HOSTEIN J, FOURNET J: **A Villous Adenoma of the Distal Duodenum Treated by Laser Therapy [letter].** *Dig Dis Sci* 1990, **35**:668.

SALENA BJ, HUNT RH: **Comparison of Endoscopic Polidocanol Injection and Nd:YAG Laser Therapy for Bleeding Peptic Ulcers [letter].** *Gastrointest Endosc* 1990, **36**:171.

SANDER R, POESL H, SPUHLER A, BRAIDA M: **The Importance of Polypectomy Prior to ● Laser Therapy in Broad-based Villous Adenomas.** *Gastrointest Endosc* 1990, **36**:318. **[22].**

SEMLER P: **Palliative Treatment of Cancer of the Colon with Laser Ablation and ● Afterloading Radiotherapy.** *Dtsch Med Wochenschr (DMW)* 1990, **115**:328–331. **[14].**

SHIMAMURA Y, GUNVEN P, ISHII M, *ET AL.*: **Endoscopic Laser Coagulation Through an ● Optical Laser Balloon.** *Lasers Surg Med* 1990, **10**:25–27. **[29].**

STRANGE EF, DYLLA J, FLEIG WE: **Laser Treatment of Upper Gastrointestinal ● Carcinoma: Determinants of Survival.** *Endoscopy* 1989, **21**:254–257. **[8].**

UNGER SW, STERN JD, ARROYO PJ, RUSSIN DJ: **Endoscopic Nd : YAG Laser Treatment ● of Colorectal Neoplasms: a Four-year Longitudinal Study.** *Am Surg* 1990, **56**:153–157. **[1].**

WENK H, LANGE V, HOHLBACH G, SCHILDBERG FW: **Endoscopic Laser Treatment of ● Bleeding Actinic Proctitis.** *Color-proctology* 1989, **12**:173–176. **[10].**

Endosonography

ANONYMOUS: **Endoscopic Ultrasonography in Achalasia [letter].** *Gastroenterology* 1990, **98**:253.

BOLONDI L, LI BASSI S, GAIANI S, CAMPIONE O, MARRANO D, BARBARA L: **Diagnosis of Islet Cell Tumor by Means of Endoscopic Ultrasonography.** *J Clin Gastroenterol* 1990, **12**:218–221. **[52].**

BOYCE GA, SIVAK MV: **Endoscopic Ultrasonography in the Diagnosis of Pancreatic ●● Tumors.** *Gastrointest Endosc* 1990, **36**:S28–S32. **[53].**

BOYCE GA, SIVAK MV JR: **Endoscopic Ultrasonography in the Diagnosis of Pancreatic Tumors.** *Gastrointest Endosc* 1990, **36 (suppl)**:S28–S32.

CALETTI GC, BROCCHI E, BARALDINI M, FERRARI A, GIBILARO M, BARBARA L: **Assessment of ●● Portal Hypertension by Endoscopic Ultrasonography.** *Gastrointest Endosc* 1990, **36**:S21–S27. **[57].**

CALETTI GC, BROCCHI E, GIBILARO M, FERRARI A, CARFAGNA L, BARBARA L: **Sensitivity Specificity and Predictive Value of Endoscopic Ultrasonography (EUS) in the Diagnosis and Assessment of Gastric Cancer.** *Gastrointest Endosc* 1990, **36**:194–195. **[32].**

CALETTI GC, GUILLINI S, BROCCHI E, BOCCIA S, GIBILARO M, CANTARINI D, FERRARI A, CARFAGNA L, BARBARA L: **Endoscopic Ultrasonography (EUS) with the Guillotine Needle Biopsy in the Diagnosis of Gastric Submucosal Tumors (GSMT).** *Gastrointest Endosc* 1990, **36**:222. **[43].**

COTTE L, PUJOL B, VALETTE PJ, GRANDJEAN JP, SOUQUET JC: **Complicated Perianorectal Fistula — Contribution of Endosonography [in French] [letter].** *Gastroenterol Clin Biol* 1990, **14**:510–511.

DEVIÉRE J, DUNHAM F, CREMER M: **Endoscopic Ultrasonography in Achalasia.** *Gastroenterology* 1990, **98**:253(L). **[23].**

FULLARTON GM, MURRAY WR: **Prediction of Rebleeding in Peptic Ulcers by Visual Stigmata and Endoscopic Doppler Ultrasound Criteria.** *Endoscopy* 1990, **22**:68–71.

GANA TJ, SOENEN GM, KOO J: **A Controlled Study of Human Resting Gastric Mucosal Blood Flow by Endoscopic Laser-Doppler Flowmetry.** *Gastrointest Endosc* 1990, **36**:264–267.

GLASER F, SCHLAG P, HERFARTH CH: **Endorectal Ultrasonography for the Assessment ● of Invasion of Rectal Tumours and Lymphnode Involvement.** *Br J Surg* 1990, **77**:883–887. **[44].**

HEINTZ A, JUNGINGER TH, BÖTTGER TH, KREITNER KF: **Endosonography for Diagnosis of Locoregional Recurrence after Anterior Rectal Dissection. Case Report.** *Colo-proctology* 1990, **12**:138–141. **[45].**

KIMMEY MB, MARTIN RW, SILVERSTEIN FE: **Endoscopic Ultrasound Probes.** *Gastrointest* ● *Endosc* 1990, **36**:S40–S46. **[5].**

LIGHTDALE CJ, BOTET JF: **Esophageal Carcinoma: Pre-operative Staging and ●● Evaluation of Anastomotic Recurrence.** *Gastrointest Endosc* 1980, **36**:S11–S16. **[18].**

NAKAMURA H, ENDO M, SHIMOJUU K, GOSEKI N, INOUE H: **Esophageal Varices Evaluated by Endoscopic Ultrasonography: Observation of Collateral Circulation During Non Shunting Operations.** *Surg Endosc* 1990, **4**:69–75. **[58].**

NICKL NJ, COTTON PB: **Clinical Application of Endoscopic Ultrasonography.** *Am J* ● *Gastroenterol* 1990, **85**:675–682. **[3].**

NISHIWAKI H, ASAI T, SOWA M, UMEYAMA K: **Endoscopic Measurement of Gastric Mucosal Blood Flow with Special Reference to the Effect of Sclerotherapy in Patients with Liver Cirrhosis.** *Am J Gastroenterol* 1990, **85**:34–37.

NIWA Y, NAKAZAWA S, YOSHINO J, NAKAMURA T, OHASHI S, TSUKAMOTO Y: **Quantification of Gastric Ulcer Healing by Endoscopic Ultrasonography.** *Gastrointest Endosc* 1990, **36**:116–122. **[35].**

PALAZZO L, GAYET B, VILGRAIN V, MOLAS G, AMOUYAL P, ROSEAU G, PONSOT P, AMOUYAL G, FEKETE F, PAOLAGGI JA: **Endoscopic Ultrasound and Esophageal Carcinoma — Results of a Prospective Study [in French].** *Gastroenterol Clin Biol* 1990, **14**:428–436.

Ponsot P, Chaussade S, Palazzo L, Amouyal P, Gaudric M, Couturier D, Paolaggi JA: **Endoscopic Ultrasonography in Achalasia.** *Gastroenterology* 1990, **98**:253. **[21].**

Rösch T, Classen M: **A New Ultrasonic Probe for Endosonographic Imaging of the**
● **Upper GI Tract.** *Endoscopy* 1990, **22**:41–46. **[4].**

Rösch T, Lorenz R, Classen M: **Endoscopic Ultrasonography in the Evaluation of Colon and Rectal Disease.** *Gastrointest Endosc* 1990, **36 (suppl)**:S33–S39.

Rösch Th, Lorenz R, Classen M: **Endoscopic Ultrasonography in the Evaluation of**
●● **Colon and Rectal Disease.** *Gastrointest Endosc* 1990, **36**:S33–S39. **[48].**

Rösch Th, Lorenz R, Suchy R, Dancygier H, Classen M: **Colonic Endoscopic**
● **Ultrasonography: First Results of a New Technique.** *Gastrointest Endosc* 1990, **36**:382–386. **[46].**

Shimizu S, Tada M, Kawai K: **Use of Endoscopic Ultrasonography for the Diagnosis of Colorectal Tumors.** *Endoscopy* 1990, **22**:31–34. **[47].**

Sivak MV Jr, Boyce GA: **Endoscopic Ultrasonography: an Introduction.** *Gastrointest Endosc* 1990, **36 (suppl)**:S1.

Sugimachi K, Ohno S, Fujishima H, Kuwano H, Mori M, Misawa T: **Endoscopic**
● **Ultrasonographic Detection of Carcinomatous Invasion and of Lymph Nodes in the Thoracic Esophagus.** *Surgery* 1990, **107**:366–371. **[15].**

Tanaka M, Bandou T, Watanabe A, Sasaki H: **A New Technique in Endoscopic**
● **Ultrasonography of the Upper Gastrointestinal Tract.** *Endoscopy* 1990, **22**:221–225. **[6].**

Tio PL, Coene PPLO, Den Hartog Jager FCA, Tytgat GNJ: **Preoperative Classification**
● **of Esophageal Carcinoma by Endosonography.** *Hepatogastroenterol* 1990, **37**:376–381. **[16].**

Tio TL: **Endosonography in Gastroenterology (in German).** *Dtsch Med Wochenschr* 1990, **115**:584–588.

Tio TL, Coene PPLO, Luiken GJHM, Tytgat GNJ: **Endosonography in the Clinical**
●● **Staging of Esophagogastric Carcinoma.** *Gastrointest Endosc* 1990, **36**:S2–S10. **[17].**

Tio TL, Coene PPLO, Luiken GJHM, Tytgat GNJ: **Endosonography in the Clinical Staging of Esophagogastric Carcinoma.** *Gastrointest Endosc* 1990, **36 (suppl)**:S2–S10.

Tio TL, Mulder CJJ, Wijers OB, Sars PRA, Tytgat GNJ: **Endosonography of Peri-anal**
● **and Peri-colorectal Fistula And/or Abscess in Crohn's Disease.** *Gastrointest Endosc* 1990, **36**:331–336. **[49].**

Tio TL, Tytgat GNJ, Cikot RJLM, Houthoff HJ, Sars PRA: **Ampullopancreatic Carcinoma: Preoperative TNM Classification with Endosonography.** *Radiology* 1990, **175**:455–461. **[50].**

Tio TL, Tytgat GNJ, Den Hartog Jager FCA: **Endoscopic Ultrasonography for the**
● **Evaluation of Smooth Muscle Tumors in the Upper Gastrointestinal Tract: an Experience with 42 Cases.** *Gastrointest Endosc* 1990, **36**:342–350. **[42].**

Yasuda K, Cho E, Nakajima M, Kawai K: **Diagnosis of Submucosal Lesions of the**
● **Upper Gastrointestinal Tract by Endoscopic Ultrasonography.** *Gastrointest Endosc* 1990, **36**:S17–S20. **[39].**

Ziegler K, Sanft C, Friedrich M, Gregor M, Riecken O: **Endosonographic Appearance**
● **of the Esophagus in Achalasia.** *Endoscopy* 1990, **22**:1–4. **[22].**

Ziegler K, Sanft C, Zeitz M, Riecken EO: **Preoperative Staging of Gastrointestinal Tumors by Endosonography.** *Surg Endosc* 1990, **4**:154–160. **[29].**

Endoscopy and pancreatic disease

Bastid C, Bernard JP, Sarles H, Payan MJ, Sahel J: **Mucinous Ductal Ectasia of the Pancreas: a Premalignant Disease and a Cause of Obstructive Pancreatitis.** *Pancreas* 1991, 6:15–22. **[23].**

Bastid C, Filho M, Sahel J: **Main Bile Duct Diameter in Chronic Calcifying Pancreatitis — Comparison of Measurement by Ultrasonography and Endoscopic Retrograde Cholangiography (in French) [letter].** *Gastroenterol Clin Biol* 1990, **14**:402.

Benage D, McHenry R, Hawes RH, O'Connor KW, Lehman GA: **Minor Papilla**
● **Cannulation and Dorsal Ductography in Pancreas Divisum.** *Gastrointest Endosc* 1990, **36**:553–557. **[33].**

Boustiere C, Ponchon T, Valette PJ, Genin G, Gagnon P, Labadie M: **Percutaneous Fine Needle Aspiration Cytology of Main Pancreatic Duct Stenosis Guided by Wirsungography.** *Gastrointest Endosc* 1990, **36**:200A. **[12].**

Carr-Locke DL: **Endoscopic Procedures in the Treatment of Pancreatic Pain.** *Acta Chir Scand* 1990, **156**:293–298.

Dabezies MA, Campana T, Friedman AC: **ERCP in the Diagnosis of Ductectatic Mucinous Cystadenocarcinoma of the Pancreas.** *Gastrointest Endosc* 1990, **36**:410–411. **[19].**

Delcenserie R: **Jaundice Due to Incurable Malignant Tumors: to Drain or not to Drain? [editorial] (in French).** *Gastroenterol Clin Biol* 1990, **14**:113–114.

Delhaye M, Vandermearen A, Gabbrielli A, Cremer MP: **Lithotripsy and Endoscopy for**
● **Pancreatic Calculi: the First 104 Patients.** *Gastroenterology* 1990, **98**:A216. **[62].**

Derfus GA, Geenen JE, Hogan WJ: **Effect of Endoscopic Pancreatic Duct Stent Placement on Pancreatic Ductal Morphology.** *Gastrointest Endosc* 1990, **36**:206A. **[69].**

Deviere J, Devaere S, Baize M, Cremer M: **Endoscopic Biliary Drainage in Chronic**
● **Pancreatitis.** *Gastrointest Endosc* 1990, **36**:96–100. **[71].**

Ebbehoj N, Borly L, Madsen P, Matzen P: **Comparison of Regional Pancreatic Tissue Fluid Pressure and Endoscopic Retrograde Pancreatographic Morphology in Chronic Pancreatitis.** *Scand J Gastroenterol* 1990, **25**:756–760.

Eskelinen M, Lipponen P, Collan Y, Marin S, Alhava E, Nordling S: **Relationship Between DNA Ploidy and Survival in Patients with Exocrine Pancreatic Cancer.** *Pancrease* 1991, 6:90–95. **[30].**

Foerster EC, Stommer P, Schneider MU, Matek W, Gerner G, Domschke W: **Transpapillary Miniscopy and Mini-biopsy of the Pancreatic Duct.** *Endoscopy* 1990, **22**:78–80. **[31].**

Foutch PG, Kerr DM, Harlan JR, Manne RK, Kummet TD, Sanowski RA: **Endoscopic**
● **Retrograde Wire-guided Brush Cytology for Diagnosis of Patients with Malignant Obstruction of the Bile Duct.** *Am J Gastroenterol* 1990, **85**:791–795. **[8].**

Gagnon P, Ponchon T, Labadie M, Berger F, Chavaillon A, Boustiere C: **Value of Endobiliary Brushing Cytology and Biopsies of Bile Duct Stenosis.** *Gastrointest Endosc* 1990, **36**:200A. **[9].**

Glaser J: **Imaging in Diseases of the Pancreas [in German] [Review].** *Dtsch Med Wochenschr* 1990, **115**:1361–1367.

Gregg JA, Stern JS, Gregg L: **Correlation of Postoperative Dorsal Duct Pancreatic Sphincter Manometry and Intraductal Secretin Tests with Relief of Pain in Pancreas Divisum.** *Am J Gastroenterol* 1990, **85**:1249A. **[37].**

Haber G, Sherman S, Miller L, Hawes R, Ponich T, Kortan R, Lehman G: **Pancreatic**
● **Duct Stones: Frequency of Successful Removal and Improvement in Symptoms.** *Gastrointest Endosc* 1990, **36**:202–203A. **[63].**

Halpert RD, Shabot JM, Heare BR, Rogers RE: **The Bifid Pancreas: a Rare Anatomical**
● **Variation.** *Gastrointest Endosc* 1990, **36**:60–61. **[5].**

Hyoty MK, Nordback IH: **Biliary Stent or Surgical Bypass in Unresectable Pancreatic Cancer with Obstructive Jaundice.** *Acta Chir Scand* 1990, **156**:391–396.

Kohler B, Kohler G, Riemann J: **Pancreoscopic Diagnosis of Intraductal Cystadenoma of the Pancreas.** *Dig Dis Sci* 1990, **35**:382–284. **[21].**

Kozarek RA: **Pancreatic Stents can Induce Ductal Changes Consistent with**
● **Chronic Pancreatitis.** *Gastrointest Endosc* 1990, **36**:93–95. **[68].**

Lans JI, Geenen JE, Johanson JF, Hogan WJ: **Endoscopic Therapy in Patients with**
●● **Pancreas Divisum and Acute Pancreatitis: a Prospective, Randomized, Controlled Clinical Trial.** *Gastroenterology* 1991, **100**:(in Press). **[35].**

Lersch C, Classen M: **Treatment Concept for Advanced Carcinoma of the Pancreas (in German).** *Dtsch Med Wochenschr* 1990, **115**:340–342.

Lorente JA, Del Arbol LR, Morelra VF, Garcia-Plaza A: **Recurrent Pancreatitis in a Young Patient Associated with a Solitary Nonopaque Concretion in the Main Pancreatic Duct.** *Gastrointest Endosc* 1990, **36**:63–65. **[58].**

Misra SP, Dwivedi M: **Pancreaticobiliary Ductal Union.** *Gut* 1990, **31**:1144–1149. **[3].**

Misra SP, Gulati P, Choudhary V, Anand BS: **Pancreatic Duct Abnormalities in Gall**
● **Stone Disease: an Endoscopic Retrograde Cholangiopancreatographic Study.** *Gut* 1990, **31**:1073–1075. **[2].**

Moreira VF, Roman AL-S, Ledo L, Merono ?, Erdozain JC: **Retroperitoneal Lymphoma Causing Pancreatic Ductal Obstruction in Endoscopic Retrograde Cholangiopancreatography.** *Gastrointest Endosc* 1990, **36**:80–81. **[16].**

Morris JB, Zollinger RM Jr, Stellato TA, Yang P: **The Pseudo-Double Duct Sign: an ERCP Finding in Pancreatic Carcinoma.** *Gastrointest Endosc* 1990, **36**:408–409. **[1].**

Nishimori I, Okazaki K, Morita M, Miyao M, Sakamoto Y, Kagiyama S, Yamamoto Y, Yamamoto Y: **Congenital Hypoplasia of the Dorsal Pancreas: with Special Reference to Duodenal Papillary Dysfunction.** *Am J Gastroenterol* 1990, **85**:1029–1033. **[6].**

Nowak A, Nowakowska-Dutawa E, Rybicka J: **Patency of the Santorini Duct and**
●● **Acute Biliary Pancreatitis: a Prospective ERCP Study.** *Endoscopy* 1990, **22**:124–126. **[53].**

Ogawa Y, Tanaka M, Matsumoto S, Yamauchi S, Ikeda S, Yoshimoto H: **Islet Cell Tumors of the Pancreas.** *Int J Pancreatol* 1990, **6**:49–60. **[13].**

Payan MJ, Xerri L, Moncada K, Bastid C, Agostini S, Sastre B, Sahel J, Choux R: **Villous**
● **Adenoma of the Main Pancreatic Duct: a Potentially Malignant Tumor?** *Am J Gastroenterol* 1990, **85**:459–463. **[24].**

Pinson CW, Munson JL, Deveney CW: **Endoscopic Retrograde Cholangiopancreatography in the Preoperative Diagnosis of Pancreatic Neoplasms Associated with Cysts.** *Am J Surg* 1990, **159**:510–513. **[17].**

Raddawi HM, Geenen JE, Hogan WJ, Dodds WJ, Venu RP, Johnson GK: **Pressure**
● **Measurements from Biliary and Pancreatic Segments of Sphincter of Oddi — Comparison Between Patients with Functional Abdominal Pain, Biliary, or Pancreatic Disease.** *Dig Dis Sci* 1991, **36**:71–74. **[46].**

Rolny P, Anderberg B, Ihse I, Lindstrom E, Olaison G, Arvill A: **Pancreatitis after**
● **Sphincter of Oddi Manometry.** *Gut* 1990, **31**:821–824. **[43].**

Rolny P, Arleback A, Funch-Jensen P, Kruse A, Jarnerot G: **Clinical Significance of**
● **Manometric Assessment of Both Pancreatic Duct and Bile Duct Sphincter in the Same Patient.** *Scand J Gastroenterol* 1989, **24**:751–754. **[47].**

Rosch T, Lorenz R, Braig C, Feuerbach S, Siewert JR, Classen M: **Endoscopic Ultrasound in the Diagnosis of Pancreatic Tumours [in German].** *Dtsch Med Wochenschr* 1990, **115**:1339–1347.

Rösch Th, Classen M: **Diagnosis of Carcinoma of the Pancreas (in German).** *Dtsch Med Wochenschr* 1990, **115**:304–308.

Satake K, Arimoto Y, Fujimoto Y, Nishiwaki H, Nishino H, Umeyama K, Inoue T, Mitsuhashi T: **Malignant T-cell Lymphoma of the Pancreas.** *Pancreas* 1991, 6:120–124. **[15].**

Schuman BM: **The Evolution of Diagnostic ERCP [editorial].** *Gastrointest Endosc* 1990, **36**:155.

Scudera PL, Koizumi J, Jacobson IM: **Brush Cytology Evaluation of Lesions**
● **Encountered During ERCP.** *Gastrointest Endosc* 1990, **36**:281–294. **[7].**

Shemesh E, Czerniak A, Nass S, Klein E: **Role of Endoscopic Retrograde Cholangiopancreatography in Differentiating Pancreatic Cancer Coexisting with Chronic Pancreatitis.** *Cancer* 1990, **65**:893–896. **[29].**

Sherman S, Lehman GA: **ERCP and Endoscopic Sphincterotomy Induced**
●● **Pancreatitis.** *Pancreas* 1991, :(in Press). **[38].**

Sherman S, Troiano FP, Hawes RH, Lehman GA: **Does Continuous Aspiration from**
● **an End and Side Port in a Sphincter of Oddi Manometry Catheter Alter Recorded Pressures?** *Gastrointest Endosc* 1990, **36**:500–502. **[44].**

Sherman S, Troiano FP, Hawes RH, Lehman GA: **Sphincter of Oddi Manometry:**
●● **Decreased Risk of Clinical Pancreatitis with the use of a Modified Aspirating Catheter.** *Gastrointest Endosc* 1990, **36**:462–466. **[45].**

Siegel JH, Ben-Zvi JS, Pullano W, Copperman A: **Effectiveness of Endoscopic Drainage for Pancreas Divisum: Endoscopic and Surgical Results in 31 Patients.** *Endoscopy* 1990, **22**:129–133. **[36].**

Silverman WB, Ruffolo TA, Sherman S, Hawes RH, Lehman GA: **Correlation of Basal Sphincter Pressure Measured from Both Bile Ducts and Pancreatic Duct in Patients with Suspected Sphincter of Oddi Dysfunction (SOD).** *Gastrointest Endosc* 1991, :in Press. **[48].**

Stanten R, Frey CF: **Pancreatitis after Endoscopic Retrograde Cholangiopancreatography - an Underreported Disease Whose Severity is Often Unappreciated.** *Arch Surg* 1990, **125**:1032–1035.

STEINBERG W: **The Clinical Utility of CA 19-9 Tumor-associated Antigen.** *Am J*
• *Gastroenterol* 1990, **85**:350–356. **[25].**
STERNLIEB J, ARONCHICK C, RETIG J, DABEZEIS M, SAUNDERS F, GOOSENBERG R, INFANTOLINO
• A, IONNA S, MAISLIN G, WRIGHT S, LIPSHUTZ W: **A Multicenter, Randomized, Controlled Trial to Evaluate the Effect of Octreotide on Post-ERCP Pancreatitis.** *Am J Gastroenterol* 1990, **85**:1259A. **[40].**
TAYLOR DH, BRODMERKEL GJ: **Role of Octreotide in ERCP Associated Pancreatitis.**
• *Am J Gastroenterol* 1990, **85**:1260A. **[41].**
WARSHAW AL, SIMEONE JF, SCHAPIRO RH, FLAVIN-WARSHAW B: **Evaluation and Treatment**
•• **of the Dominant Dorsal Duct Syndrome (Pancreas Divisum Redefined).** *Am J Surg* 1990, **159**:59–66. **[34].**
ZERA RT: **Is Pancreatic Cancer Hopeless?** *Gastrointest Endosc* 1990, **36**:161. **[26].**
ZERA RT: **Is Pancreatic Cancer Hopeless? [letter].** *Gastrointest Endosc* 1990, **36**:161.
ZIMMON D, RANSON JHC: **What is the Role of Endoscopy in the Management of**
• **Biliary Pancreatitis and when Should it be Utilized?** *Am J Gastroenterol* 1990, **85**:9–11. **[56].**

Endoscopic management of gallstone disease

ANONYMOUS: **Choledochoscopy Via the Cystic Duct: Evaluation of a New Ultrathin Disposable Choledochoscope.** *Ann R Coll Surg Engl* 1990, **72**:147.
ANONYMOUS: **Early Postoperative Endoscopic Sphincterotomy for Retained Common Duct Stones.** *Ann R Coll Surg Engl* 1990, **72**:147.
APELGREN KN, ZAMBOS JM, VARGISH T: **Intraoperative Flexible Videocholedochoscopy: an Improved Technique for Evaluating the Common Duct.** *Am Surg* 1990, **56**:178–181.
BAILLIE J, CAIRNS SR, COTTON PB: **Endoscopic Management of Choledocholithiasis**
• **During Pregnancy.** *Surg Gynecol Obstet* 1990, **171**:1–4. **[20].**
BERCI G: **Extra Corporeal Shock Wave Lithotripsy of Gallstones and the**
•• **Importance of Operative Cholangiography During Laparoscopic Cholecystectomy.** *Surg Endosc* 1990, **4**:131–132. **[31].**
BERCI G, HAMLIN JA, DAYKHOVSKY L, PAZ-PARTLOW M: **Common Bile Duct Laser**
• **Lithotripsy.** *Gastrointest Endosc* 1990, **36**:137–138. **[7].**
BERCI G, HAMLIN JA, GRUNDFEST W, DAYHKHOVSKY L, PAZ-PARTLOW M: **Percutaneous**
• **Endoscopic Laser Lithotripsy of Retained Stone in the Left Hepatic Duct.** *Surg Endosc* 1990, **4**:36–38. **[8].**
BERKOWITZ I, BORNMAN PC, KOTTLER RE: **Cystic Duct Entry — Another Cause of Pseudocalculus.** *Endoscopy* 1990, **22**:85–87.
BRATZKE H, RAUCH E: **Fatal Complication of Endoscopic Papillotomy (in German).** *Dtsch Med Wochenschr* 1990, **115**:300–303.
DESA LA, GRACE PA, HENDERSON B, THOMPSON JN, VIPOND MN: **Gallbladder Function**
• **after Endoscopic Sphincterotomy.** *Br Med J* 1990, **300**:1111. **[30].**
DICKENS CM, HESELTINE D, WALTON S, BENNETT JR: **The Oesophagus in Lichen Plants: an Endoscopic Study.** *Br Med J [Clin Res]* 1990, **300**:84.
DITZEL H, DE MUCKADELL OBS: **Endoscopic Sphincterotomy in Acute Cholantitis**
• **Due to Choledocholithiasis.** *Hepatogastroenterology* 1990, **37**:204–207. **[17].**
FLOWERS BF, SASLAWSKY MJ, MATHES GL, TONKIN AK: **Use of the Pulsed Dye Laser and**
• **Ultrasonic Lithotriptor for Removal of Multiple Intrahepatic Gallstones.** *Surg Gynecol Obstet* 1990, **170**:443–444. **[9].**
HEARNE SE, STUMP DL: **Endoscopic Removal of Proline Sutures from the Common**
• **Bile Duct During Endoscopic Retrograde Cholangiography.** *Gastrointest Endosc* 1990, **36**:301. **[23].**
HILL J, MARTIN DF, TWEEDLE DEF: **What are the Risks of Leaving the Gallbladder *in Situ* after Endoscopic Sphincterotomy for Bile Duct Stones.** *Br J Surg* , :(in Press). **[27].**
HORTON R, LAURI A, ARNOLD JD *ET AL*; DESA LA *ET AL*: **Gall Bladder Function after Endoscopic Sphincterotomy [letter].** *Br Med J [Clin Res]* 1990, **300**:1584.
KOHLBERGER EJ, RADECKE J, SALM R, WANINGER J: **Large-Bile-Duct Stones—Extracorporeal**
• **Piezoelectric Lithotripsy as Adjuvant Measure for Endoscopic Basket Extraction.** *Surg Endosc* 1990, **4**:20–22. **[12].**
LANDRENEAU RJ, MCCLELLAND RN: **Impaction of the Endoscopic Basket.** *Am Surg* 1990,
• **56**:388–393. **[22].**
LEUNG JWC, BANEZ VP, CHUNG SCF: **Precut (needle Knife) Papillotomy for**
•• **Impacted Common Bile Duct Stone at the Ampulla.** *Am J Gastroenterol* 1990, **85**:991–993. **[15].**
MACFADYEN BV JR, SANDLER CM: **Percutaneous Cholecystostomy and Lithotripsy of Gallstones.** *Am Surg* 1990, **56**:226–231.
MALONE DE, BURHENNE HJ: **Technical Problems: Impacted Retained Distal**
• **Common Duct Stone.** *Clin Radiol* 1990, **41**:130–133. **[6].**
MARTIN DF, TWEEDLE DEF: **Retroperitoneal Perforation During Ercp and Endoscopic Sphincterotomy - Causes, Clinical Features and Management.** *Endoscopy* 1990, **22**:174–175.
MCCARTHY JH, MILLER GL, LAURENCE BH: **Cannulation of the Cystic Duct and**
• **Gallbladder.** *Endoscopy* 1990, **22**:191. **[29].**
MERRETT M, DESMOND P: **Removal of Impacted Endoscopic Basket and Stone from**
• **the Common Bile Duct by Extra Corporeal Shock Waves.** *Endoscopy* 1990, **22**:92. **[21].**
NAGORNEY DM, LOHMULLER JL: **Choledochoscopy: a Cost-minimization Analysis.** *Ann Surg* 1990, **211**:354–359.
NG SK, YIP WC, CHOW WC, CHOI TK: **Removal of Intrahepatic Stone by Rigid Ultrasonic Lithotripter Through a Choledochotomy Tract.** *Gastrointest Endosc* 1990, **36**:402–404.
PONSKY JL, SCHEERES DE, SIMON I: **Endoscopic Retrograde Cholangioscopy.** *Am Surg*
• 1990, **56**:235–237. **[11].**
PONSKY JL, SCHEERES DE, SIMON I: **Endoscopic Retrograde Cholangioscopy: an Adjunct to Endoscopic Exploration of the Common Bile Duct+.** *Am Surg* 1990, **56**:235–237.
REDDICK EJ, OLSEN D, ALEXANDER W, BAILEY A, BAIRD D, PRICE N, PRUITT R: **Laparoscopic**
•• **Laser Cholecystectomy and Choledocholithiasis.** *Surg Endosc* 1990, **3**:133–135. **[1].**
SAKAI P, ISHIOKA S, ZAMBRANO M, MARONE P, ZITRON C: **Endoscopic Removal of an**
• **Atypical Common Bile Duct Foreign Body.** *Endoscopy* 1990, **22**:93. **[24].**
SCHER KS, GARDNER SA, PEOPLES JB: **Assessing the Role of Routine Choledochoscopy During Exploration of the Bile Duct.** *Surg Gynecol Obstet* 1990, **171**:9–12.
SCHULZ H-J: **Non-surgical Gallstone Therapy.** *Z Klin Med* 1990, **45**:101–102.
SCHUMAN BM: **The Evolution of Diagnostic ERCP [editorial].** *Gastrointest Endosc* 1990, **36**:155.
SCHWARTZ HM, BARKIN JS: **Wire Guided Basket Extraction of Common Bile Duct**
• **Stones.** *Gastrointest Endosc* 1990, **36**:296–298. **[5].**
SHEMESH E, KLEIN E, CZERNIAK A, CORET A, BAT L: **Endoscopic Sphincterotomy in**
• **Patients with Gallbladder in Situ: the Influence of Periampullary Duodenal Diverticula.** *Surgery* 1990, **107**:163–166. **[26].**
SIEGEL JH, BEN-ZVI JS, PULLANO WE: **Mechanical Lithotripsy of Common Duct Stones.**
•• *Gastrointest Endosc* 1990, **36**:351–356. **[4].**
SIEGEL JH, BEN-ZVI JS, PULLANO WE: **Endoscopic Electrohydraulic Lithotripsy.**
• *Gastrointest Endosc* 1990, **36**:134–136. **[10].**
SOEHENDRA N, SCHULZ H, NAM V. CH *ET AL*: **ESWL and Gallstone Dissolution with**
•• **MTBE Via a Naso-Vesicular Catheter.** *Endoscopy* 1990, **22**:176–179. **[28].**
SOOMERS AJ, NAGENGAST FM, YAP SH: **Endoscopic Placement of Biliary**
• **Endoprostheses in Patients with Endoscopically Unextractable Common Bile Duct Stones.** *Endoscopy* 1990, **22**:24–26. **[13].**
TWEEDLE DEF, MARTIN DF: **Pre-Cut Papillotomy for Endoscopic Sphincterotomy and Cholangiography.** *Gastrointest Endosc* , :(in Press). **[16].**
VON SANDEN H, SCHMITT W, OTTENJANN R: **Single-Step Percutaneous Transhepatic Cholecystoscopy.** *Endoscopy* 1990, **22**:149–150.
WHEELER BR, ANIGIAN G, STEPHENS G, LARSON GM: **Choledochoscopy and Common Bile Duct Exploration.** *Am Surg* 1990, **56**:182–184.
WORTHLEY CS, TOOULI J: **Endoscopic Decompression for Acute Cholangitis Due to**
• **Stones.** *Aust NZ J Surg* 1990, **60**:355–359. **[18].**

Endoscopic management of biliary strictures

AKIYAMA H, OKAZAKI T, TAKASHIMA I, SATOH S, RYAN T, IWAMORI S, HIDAKA T, MORIO K,
• OKUHARA T: **Percutaneous Treatments for Biliary Diseases.** *Radiology* 1990, **176**:25–30. **[16].**
ALCANTARA M, CARROBLES JM, POTENCIANO JLM, CHACON JM, GARCIA L, CUESTA MA: **Morrhage in the Upper Digestive Tract Caused by an Aorto- Esophageal Fistula.** *Endoscopy* 1990, **22**:51–53.
ANDERSSON R, TRANHERG KG, BENGMARK S: **Role of Bile and Bacteria in Biliary**
• **Peritonitis.** *Br J Surg* 1990, **77**:36–39. **[59].**
ANONYMOUS: **Ampullary Neoplasia: an Endoscopic Approach.** *Gastroenterology* 1990, **98**:539–541.
BANEZ VP, LEUNG JWC, LAU WY: **Endoscopic Management of an Unusual Intrabiliary Foreign Body.** *Br J Surg* 1990, **77**:882.
BICKERSTAFF KI, BERRY AR, CHAPMAN RW, BRITTON BJ: **Endoscopic Sphincterotomy and**
• **Ampullary Carcinoma.** *Br J Surg* 1990, **77**:160–162. **[24].**
BREM H, GIBBONS GD, COBB G, EDGIN RA, ELLISON EG, CAREY LC: **The use of**
• **Endoscopy to Treat Bronchobiliary Fistula Caused by Choledocholithiasis.** *Gastroenterology* 1990, **98**:490–492. **[55].**
BROWN PE, MCCLAVE SA: **Randomized Trial of Endoscopic Endoprosthesis Versus Operative Bypass in Malignant Obstructive Jaundice.** *Gastrointest Endosc* 1990, **36**:86.
CHOSKI AP, DESSAI EG: **ERCP Without Fluoroscopy.** *Endoscopy* 1990, **22**:91.
COENE PPLO, GROEN AK, CHENG J, OUT MMJ, TYTGAT GNJ, HUIBREGTSE K: **Cloning of**
•• **Biliary Endoprotheses: a New Perspective.** *Gut* 1990, **31**:913–917. **[44].**
COTTON PB: **Management of Malignant Bile Duct Obstruction.** *J Gastroenterol*
•• *Hepatol* 1990, **Suppl 1**:63–77. **[27].**
CREMER M, DEVIERE J, SUGAI B, BAIZE M: **Expandable Biliary Metal Stents for**
• **Malignancies: Endoscopic Insertion and Diathermic Cleaning for Tumor Ingrowth.** *Gastrointest Endosc* 1990, **36**:451–457. **[52].**
DELCENSERIE R: **Jaundice Due to Incurable Malignant Tumors: to Drain or not to Drain? [editorial] (in French).** *Gastroenterol Clin Biol* 1990, **14**:113–114.
DOMSCHKE W, FOERSTER E: **Endoscopic Implantation of Large Bore Self-expanding**
• **Biliary Mesh Stent.** *Gastrointest Endosc* 1990, **36**:55–57. **[51].**
EVANS RA, RABY ND, O'GRADY JG, KARANI JB, NUNNERLEY HB, CALNE RY, WILLIAMS R: **Biliary**
• **Complications Following Orthotopic Liver Transplantation.** *Clin Radiol* 1990, **41**:190–194. **[72].**
FINCH MD, BUTLER JA: **Palliation for Non-pancreatic Malignant Obstruction of the**
• **Biliary Tract.** *Surg Gyn Obst* 1990, **170**:437–440. **[32].**
FOUTCH PG, KERR DM, HARLAN JR, MANNE RK, KUMMET TD, SANOWSKI RA: **Endoscopic**
• **Retrograde Wire-guided Brush Cytology for Diagnosis of Patients with Malignant Obstruction of the Bile Duct.** *Am J Gastroenterol* 1990, **85**:791–795. **[10].**
FOUTCH PG, SAWYER RL, SANOWSKI RA: **The Biliograstric Shunt: a Method for**
• **Simultaneous Internal Diversion of Bile and Enteric Feeding in Patients with Cancer.** *Gastrointest Endosc* 1990, **36**:440–443. **[18].**
FULLARTON GM, HILDITCH T, CAMPBELL A, MURRAY WR: **Clinical and Scintigraphic Assessment of the Role of Endoscopic Sphincterotomy in the Treatment of Sphincter of Oddi Dysfunction.** *Gut* 1990, **31**:231–235.
GILLAMS A, DICK R, DOOLEY JS, WALLSTEN H, EL-DIN A: **Self-expandable Stainless Steel**
• **Braided Endoprosthesis for Biliary Strictures.** *Radiology* 1990, **174**:137–140. **[53].**
GOLDIN E, KATZ E, WENGROWER D, KLUGER Y, KASKEL L, SHILONI E, LIBSON E: **Treatment of**
• **Fistulas of the Biliary Tract by Endoscopic Insertion of Endoprostheses.** *Surg Gynecol Obstet* 1990, **170**:418–423. **[61].**
GYA D, SALI A, HENNESSY O, KUNE GA: **Balloon Dilatation of Biliary Strictures:**
• **Experience and Review of the Literature.** *Aust NZ J Surg* 1990, **60**:361–364. **[67].**
HAGEGE H, DE MONTIGNY S, INK O FRITSCH J, CHOURY AD, LIGUORY C, ÉTIENNE JP: **Obstructive Jaundice in Patients with Hepatic Tumor: Result of Non Surgical Biliary Drainage (in French).** *Gastroenterol Clin Biol* 1990, **14**:115–119.
HALL RI, DENYER ME, CHAPMAN AH: **Percutaneous-endoscopic Placement of**
• **Endoprostheses for Relief of Jaundice Caused by Inoperable Bile Duct Strictures.** *Surg* 1990, **107**:224–227. **[19].**
HATFIELD ARW: **Palliation of Malignant Obstructive Jaundice — Surgery or Stent?**
• *Gut* 1990, **31**:1339–1340. **[36].**

Hearne SE, Stump DL: **Endoscopic Removal of Prolene Sutures from the Common Bile Duct During Endoscopic Retrograde Cholangiography.** *Gastrointest Endosc* 1990, **36**:301–303.

● Heit P, McKinley M, Javors B: **Mucoid Biliary Obstruction: Direct Endoscopic Visualization of Mucine-hypersecreting Bile Duct Tumor.** *Gastrointest Endosc* 1990, **36**:164–166. **[3].**

● Hoffman BJ, Cunningham JT, Marsh WH: **Endoscopic Management of Biliary Fistulas with Small Calibre Stents.** *Am J Gastroenterol* 1990, **85**:705–707. **[62].**

● Hsu D: **Recanalization of Clogged Biliary Stent.** *Gastrointest Endosc* 1990, **36**:322–323. **[47].**

● Huibregtse K: **Endoscopic Palliation in Malignant Bile Duct Strictures: the Amsterdam Experience.** *Dig Endosc* 1990, **2**:203–206. **[13].**

● Hyoty MK, Nordback IH: **Biliary Stent or Surgical Bypass in Unresectable Pancreatic Cancer with Obstructive Jaundice.** *Acta Chir Scand* 1990, **156**:301–396. **[31].**

● Jackson JE, Roddie ME, Yeung YC, Benjamin IS, Adam A: **Biliary Endoprosthesis Dysfunction in Patients with Malignant Hilar Tumors: Successful Treatment by Percutaneous Replacement of the Stent.** *AJR* 1990, **155**:391–395. **[22].**

● Jacobs M: **Endoscopic Biliary Decompression Aided by a Different Technique of Percutaneous Transhepatic Access.** *Gastrointest Endosc* 1990, **36**:503–505. **[20].**

● Jeng KS, Yang FS, Ohrta I, Chiang HJ: **Dilatation of Intrahepatic Biliary Strictures in Patients with Hepatolithiasis.** *World J Surg* 1990, **14**:587–593. **[73].**

● Kauffmann GW, Roeren T, Friedl P, Brambs HJ, Richter GM: **Interventional Radiological Treatment of Malignant Biliary Obstruction.** *Europ J Surg Oncol* 1990, **16**:397–403. **[17].**

● Krige JEJ, Bornman PC, Beningfield SJ, Nieuwouldt JHM, Terblanche J: **Endoscopic Embolization of ExternalBiliary Fistula.** *Br J Surg* 1990, **77**:581–583. **[64].**

● Kubota Y, Seki T, Junieda K, Nakahashi Y, Yamaguchi T, Tateiwa J, Mizuno T, Shiozaki Y, Sameshima Y: **Long Term Efficacy of Percutaneous Transhepatic Choledochoscopic YAG Laser Therapy for Malignant Biliary Obstruction.** *Dig Endosc* 1990, **2**:156–163. **[30].**

● Lau WY, Leung JWC, Li AKC: **Management of Patients with Hepatocellular Carcinoma Presenting as Obstructive Jaundice.** *Am J Surg* 1990, **160**:280–282. **[2].**

● Lebovics E, Mittelman A, Del Guercio LRM, Hilaris B, Moorthy C, Puccio C, Rosenthal WS: **Pancreaticobiliary Fistula and Obstructive Jaundice Complicating 125 I Interstitial Implants for Pancreatic Cancer: Endoscopic Diagnosis and Management.** *Gastrointest Endosc* 1990, **36**:610–611. **[56].**

● Lee MJ, Mueller PR, Saini S, Morrison MC, Brink JA, Hahn PF: **Occlusion of Biliary Endoprostheses: Presentation and Management.** *Radiology* 1990, **176**:531–534. **[23].**

● Leung JWC, Banez VP: **Clogging of Biliary Stents: Mechanisms and Possible Solution.** *Dig Endosc* 1990, **2**:97–104. **[40].**

Leung JWC, Banez VP, Lam K, Cotton PB, Costerton JW: **Mechanisms of Clogging and the Role of Biocide Impregnation in Preventing Stent Clogging.** *Gastrointest Endosc* 1990, **36**:160 (abstract). **[42].**

● Leung JWC, Banez VP, Sung JY, Wu ZM, Agas FV, Chung SCS: **Endoscopic Cholangiopancreatography in Hepatic Clonorchiasis — a Follow-up Study.** *Gastrointest Endosc* 1990, **36**:. **[65].**

●● Leung JWC, Chan RCY, Cheung SW, Sung JY, Chung SCS, French GL: **The Effect of Obstruction on Biliary Excretion of Cefoperazone and Ceftazidime.** *J Antimicrobial Chemo* 1990, **25**:399–406. **[15].**

● Levine GJ, Botet J, Kurtz RC: **Microbiological Analysis of Sepsis Complicating Non-surgical Biliary Drainage in Malignant Obstruction.** *Gastrointest Endosc* 1990, **36**:364–368. **[14].**

● Liguory C, Vitale GC: **Biliary Perestroika.** *Am J Surg* 1990, **160**:237–238. **[75].**

Liguory C, Vitale GC: **Biliary Perestroika [Editorial].** *Am J Surg* 1990, **160**:237–238.

● Lygidakis NJ, Carlei F: **Structural and Functional Biliary Tree Changes Secondary to Extrahepatic Biliary Obstruction.** *Endoscopy* 1990, **21**:321–323. **[11].**

● Marshall T, Kamalvand K, Cairns SR: **Endoscopic Treatment of Biliary Enteric Fistula.** *Br Med J* 1990, **300**:1176. **[54].**

McCarthy JH, Miller GL, Laurence BH: **Cannulation of the Biliary Tree, Cystic Duct and Gallbladder Using a Hydrophilic Polymer-Coated Steerable Guide Wire.** *Gastrointest Endosc* 1990, **36**:386–389.

Münster B, Schulz H-J, Münster W: **Extrahepatic Cholestatis — Indications for a Direct Cholangiography.** *Z Klin Med* 1990, **45**:619–628.

Neuhaus H, Hagenmuller F, Griebel M, Rotter M, Classen M: **Endoscopic and Percutaneous Implantation of Self-Expanding Stents for Biliary Stenoses [in German].** *Dtsch Med Wochenschr* 1990, **115**:1299–1306.

● Ohshio G, Manabe T, Tamura K, Kudo H, Yoshioka H, Tobe T: **Effects of Percutaneous Transhepatic Biliary Drainage on Blood-Bile Permeability and Selective IgA Transport in Patients with Biliary Obstruction.** *Ann Surg* 1990, **211**:428–432. **[12].**

Patel SA, Borges MC, Batt MD, Rosenblate HJ: ***Trichosporon* Cholangitis Associated with Hyperbilirubinemia, and Findings Suggesting Primary Sclerosing Cholangitis on Endoscopic Retrograde Cholangiopancreatography.** *Am J Gastroenterol* 1990, **85**:84–87.

● Pua SC, Fuji T, Aibe T, Akiyama T, Noguchi T, Tanaka S, Harima K, Sasaki T, Kondon S, Adachi K, Tanaka H, Okita K: **Hepatocellular Carcinoma with Invasion of the Right Intrahepatic Bile Duct Observed by Peroral Cholangioscopy.** *Dig Endosc* 1990, **2**:329–334. **[9].**

Railey DJ, Barkin JS: **Randomized Trial of Endoscopic Endoprosthesis Versus Operative Bypass in Malignant Obstructive Jaundice [letter].** *Gastrointest Endosc* 1990, **36**:169.

● Rao KJM, Blake H, Thoedossi A: **Use of a Modified Angioplasty Balloon Catheter in the Dilatation of Tight Biliary Strictures.** *Gut* 1990, **31**:565–567. **[68].**

Richieri JP: **Early Postendoscopic Sphincterotomy Stenosis [letter].** *Endoscopy* 1990, **22**:98.

Riesenfeld V, Hagerstrand I, Lunderquist A: **Balloon Dilatation of the Ampulla of Vater - an Experimental Study in the Rabbit.** *Acta Radiol* 1990, **31**:222–224.

● Rosengart TK, Rotterdam H, Ranson JHC: **Eosinophilic Cholangitis: a Self-limited Cause of Extrahepatic Biliary Obstruction.** *Am J Gastroenterol* 1990, **85**:582–585. **[4].**

● Rossi P, Bezzi M, Salatori FM, Maccioni F, Porcaro ML: **Recurrent Benign Biliary Strictures: Management with Self-expanding Metallic Stents.** *Radiology* 1990, **175**:661–665. **[71].**

● Schultze K, Hentschel R, Dufek W: **Malignant Bile Duct Obstruction by Tumour Embolism.** *Endoscopy* 1990, **22**:197–198. **[1].**

Schutze K, Hentschel E, Dufek W: **Malignant Bile Duct Obstruction by Tumor Embolism [letter].** *Endoscopy* 1990, **22**:197–198.

● Shemesh E, Nass S, Czerniak A: **Endoscopic Sphincterotomy and Endoscopic Fulguration in the Management of Adenoma of the Papilla of Vater.** *Surg Gyn Obst* 1990, **169**:445–448. **[25].**

●● Sung JY, Olsen ME, Leung JWC, Lundberg MS, Costerton JW: **Microbial Flora of the Gastrointestinal and Biliary System in Cats.** *Microbial Ecology in Health and Diseases* 1990, **3**:199–207. **[45].**

● Szauter KM, Mullen KD, Marshall JB: **Gastrosto-biliary Irrigation for Maintenance of Stent Patency.** *Gastrointest Endosc* 1990, **36**:597–598. **[49].**

● Tam PC, Lai ESC, Hui WM, Chan SCH: **Pitfalls of Percutaneous-endoscopic Biliary Stent Placement.** *Am J Gastroenterol* 1990, **85**:207–209. **[21].**

● Tartar VM, Balfe DM: **Lymphoma in the Wall of the Bile Ducts: Radiologic Imaging.** *Gastrointest Radiol* 1990, **15**:53–57. **[6].**

Theilmann L, Stiehl A: **Detection of Large Intrahepatic Cholangiectases in Patients with Primary Sclerosing Cholangitis by Endoscopic Retrograde Cholangiography.** *Endoscopy* 1990, **22**:49–50.

● Urban MS, Siegel JH, Pavlou W, Tuvia J, Gelb AM, Vikram B, Aubrey R: **Treatment of Malignant Biliary Obstruction with a High-dose Rate Remote Afterloading Device Using a 10 F Nasobiliary Tube.** *Gastrointest Endosc* 1990, **36**:292–296. **[29].**

Vignote ML, Mino G, De La Mata M, De Dios JF, Gomez F: **Endoscopic Sphincteromy in Hepatic Hydatid Disease Open to the Biliary Tree.** *Br J Surg* 1990, **77**:30–31.

von Sanden H, Schmitt W, Ottenjann R: **Single-Step Percutaneous Transhepatic Cholecystoscopy.** *Endoscopy* 1990, **22**:149–150.

● Wengrower D, Goldin E: **Balloon Retrieval of Biliary Stents.** *Gastrointest Endosc* 1990, **36**:639–640. **[46].**

● Yamaguchi K, Enjoji M, Kitamura K: **Endoscopic Biopsy Has Limited Accuracy in Diagnosis of Ampullary Tumors.** *Gastrointest Endosc* 1990, **36**:588–592. **[7].**

Laparoscopy

●● Airan MC: **Letter to the Editor. Laparoscopic Cholecystectomy.** *Am J Surg* 1990, **159**:619. **[3].**

● Al-Hadeedi S, Walia HS, Al-Sayer HM: **Abdominal Tuberculosis.** *CJS* 1990, **33**:233–237. **[13].**

Auguste LJ: **Laparoscopy-guided Percutaneous Cholecystostomy.** *Gastrointest Endosc* 1990, **36**:58–59.

Cava A, Roman J, Quintela AG, Martin F, Aramburo P: **Subcutaneous Metastasis Following Laparoscopy in Gastric Adenocarcinoma.** *Eur J Surg Oncol* 1990, **16**:63–67. **[6].**

● Cohen SM, Franklin RR, Haney AF, et al.: **Prevention of Postsurgical Adhesions by INTERCEED(TC7), an Absorbable Adhesion Barrier: a Prospective, Randomized Multicenter Clinical Study.** *Fertility and Sterility* 1989, **51**:933–938. **[35].**

● Contractor QQ, Benson L, Contractor TQ, Kher YR: **Laparoscopic Appearance of the Liver in *Schistosoma Mansoni* Infection.** *Endoscopy* 1990, **22**:137–139. **[9].**

● Cuschieri A, Abd El Ghany AA, Holley MP: **Successful Chemical Cholecystectomy: a Laparoscopic Guided Technique.** *Gut* 1989, **30**:1786–1794. **[37].**

● Cuschieri A, Berci G, McSherry CK: **Laparoscopic Cholecystectomy.** *Am J Surg* 1990, **159**:273. **[1].**

●● Cuschieri A, Terblanche J: **Laparoscopic Cholecystectomy: Evolution, not Revolution.** *Surg Endosc* 1990, **4**:125–126. **[2].**

● Domingo M, Grau J, Vazquez A, Diez A, Coll J, Vivancos J: **Septic Shock and Bacteremia Associated with Laparoscopic Guided Liver Biopsy, Report on Two Cases.** *Endoscopy* 1989, **21**:240–241. **[8].**

●● Dubois F, Berthelot G, Levard H: **Cholecystectomy Under Celioscopy.** *Ann Chir* 1990, **44**:206. **[26].**

● Ger R, Monroe K, Duvivier R, Mishrick A: **Management of Indirect Inguinal Hernias by Laparoscopic Closure of the Neck of the Sac.** *Am J Surg* 1990, **159**:370–373. **[31].**

Gibson DH, Heasley RN, Price JH, Doherty CC, Douglas JF: **Laparoscopic Repositioning of Blocked Peritoneal Dialysis Catheters in Patients on CAPD.** *Clinical Nephrology* 1990, **33**:208. **[23].**

●● Gordon SC, Watts JC, Veneri RJ, Chandler FW: **Focal Hepatic Candidiasis with Perihepatic Adhesions: Laparoscopic and Immunohistologic Diagnosis.** *Gastroenterology* 1990, **98**:214–217. **[14].**

●● Gotz F, Pier A, Bacher C: **Modified Laparoscopic Appendectomy in Surgery. A Report on 388 Operations.** *Surg Endosc* 1990, **4**:6–9. **[29].**

● Hanafusa T, Miyazaki A, Miyagawa J, et al: **Examination of Islets in the Pancreas Biopsy Specimens from Newly Diagnosed Type 1 (Insulin-dependent) Diabetic Patients.** *Diabetologia* 1990, **33**:105–111. **[36].**

● Hasan FA, Jeffers LJ, Welsh SW, Reddy KR, Schiff ER: **Hepatic Involvement as the Primary Manifestation of Kaposi's Sarcoma in the Acquired Immune Deficiency Syndrome.** *Am J Gastroenterol* 1989, **84**:1449–1451. **[11].**

● Inui Y, Kawata S, Tarui S: **Laparoscopic Findings of Fatty Liver Using Multiple Regression Analysis.** *Endoscopy* 1990, **22**:27–30. **[19].**

● Jarrett JC II: **Laparoscopy: Direct Trocar Insertion Without Pneumoperitoneum.** *Obstet Gynecol* 1990, **75**:725–727. **[4].**

Liguory C, Vitale GC: **Biliary Perestroika [Editorial].** *Am J Surg* 1990, **160**:237–238.

● Mage G, Canis M, Manhes H, Pouly J-L, Bruhat M-A: **Laparoscopic Management of Adnexal Torsion. A Review of 35 Cases.** *J Reprod Med* 1989, **34**:520–524. **[24].**

● Marti Vicente A, Sainz S, Soriano G, Ojeda B, Mendez C, Alonso C, Cusso X: **Utilidad De La Laparoscopia Como Metodo De Second-look En Las Neoplasias De Ovario.** *Rev Esp Enf Digest* 1990, **77**:275–278. **[22].**

MICHITAKA K, ONJI M, HORIIKE N, NADANO S, OHTA Y: **Hepatitis B Virus Replication in Dark Reddish Patchy Markings Appearing on the Hepatic Surface.** *Gastrointest Endosc* 1990, **36**:15–18.

• NATHANSON LK, CUSCHIERI A: **The Falciform Lift: a Simple Method for Retraction of the Falciform Ligament During Laparoscopic Cholecystectomy.** *Surg Endosc* 1990, **4**:186. **[28].**

• O'REGAN PJ, SCARROW GD: **Laparoscopic Jejunostomy.** *Endoscopy* 1990, **22**:39–40.**[33].**

•• ORLANDO R, LIRUSSI F, OKOLICSANYI L: **Laparoscopy and Liver Biopsy: Further Evidence that the Two Procedures Improve the Diagnosis of Liver Cirrhosis.** *J Clin Gastroenterol* 1990, **12**:47–52. **[16].**

PASCUAL JB, BARANDA MM, TARRERO MT, GUTIERREZ MFM, GARRIDO IM, ERRASTI CA: **Subcutaneous Emphysema, Pneumomediastinum, Bilateral Pneumothorax and Pneumopericardium after Laparoscopy.** *Endoscopy* 1990, **22**:59. **[7].**

•• PERISSAT J, COLLET D, BELLIARD R: **Gallstones: Laparoscopic Treatment — Cholecystectomy, Cholecystostomy, and Lithotripsy.** *Surg Endosc* 1990, **4**:1–5. **[27].**

• PETERSON HB, HULKA JF, PHILLIPS JM: **American Association of Gynecologic Laparoscopists' 1988 Membership Survey on Operative Laparoscopy.** *J Reprod Med* 1990, **35**:587–589. **[34].**

• POPP LW: **Endoscopic Patch Repair of Inguinal Hernia in a Female Patient.** *Surg Endosc* 1990, **4**:10–12. **[32].**

•• SALKY BA: **Laparoscopic Cholecystectomy.** *In Laparoscopy for Surgeons: Igaku-Shoin, New York, , :*p 136. **[25].**

• SCHIER F, WALDSCHMIDT J: **Experience with Laparoscopy for the Evaluation of Cholestasis in Newborns.** *Surg Endosc* 1990, **4**:13–14. **[20].**

• SCZIGETVARI I, FEINMAN M, BARAD D, BARTFAI G, KAALI SG: **Association of Previous Abdominal Surgery and Significant Adhesions in Laparoscopic Sterilization Patients.** *J Reprod Med* 1989, **34**:465–466. **[5].**

STELLATO TA, PETERSON DK, BUEHNER P, NOCHOMOVITZ ML, MORTIMER JT: **Taking the Laparoscope to the Laboratory for Ventilatory Research.** *Am Surg* 1990, **56**:131–133.

•• TAMEDA Y, YOSHIZAWA N, TAKASE K, NAKANO T, KOSAKA Y: **Prognostic Value of Peritoneoscopic Findings in Cirrhosis of the Liver.** *Gastroinstest Endosc* 1990, **36**:34–38. **[15].**

•• VAN GELDER T, HOOGSTEDEN HC, VERSNEL MA, DE BEER PH, VANDENBROUCKE JP, PLANTEYDT HT: **Malignant Peritoneal Mesothelioma: a Series of 19 Cases.** *Digestion* 1989, **43**:222–227. **[12].**

•• VERCELLINI P, FEDELE L, ARCAINI L, BIANCHI S, ROGNONI MT, CANDIANI GB: **Laparoscopy in the Diagnosis of Chronic Pelvic Pain in Adolescent Women.** *J Reprod Med* 1989, **34**:827–830. **[10].**

VICENTE AM, SAINZ S, SORIANO G, OJEDA B, MENDEZ C, ALONSO C, CUSSO X: **Usefulness of Laparoscopy as a 2nd Look Method in Cancer of the Ovaries [in Spanish].** *Rev Esp Enferm Dig* 1990, **77**:275–278.

•• WARSHAW AL, GU Z, WITTENBERG J, WALTMAN AC: **Preoperative Staging and Assessment of Resectability of Pancreatic Cancer.** *Arch Surg* 1990, **125**:230–233. **[21].**

Endoscopic instrumentation

BARDE CJ: **New Computer Simulation Study Group Formed [letter].** *Gastrointest Endosc* 1990, **36**:417.

COENE PP, GROEN AK, CHENG J, OUT MM, TYTGAT GN: **Clogging of Biliary Endoprostheses: a New Perspective.** *Gut* 1990, **31**:913–917. **[18].**

COTTON PB, KOZAREK RA, SCHAPIRO RH, *ET AL*: **Endoscopic Laser Lithotripsy of Large Bile Duct Stones.** *Gastroenterology* 1990, **99**:1128–1133. **[16].**

CREMER M, DEVIERE J, BAIZE M, MATOS C: **New Device for Endoscopic Cystoenterostomy.** *Endoscopy* 1990, **22**:76–77. **[25].**

• CREMER M, DEVIERE J, SUGAI B, *ET AL*: **Expandable Biliary Metal Stents for Malignancies: Endoscopic Insertion and Diathermic Cleaning for Tumor Ingrowth.** *Gastrointest Endosc* 1990, **36**:451–457. **[20].**

• DE KNYRIM K, SEIDLITZ H, VAKIL N, *ET AL*: **Perspectives in 'Electronic Endoscopy'.** *Endoscopy* 1990, **22**:2–8. **[1].**

DE REUCK M, RAMDANI B, JONAS C, *ET AL*: **A Randomized Multi-Observer, Comparative Evaluation of Conventional Fiberendoscopy and Videoendoscopy in the Upper GI Tract.** *Endoscopy* 1990, **22**:9–12. **[2].**

DOMSCHKE W, FOERSTER E: **Endoscopic Implantation of Large-bore Self-expanding Biliary Mesh Stent.** *Gastrointest Endosc* 1990, **36**:55–57. **[19].**

DOMSCHKE W, FOERSTER EC, MATEK W, RODL W: **Self-expanding Mesh Stent for Esophageal Cancer Stenosis.** *Endoscopy* 1990, **22**:134–136. **[23].**

• FOUTCH PG, KERR DM, HARLAND JR, MANNE RU, KUMMET TD, SANOWSKI RA: **Endoscopic Retrograde Wire-guided Brush Cytology for Diagnosis of Patients with Malignant Obstruction of the Bile Duct.** *Amer J Gastroenterol* 1990, **85**:791–795. **[21].**

FRANCESCHI D, STELLATO TA: **Microcomputer Image Processing in Gastrointestinal Endoscopy.** *Am Surg* 1990, **56**:128–130. **[4].**

•• FULLARTON GM, MURRAY WR: **Prediction of Rebleeding in Peptic Ulcers by Visual Stigmata and Endoscopic Doppler Ultrasound Criteria.** *Endoscopy* 1990, **22**:68–71. **[10].**

GOLDBERG BB, LIU JB, MERTON DA, KURTZ AB: **Endoluminal US: Experiments with Nonvascular uses in Animals.** *Radiology* 1990, **175**:49–43. **[8].**

KIMMEY MB, MARTIN RW, SILVERSTEIN FE: **Endoscopic Ultrasound Probes.** *Gastrointest Endosc* 1990, **36**:S40–S46. **[9].**

LIN HJ, LEE FY, CHAN CY, HUANG ZC, KANG WM, LEE CH, LEE SD, TSAI YT: **Heat Probe Thermocoagulation as a Substitute for Surgical Intervention to Arrest Massive Peptic Ulcer Hemorrhage - an Experience in 153 Cases.** *Surgery* 1990, **108**:18–21.

•• MCCARTHY JH, MILLER GL, LAURENCE BH: **Cannulation of the Biliary Tree, Cystic Duct and Gallbladder Using a Hydrophilic Polymer-coated Steerable Guidewire.** *Gastrointest Endosc* 1990, **36**:386–391. **[17].**

RÖSCH T, LORENZ R, SUCHY R, DANCYGIER H, CLASSEN M: **Colonic Endoscopic Ultrasonography: First Results of a New Technique.** *Gastrointest Endosc* 1990, **36**:382–386. **[5].**

RÖSCH TH, CLASSEN M: **A New Ultrasonic Probe for Endosonographic Imaging of the Upper GI Tract.** *Endoscopy* 1990, **22**:41–46. **[7].**

SAEED AZ, MICHALETZ PA, FEINER SD, *ET AL*: **A New Endoscopic Method for Managing Food Impaction in the Esophagus.** *Endoscopy* 1990, **22**:226–228. **[13].**

SAEED ZA, MICHALETZ PA, WINCHESTER CB, *ET AL*: **Endoscopic Variceal Ligation in Patients Who have Failed Endoscopic Sclerotherapy.** *Gastrointest Endosc* 1990, **36**:572–574. **[12].**

•• SHAW MJ, DORSHER PJ, VENNES JA: **A New Mechanical Lithotripter for the Treatment of Large Common Bile Duct Stones.** *Amer J Gastroenterol* 1990, **85**:796–798. **[15].**

• SHIMIZU S, TADA M, KAWAI K: **Use of Endoscopic Ultrasonography for the Diagnosis of Colorectal Tumors.** *Endoscopy* 1990, **22**:31–34. **[6].**

STARK GA, CASTELL DO, RICHTER JE, WU WC: **Prospective Randomized Comparison of Brown-McHardy and Microvasive Balloon Dilators in Treatment of Achalasia.** *Am J Gastroenterol* 1990, **85**:1322–1326. **[24].**

• STIEGMANN G, GOFF J, MICHALETZ P, KORULA J, LIEBERMAN D, REVEILLE M, SUN J: **Endoscopic Variceal Ligation Vs. Sclerotherapy for Rebleeding Esophageal Varices: Early Results of a Prospective Randomized Trial.** *Gastrointest Endosc* 1990, **36**:189. **[11].**

STROEHLEIN JR, BARROSO A, GLOMBICKI A, SACHS I: **Documentation of Fluoroscopic and Endoscopic Images Using a Color Video Printer.** *Gastrointest Endosc* 1990, **36**:392–394. **[3].**

TUCKER RD, PLATZ CE, SIEVERT CE, VENNES JA, SILVIS SE: ***In Vivo* Evaluation of Monopolar Versus Bipolar Electrosurgical Polypectomy Snares.** *Am J Gastroenterol* 1990, **85**:1386–1390. **[26].**

TUCKER RD, SIEVERT CE, VENNES JA, SILVIS SE: **Endoscopic Radio Frequency Electrosurgery [Editorial].** *Gastrointest Endosc* 1990, **36**:412–413.

VENU RP, GEENEN JE, KINI M, HOGAN WJ, PAYNE M, JOHNSON GK, SCHMALZ MJ: **Endoscopic Retrograde Brush Cytology.** *Gastroenterology* 1990, **99**:1475–1479. **[22].**

YANG R, VUITCH F, WRIGHT K,: **Adequacy of Disposable Biopsy Forceps for Gastrointestinal Endoscopy: a Direct Comparison with Reusable Forceps.** *Gastrointest Endosc* 1990, **36**:379–381. **[14].**

Pediatric endoscopy

• BORGSTEIN ES, HUNTER DS, YOUNGSON GG: **Endoscopic Restoration of Esophageal Continuity.** *J Pediatr Surg* 1990, **25**:1222–1223. **[10].**

•• BUCKLEY A, CONNON JJ: **The Role of ERCP in Children and Adolescents.** *Gastrointest Endosc* 1990, **36**:369–372. **[1].**

•• CROMBLEHOLME TM, DELORIMIER AA, ADZICK NS, LONGAKER MT, HARRISON MR, COX KL, HEYMAN MB: **Mediastinal Pancreatic Pseudocysts in Children.** *J Pediatr Surg* 1990, **25**:843–845. **[7].**

• CROMBLEHOLME TM, DELORIMIER AA, WAY LW, ADZICK NS, LONGAKER MT, HARRISON MR: **The Modified Puestow Procedure for Chronic Relapsing Pancreatitis in Children.** *J Pediatr Surg* 1990, **25**:749–753. **[8].**

• HOLMQUIST L, AHREN C, FALLSTROM SP: **Clinical Disease Activity and Inflammatory Activity in Relation to Mucosal Inflammation Assessed by Colonoscopy: a Study of Children and Adolescents with Chronic Inflammatory Bowel Disease.** *Acta Paediatr Scand* 1990, **79**:527–534. **[14].**

•• MASILLAH C, GALMICHE J-P, CLOAREC D, GERARD P, CZERNICHOW P, BRULEY DES VARANNES S: **Twenty-four Hour Oesophageal PH Monitoring in Infants with Suspected Gastro-Oesophageal Reflux Disease: Relationships with Symptoms, Endoscopy and Evolution.** *Eur J Gastroenterol Hepatol* 1990, **2**:137–142. **[13].**

NELSON AM: **Delayed Hemorrhage Following Hot Biopsy of a Diminutive Colonic Polyp [letter].** *Gastrointest Endosc* 1990, **36**:418.

• RESCORLA FJ, CORY D, VANE DW, WEST KW, GROSFELD JL: **Failure of Percutaneous Drainage in Children with Traumatic Pancreatic Pseudocysts.** *J Pediatr Surg* 1990, **25**:1038–1042. **[9].**

• TSANG T-M, SAING H, YEUNG C-K: **Peptic Ulcer in Children.** *J Pediatric Surg* 1990, **25**:744–748. **[11].**

Colonoscopy: polyps and cancer

ACHKAR E: **A Hyperplastic Polyp is Discovered on Flexible Sigmoidoscopy — is a Full Colonoscopy Indicated?** *Am J Gastroenterol* 1990, **85**:367–368.

ADAMSEN S: **The Value of Haemoccult [letter].** *Endoscopy* 1990, **22**:90.

• AGREZ MV, REDMAN S, SANSON-FISHER R, HENNRIKUS D: **Feasibility of Sigmoidoscopic Screening for Colorectal Cancer in the Hunter Region.** *Dis Col Rectum* 1990, **33**:87–92. **[9].**

• ARNAUD JP, BERGAMASCHI R, SCHLOEGEL M, OLLIER JC, HAEGELE P, GROB JC, ADLOFF M: **Progress in the Assessment of Lymphatic Spread in Rectal Cancer. Rectal Endoscopic Lymphoscintigraphy.** *Dis Col Rectum* 1990, **33**:398–401. **[41].**

BARILLARI P, RAMACCIATO G, DE ANGELIS R, GOZZO P, INDINNIMEO M, VALABREGA S, AURELLO P, FEGIZ G: **Effect of Preoperative Colonoscopy on the Incidence of Synchronous and Metachronous Neoplasms.** *Acta Chir Scand* 1990, **156**:163–166.

BERRY AR, SOUTER RG, CAMPBELL WB, MORTENSEN NJMC, KETTLEWELL MGW: **Endoscopic Transanal Resection of Rectal Tumours — a Preliminary Report of Its Use.** *Br J Surg* 1990, **77**:134–137. **[45].**

• BRAVERMAN DZ, STANKIEWICZ H, GOLDSTEIN R, PATZ JK, MORALI GA, JACOBSOHN WZ: **Ornithine Decarboxylase —an Unreliable Marker for the Identification of Population Groups at Risk for Colonic Neoplasia.** *Am J Gastroenterol* 1990, **85**:723–726. **[35].**

• BRENNA E, SKREDEN K, WALDUM HL, MARVIK R, DYBDAHL JH, KLEVELAND PM, SANDVIK AK, HALVORSEN T, MYRVOLD HE, PETERSEN H: **The Benefit of Colonoscopy.** *Scand J Gastroenterol* 1990, **25**:81–88. **[16].**

•• BRUNETAUD JM, MAUNOURY V, COCHELARD D, ADENIS A, BONIFACE B, CORTOT A, PARIS JC: **Lasers in Rectosigmoid Cancers: Factors Affecting Immediate and Long-term Results.** *In Ballieres Clinical Gastroenterology* 1990, :615–625. **[42].**

CHOKSI AP, DESSAI HG: **Ercp Without Fluoroscopy [letter].** *Endoscopy* 1990, **22**:91.

CHRISTIE JP: **The Removal of Lipomas.** *Gastrointest Endosc* 1990, **36**:532. **[49].**

• COLLIN GR, RUSSELL JC: **Endometriosis of the Colon — Its Diagnosis and Management.** *Am Surg* 1990, **56**:275–279. **[50].**

● COTHREN RM, RICHARDS-KORTUM R, SIVAK MJ, FITZMAURICE M, RAVA RP, BOYCE GA, DOZTADER M, BLACKMAN R, IVANC TB, HAYES GB, FELD MS, PETRAS RE: **Gastrointestinal Tissue Diagnosis by Laser-induced Fluorescence Spectroscopy at Endoscopy.** *Gastrointestinal Endoscopy* 1990, **36**:105–111. **[36]**.

● DEMERS RY, NEALE AV, BUDEV H, SCHADE WJ: **Pathologist Agreement in the Interpretation of Colorectal Polyps.** *Am J Gastronterol* 1990, **85**:417–421. **[5]**.

DROSSEL R, SCHULZ H-J, JACOBASCH K-H: **Palliative Laser Therapy in Case of Rectosigmois Tumours.** *Z Klin Med* 1990, **45**:1709–1712.

● DUPHARE H, NIJHAWAN S, RANA S, BHARGAVA DK: **Heterotopic Gastric and Pancreatic Tissue in Large Bowel.** *Am J Gastroenterol* 1990, **85**:68–71. **[52]**.

● FANTINI GA, DECOSSE JJ: **Surveillance Strategies after Resection of Carcinoma of the Colon and Rectum.** *Surg Gynecol Obstet* 1990, **171**:267–273. **[17]**.

FARR CM, RAJALA WP: **Carcinoid Tumor Complicating Ulcerative Colitis [letter].** *Gastrointest Endosc* 1990, **36**:315–316.

FOERSTER EC, MATEK W, HOEPFFNER N, DOMSCHKE W: **Retrograde Endoscopic Implantation of a Self-expanding Stent in Malignant Stenosis of the Common Bile Duct [in German].** *Dtsch Med Wochenschr* 1990, **115**:648–652.

● HARDCASTLE JD, THOMAS WM: **Screening an Asymptomatic Population for Colorectal Cancer.** *Balliere's Clinical Gastroenterology* 1989, **3**:543–566. **[8]**.

●● HILDEBRANDT U, FEIFEL G, ECKER KTW: **Rectal Endosonography.** *In Ballieres Clinical Gastroenterology* 1990, :531–541. **[37]**.

● HOULSTON RS, MURDAY V, HAROCOPOS C, WILLIAMS CB, SLACK J: **Screening and Genetic Counselling for Relatives of Patients with Colorectal Cancer in a Family Cancer Clinic.** *Br Med J* 1990, **2**:366–368. **[26]**.

● HOWARD ML, GREENE PL: **The Effect of Preoperative Endoscopy on Recurrence and Survival Following Surgery for Colorectal Carcinoma.** *Am Surg* 1990, **56**:124–127. **[19]**.

● HUNT DR, CHERIAN M: **Endoscopic Diagnosis of Small Flat Carcinoma of the Colon. Report of Three Cases.** *Dis Col Rectum* 1990, **33**:143–147. **[29]**.

● JOHNSON DA, GURNEY MS, VOLPE RJ, JONES DM, VANNESS MM, CHOBANIAN SJ, AVALOS JC, BUCK JL, KOOYMAN G, CATTAU EL: **A Prospective Study of the Prevalence of Colonic Neoplasms in Asymptomatic Patients with an Age-related Risk.** *Am J Gastroenterol* 1990, **85**:969–974. **[3]**.

● JUHL G, LARSON GM, MULLINS R, BOND S, ROLK HC: **Six-year Results of Annual Colonoscopy after Resection of Colorectal Cancer.** *World J Surg* 1990, **14**:255–261. **[18]**.

KHUBCHANDANI IT: **Colonoscopy in Patients with a Primary Family History of Colon Cancer [editorial Comment].** *Dis Colon Rectum* 1990, **33**:107.

● KIMMEY MB, MARTIN RW, SILVERSTEIN FE: **Endoscopic Ultrasound Probes.** *Gastrointest Endosc* 1990, **36**:S40–S46. **[40]**.

KIMMIG JM: **Negative Haemoccult Test in Malignant and Premalignant Lesions of the Colon — Reply [letter].** *Endoscopy* 1990, **22**:89.

● KOTHUR R, MARSH F, POSNER G, DOSIK H: **Endoscopic Leukemic Polyposis.** *Am J Gastroenterol* 1990, **85**:884–886. **[51]**.

● KURAMOTO S, IHARA O, SAKAI S, SHUMAZU R, KAMINISHI M, OOHARA T: **Depressed Adenoma in the Large Intestine. Endoscopic Features.** *Dis Col Rectum* 1990, **33**:108–112. **[28]**.

LAINE L, AMERIAN J, RARICK M, HARB M, GILL PS: **The Response of Symptomatic Gastrointestinal Kaposi Sarcoma to Chemotherapy - a Prospective Evaluation Using an Endoscopic Method of Disease Quantification.** *Am J Gastroenterol* 1990, **85**:959–961.

● LANSPA SJ, LYNCH HT, SMYRK TC, STRAYHORN P, WATSON P, LYNCH JF, JENKINS JX, APPELMAN HD: **Colorectal Adenomas in the Lynch Syndromes. Results of a Colonoscopy Screening Program.** *Gastroenterology* 1990, **98**:1117–1122. **[23]**.

LANSPA SJ, SMYRK TC, LYNCH HT: **The Colonoscopist and the Lynch Syndromes.** *Gastrointest Endosc* 1990, **36**:156–158. **[22]**.

●● LEPPERT M, BURT B, HUGHES JP, SAMOWITZ W, NAKAMURA Y, WOODWARD S, GARDNER E, LALOUEL JM, WHITE R: **Genetic Analysis of an Inherited Predisposition to Colon Cancer in a Family with a Variable Number of Adenomatous Polyps.** *N Engl J Med* 1990, **322**:904–908. **[21]**.

● LIEBERMAN DA: **Colon Cancer Screening: the Dilemma of Positive Screening Tests.** *Arch Intern Med* 1990, **150**:740–744. **[14]**.

● LONGACRE TA, FENOGLIO-PREISER CM: **Mixed Hyperplastic Adenomatous Polyps/Serrated Adenomas. A Distinct Form of Colorectal Neoplasia.** *Am J Surg Pathol* 1990, **14**:524–537. **[6]**.

MARINI E, FRIGO F, CAVARZERE L, CUTOLO S, PALAZZIN L, ORCALLI F: **Palliative Treatment of Carcinoma of the Rectum by Endoscopic Injection of Polidocanol.** *Endoscopy* 1990, **22**:171–173. **[46]**.

● MATSUMOTO T, IIDA M, MATSUI T, HIRAKAWA M, SHIRAISHI A, YAO T, FUJISHIMA M: **Submucosal Tumors of the Terminal Ileum Managed by Endoscopic Polypectomy.** *Gastroint Endosc* 1990, **36**:505–509. **[48]**.

MATSUMOTO T, IIDA M, MATSUI T, YAO T, FUJISHIMA M: **A Large Brunners Gland Adenoma Removed by Endoscopic Polypectomy [letter].** *Endoscopy* 1990, **22**:192–193.

MCCONNELL JC: **Colonoscopy in Patients with a Primary Family History of Colon Cancer [letter].** *Dis Colon Rectum* 1990, **33**:259.

● MCCONNELL JC, NIZIN JS, SLADE M: **Colonoscopy in Patients with a Primary Family History of Colon Cancer.** *Dis Col Rectum* 1990, **33**:105–107. **[25]**.

● MORSON BC, WILLIAMS CB, FRUHMORGEN P, GRIGIONI W, KRONBORG O, ATKINS W, WINAWER SJ: **Colorectal Adenomas: Risk of Cancer and Results of Follow-up (Working Team Report — Rome European Congress).** *Gastroenterol Internat* 1990, **3**:57–62. **[7]**.

● NUESSLE WR, MAGILL TR: **Leiomyosarcoma of the Transverse Colon — Report of a Case with Discussion.** *Dis Col Rectum* 1990, **33**:323–326. **[53]**.

●● O'BRIEN MJ, WINAWER SJ, ZAUBER AG, GOTTLIEB LS, STERNBERG SS, DIAZ B, DICKERSIN GR, EWING S, GELLER S, KASIMIAN D, KOMOROWSKI R, SZORN A: **The National Polyps Study: Patients and Polyp Characteristics Associated with High-grade Dysplasia in Colorectal Adenomas.** *Gastroenterology* 1990, **98**:371–379. **[4]**.

● OKAMURA S, ASAI T, YAMAGUCHI H, HAMAJIMA E, KATOH T, SHIMODAIRA M, ITOH H: **A Clinicopathological Study of IIa + LLc Type Early Colorectal Cancer with Massive Submucosal Invasion.** *Dig Endosc* 1990, **2**:148–155. **[30]**.

● ORROM WJ, BREZEZINSKI WS, WIENS EW: **Heredity and Colorectal Cancer. A Prospective, Community-based, Endoscopic Study.** *Dis Col Rectum* 1990, **33**:490–493. **[27]**.

PASCAL RR, HERTZLER G, HUNTER S, GOLDSCHMID S: **Pseudoinvasion with High-Grade Dysplasia in a Colonic Adenoma — Distinction from Adenocarcinoma.** *Am J Surg Pathol* 1990, **14**:694–697.

● PATRICE T, FOULTIER MT, YACTAYO S, ADAM F, GALMICHE JP, DOUET MC, LE BODIC L: **Endoscopic Photodynamic Therapy with Hematoporphyrin Derivatives for Primary Treatment of Gastrointestinal Neoplasms in Inoperable Patients.** *Dig Dis Sci* 1990, **35**:535–552. **[44]**.

● PFEIL SA, WEAVER MG, ABUDULKARIM FW, YANG P: **Colonic Lipomas — Outcome of Endoscopic Removal.** *Gastrointest Endosc* 1990, **36**:435–438. **[47]**.

● PINES A, BAT L, SHEMESH E, RON E, HOROWITZ A, CHETRIT A, BUBIS JJ: **Invasive Colorectal Adenomas: Surgery Versus Colonoscopic Polypectomy.** *J Surg Oncol* 1990, **43**:53–55. **[33]**.

●● RANSOHOFF DF, LANG CA: **Small Adenomas Detected During Decal Occult Blood Test Screening for Colorectal Cancer. The Impact of Serendipity.** *JAMA* 1990, **264**:76–78. **[12]**.

● REILLY JM, BALLANTYNE GH, FLEMING FX, ZUCKER KA, MODLIN IM: **Evaluation of the Occult Blood Test in Screening for Colorectal Neoplasms. A Prospective Study Using Flexible Endoscopy.** *Am Surg* 1990, **56**:119–123. **[11]**.

● RIFF ER, DEHAAN K, GAREWAL GS: **The Role of Sigmoidoscopy for Asymptomatic Patients. Results of Three Annual Screening Sigmoidoscope, Polypectomy, and Subsequent Surveillance Colonoscopy in a Primary Care Setting.** *Cleveland Clin J Med* 1990, **57**:131–136. **[10]**.

● ROSCH T, LORENZ R, CLASSEN M: **Endoscopic Ultrasonography in the Evaluation of Colon and Rectal Disease.** *Gastrointest Endosc* 1990, **36**:S33–S39. **[39]**.

● ROSCH TH, LOREZ R, SUCHY R, DANCYGIER H, CLASSEN M: **Colonic Endoscopic Ultrasonography: First Results of a New Technique.** *Gastrointest Endosc* 1990, **36**:382–386. **[38]**.

ROZEN P: **Colorectal Adenomas in a tropical Country.** *Gastrointest Endosc* 1990, **36**:88.

● SARDELLA W, ROSEN L, SHEETS JA, STASIK JJ, RIETHER RD, OLENWINE J, NOLAN P, KHUBCHANDANI IT: **The Value of Colonoscopic Screening in Patients with a Family History of Colon and Rectal Neoplasia.** *Coloproctology* 1990, **5**:265–268. **[24]**.

● SAWADA T, HOJO K, MORIYA Y: **Colonoscopic Management of Focal and Early Colorectal Carcinoma.** *In Ballieres Clinical Gastroenterology* 1990, :627–645. **[31]**.

● SCHUMAN BM, SIMSEK H, LYONS RC: **The Association of Multiple Colonic Adenomatous Polyps with Cancer of the Colon.** *Am J Gastroenterol* 1990, **85**:846–849. **[2]**.

● SIMON JB: **Colonic Polyps, Occult Blood, and Chance.** *JAMA* 1990, **264**:84–85. **[13]**.

● SMITH JA, BHATAL PS, CUTHBERTSON AM: **Angiosarcoma of the Colon — Report of a Case with Long-term Survival.** *Dis Col Rec* 1990, **33**:330–333. **[54]**.

● UNGER SW, STERN JD, ARROYO PJ, RUSSIN DJ: **Endoscopic Nd-YAG Laser Treatment of Colorectal Neoplasms. A Four-year Longitudinal Study.** *Am Surg* 1990, **56**:153–157. **[43]**.

● WHALEN E: **Colon Cancer — Diagnosis in an Era of Cost Containment — ACR Conference, November 8, 1989.** *Am J Roentgenol* 1990, **154**:875–881. **[15]**.

●● WILLIAMS CB, BEDENNE L: **Quadrennial Review: Management of Colonic Polyps — is All the Effort Worthwhile?** *Gastronterol Hepatol* 1990, **5**:144–165. **[1]**.

● WILSON RG, SMITH AN, BIRD CC: **Immunohistochemical Detection of Abnormal Cell Proliferation in Colonic Mucosa of Subjects with Polyps.** *J Clin Pathol* 1990, **43**:744–747. **[34]**.

WINAWER SJ: **A Hyperplastic Polyp is Discovered on Flexible Sigmoidoscopy — is a Full Colonoscopy Indicated?** *Am J Gastroenterol* 1990, **85**:368–370.

WINDELER J: **Negative Haemoccult Test in Malignant and Premalignant Lesions of the Colon, Validation of the Haemoccult Test with Total Colonoscopy [letter].** *Endoscopy* 1990, **22**:88.

● WOLFF WL, SHINYA H, CWERN M, HSU M: **Cancerous Colonic Polyps 'hands On' or 'hands Off?'.** *Am Surg* 1990, **56**:148–152. **[32]**.

● WOOLFSON IK, ECKHOLDT GJ, WETZEL CR, GATHRIGHT JB, RAY JE, HICKS TC, TIMMCKE AE, FERRARI BT: **Usefulness of Performing Colonoscopy One Year after Endoscopic Polypectomy.** *Dis Col Rectum* 1990, **33**:389–393. **[20]**.

Colonoscopy and sigmoidoscopy

AGREZ MV, REDMAN S, SANSON-FISHER R, HENNRIKUS D: **Feasibility of Sigmoidoscopic Screening for Colorectal Cancer in the Hunter Region.** *Aust N Z J Surg* 1990, **60**:87–92.

● ANDORSKY RI: **Pneumatosis Cystoides Intestinalis after Organ Transplantation.** *Am J Gastroenterol* 1990, **85**:189–194. **[51]**.

ANONYMOUS: **Colonoscopic Diagnosis of Paraprosthetic-enteric Fistula [letter].** *Gastrointest Endosc* 1990, **36**:166–167.

ANONYMOUS: **Diagnostic and Therapeutic Technology Assessment (Datta) — Rigid and Flexible Sigmoidoscopies [letter].** *JAMA* 1990, **264**:89–92.

● BERTONI G, CONIGLIARO R, RICCI E, MORTILLA MG, BEDOGNI G, FORNACIARI G: **Endoscopic Injection Hemostasis of Colonic Diverticular Bleeding — a Case Report.** *Endoscopy* 1990, **22**:154–155. **[62]**.

● BILOTTA JJ, FLOYD JL, WAYE JD: **Arterial Oxygen Desaturation During Ambulatory Colonoscopy: Predictability, Incidence, and Clinical Insignificance.** *Gastrointest Endosc* 1990, **36**:S5–S8. **[24]**.

● BOLEY SJ: **Colonic Ischemia — 25 Years Later.** *Am J Gastroenterol* 1990, **84**:931–934. **[72]**.

● BOZDECH JM, FARMER RG: **Diagnosis of Crohn's Disease.** *Hepatogastroenterol* 1990, **37**:8–17. **[69]**.

● BRENNA E, SKREDEN K, WALDUM HL, *ET AL*: **The Benefit of Colonoscopy.** *Scand J Gastroenterol* 1990, **25**:81–88. **[57]**.

● CALLON RA JR, BRADY PG: **Toothpick Perforation of the Sigmoid Colon: an Unusual Case Associated with Erysipelothrix Rhusiopathiae Septicemia.** *Gastrointest Endosc* 1990, **36**:141–143. **[52]**.

● CAPPELL MS, GUPTA AM: **Colonic Lesions Associated with Henoch-Schonlein Purpura.** *Am J Gastroenterol* 1990, **85**:1186–1188. **[31]**.

CHRISTIE JP: **The Removal of Lipomas.** *Gastrointest Endosc* 1990,
• 36:532–533. [105].
COLARIAN J, CALZADA R, JASZEWSKI R: **Nodular Lymphoid Hyperplasia of the Colon in**
• **Adults — is it Common.** *Gastrointest Endosc* 1990, 36:421–422. [26].
COLEMONT LJ, PEN JH, PELCKMANS PA, DEGRYSE HR, PATTYN SR, VAN MAERCKE YM:
• **Herpes Simplex Virus Type 1 Colitis: an Unusual Cause of Diarrhea.** *Am J Gastroenterol* 1990, 85:1182–1185. [87].
COLLIN GR, RUSSELL JC: **Endometriosis of the Colon — Its Diagnosis and**
• **Management.** *Am Surg* 1990, 56:275–279. [54].
CONNOLLY GM, FORBES A, GLEESON JA, GAZZARD BG: **The Value of Barium Enema and**
• **Colonoscopy in Patients Infected with HIV.** *AIDS* 1990, 4:687–689. [91].
COTHREN RM, RICHARDS KORTUM R, SIVAK MV JR, *ET AL*: **Gastrointestinal Tissue**
• **Diagnosis by Laser-induced Fluorescence Spectroscopy at Endoscopy.** *Gastrointest Endosc* 1990, 36:105-111. [35].
DARK DS, CAMPBELL DR, WESSELIUS LJ: **Arterial Oxygen Desaturation During**
• **Gastrointestinal Endoscopy.** *Am J Gastroenterol* 1990, 85:1317. [21].
DENT OF, GOULSTON KJ, TENNANT CC, *ET AL*: **Rectal Bleeding — Patient Delay in**
• **Presentation.** *Dis Col Rectum* 1990, 33:851. [58].
DIFEBO G, GIZZI G, CALO G, SIRINGO S, BRUNETTI G: **Comparison of a New Colon**
• **Lavage Solution (ISO-Giuliani) with a Standard Preparation for Colonoscopy — a Randomized Study.** *Endoscopy* 1990, 22:214–217. [8].
DIFEBO G, MIGLIOLI M, LAURI A, *ET AL*: **Endoscopic Assessment of Acute**
• **Inflammation of the Ileal Reservoir after Restorative Ileo-anal Anastomosis.** *Gastrointest Endosc* 1990, 36:6–9. [71].
DIPALMA JA, MARSHALL JB: **Comparison of a New Sulfate-free Polyethylene Glycol**
• **Electrolyte Lavage Solution Versus a Standard Solution for Colonoscopy Cleansing.** *Gastrointest Endosc* 1990, 36:285–289. [7].
DUCE AM, BADIA-DE-YEBENES A, GARCES G: **Instrument for Dilation of Stenotic**
• **Colorectal Anastomosis.** *Dis Col Rectum* 1990, 33:160–161. [39].
DUPHARE H, NIJHAWAN S, RANA S, BHARGAVA DK: **Heterotopic Gastric and Pancreatic**
• **Tissue in Large Bowel.** *Am J Gastroenterol* 1990, 85:68–71. [30].
EMILIANI VJ, CHODOS JE, COMER GM, HOLNESS LG, SCHWARTZ AJ: **Streptococcus Bovis**
• **Brain Abscess Associated with an Occult Colonic Villous Adenoma.** *Am J Gastroenterol* 1990, 85:78–80. [85].
FENNERTY MB, EARNEST DL, HUDSON PB, SAMPLINER RE: **Physiologic Changes During**
• **Colonoscopy.** *Gastrointest Endosc* 1990, 36:22–25. [22].
FINE JM: **Is Brief Arterial Oxygen Desaturation During Endoscopy Dangerous.**
• *Am J Gastroenterol* 1990, 85:1314. [18].
FLESHNER PR, ACKROYD FW, SHELLITO PC: **The Freckle Sign — an Endoscopic Feature**
• **of the Cecum.** *Dis Col Rectum* 1990, 33:836–839. [25].
FORDTRAN JS, SANTA-ANA CA, CLEVELAND MB: **A Low-sodium Solution for**
• **Gastrointestinal Lavage.** *Gastroenterology* 1990, 98:11–16. [6].
FREGONESE D, DIFALCO G, DITOMA F: **Balloon Dilatation of Anastomotic Intestinal**
• **Stenoses: Long-term Results.** *Endoscopy* 1990, 22:249–253. [42].
FULP SR, GILLIAM JH III: **Beware of the Incarcerated Hernia [letter].** *Gastrointest*
• *Endosc* 1990, 36:318–319. [100].
GIARDIELLO FM, HANSEN FC III, LAZENBY AJ, *ET AL*: **Collagenous Colitis in Setting of**
• **Nonsteroidal Antiinflammatory Drugs and Antibiotics.** *Dig Dis Sci* 1990, 35:257–260. [75].
GIZZI G, VILLANI V, BRANDT G, PAGANELLI GM, DIFEBO G, BIASCO G: **Ano-rectal Lesions in**
• **Patients Taking Suppositories Containing Non-steroidal Anti-inflammatory Drugs (NSAID).** *Endoscopy* 1990, 22:146–148. [80].
GOLDENBERG SP, MARIGNANI P: **The Endoscopic Diagnosis of Colonic Enterobiasis.**
• *Gastrointest Endosc* 1990, 36:309–310. [92].
GRIFFIN PM, OLMSTEAD LC, PETRAS RE: ***Escherichia Coli* 0157-H7-associated Colitis — a**
• **Clinical and Histological Study of 11 Cases.** *Gastroenterology* 1990, 99:142–149. [86].
GROSS JB, LONG WB: **Nasal Oxygen Alleviates Hypoxemia in Colonoscopy Patients**
• **Sedated with Midazolam and Meperidine.** *Gastrointest Endosc* 1990, 36:26–29. [19].
GROSSMANN R, KITTNER I, BERGBAUER M, BORSCH G, RICKEN D: **Cardiovascular Effects**
• **of Electrolyte and Polyethlene Glycol Lavage as a Method of Bowel Preparation for Colonoscopy.** *Die Med Welt* 1990, 41:365–370. [5].
GUPTA SC, GOPALSWAMY N, SARKAR A, SURYAPRASAD AG, MARKERT RJ: **Cardiac**
• **Arrhythmias and Electrocardiographic Changes During Upper and Lower Gastrointestinal Endoscopy.** *Milit Med* 1990, 155:9–11. [23].
HAAS PA, FOX TA JR, SZILAGY EJ: **Endoscopic Examination of the Colon and Rectum**
• **Distal to a Colostomy.** *Am J Gastroenterol* 1990, 85:850–854. [49].
HART R, CLASSEN M: **Complications of Diagnostic Gastrointestinal Endoscopy.**
• *Endoscopy* 1990, 22:229. [95].
HERMAN FN: **Avoidance of Sedation During Total Colonoscopy.** *Dis Colon Rectum*
• 1990, 33:70–72. [15].
HERMAN FN: **Avoidance of Sedation During.** *Dis Colon Rectum* 1990,
• 33:540–541. [16].
HICKSON DE, COX JG, TAYLOR RG, BENNETT JR: **Enema or Picolax as Preparation for**
• **Flexible Sigmoidoscopy.** *Postgrad Med J* 1990, 66:210–211. [9].
HOLLOWAY AM, LOGAN DA: **Pain Relief for Outpatient Colonoscopy: a Comparison**
• **of Alfentanil with Fentanyl.** *Anaesth Intensive Care* 1990, 18:210–213. [13].
HOLMQUIST L, AHREN C, FALLSTROM SP: **Clinical Disease Activity and Inflammatory**
• **Activity in the Rectum in Relation to Mucosal Inflammation Assessed by Colonoscopy. A Study of Children and Adolescents with Chronic Inflammatory Bowel Disease.** *Acta Paediatr Scand* 1990, 79:527–534. [65].
INDUDHARA R, KOCHHAR R, MEHTA SK, CHUGH KS, YADVA RVS: **Acute Colitis in Renal**
• **Transplant Recipients.** *Am J Gastroenterol* 1990, 85:964–968. [73].
KAPADIA CR, CUTRUZZOLA FW, O'BRIEN KM, STETZ ML, ENRIQUEZ R, DECKELBAUM LI: **Laser-**
• **induced Fluorescence Spectroscopy of Human Colonic Mucosa. Detection of Adenomatous Transformation.** *Gastroenterology* 1990, 99:150–157. [34].
KEEFFE EB, OCONNOR KW: **1989 A/S/G/E Survey of Endoscopic Sedation and**
• **Monitoring Practices.** *Gastrointest Endosc* 1990, 36:S13–S18. [17].
KELLER KM, BENDER SW, KIRCHMANN H, *ET AL*: **Diagnostic Significance of Epithelioid**
• **Granulomas in Crohn's Disease in Children. Multicenter Paediatric Crohn's Disease Study Group.** *J Pediatr Gastroenterol Nutr* 1990, 10:27–32. [68].
KHUROO MS, MAHAJAN R, ZARGAR SA, *ET AL*: **The Colon in Shigellosis: Serial**
• **Colonoscopic Appearances in Shigella Dysenteriae I.** *Endoscopy* 1990, 22:35–38. [83].
KOHLER L, VESTWEBER KH, MENNIGEN R, SOMMER H, TROIDL H: **Whole Gut Irrigation and**
• **Prepacol Laxative Preparation for Colonoscopy: a Comparison.** *Br J Surg* 1990, 77:527–529. [4].
KOMOROWSKI RA: **Histologic Spectrum of Diversion Colitis.** *Am J Surg Pathol* 1990,
• 14:548–554. [48].
KONERU B, SELBY R, OHAIR DP, TZAKIS AG, HAKALA TR, STARZL TE: **Nonobstructing**
• **Colonic Dilatation and Colon Perforations Following Renal Transplantation.** *Arch Surg* 1990, 125:610–613. [53].
LANCASTER JF, GOTLEY D, BARTOLO DC, LEAPER DJ: **Hypoxia and Hypotension During**
• **Endoscopy and Colonoscopy.** *Aust NZ J Surg* 1990, 60:271–273. [20].
LANGDON DE: **Extended Colonoscopy.** *Gastrointest Endosc* 1990,
• 36:637. [43].
LANSPA SJ, SMYRK TC, LYNCH HT: **The Colonoscopist and the Lynch Syndromes [editorial].** *Gastrointest Endosc* 1990, 36:156–158.
LASHNER BA, WINANS CS, BLACKSTONE MO: **Randomized Clinical Trial of Two**
• **Colonoscopy Preparation Methods for Elderly Patients.** *J Clin Gastroenterol* 1990, 12:405–408. [2].
LEISSER A, DELPRE G, KADISH U: **Colonoscope Incarceration — an Avoidable Event.**
• *Gastrointest Endosc* 1990, 36:637–638. [99].
LEPINSKI SM, HAMILTON JW: **Isolated Cytomegalovirus Ileitis Detected by**
• **Colonoscopy.** *Gastroenterology* 1990, 98:1704–1706. [88].
MARK JS, SPIRO H: **Informed Consent for Colonoscopy. A Prospective Study.** *Arch*
• *Intern Med* 1990, 150:777–780. [107].
MARSHALL JB, HOYT TS, SEGER RM, REID JC, BEYER KL, BUTT JH: **Air-contrast Barium**
• **Enema Studies after Flexible Proctosigmoidoscopy: Randomized Controlled Clinical Trial.** *Radiology* 1990, 176:549–551. [47].
MASHAKO MN, SONSINO E, NAVARRO J, *ET AL*: **Microscopic Colitis: a New Cause of**
• **Chronic Diarrhea in Children.** *J Pediatr Gastroenterol Nutr* 1990, 10:21–26. [77].
MATSUMOTO T, IIDA M, MATSUI T, *ET AL*: **Endoscopic Findings in Yersinia-**
• **enterocolitica Enterocolitis.** *Gastrointest Endosc* 1990, 36:583–587. [84].
MCCOLLISTER DL, HAMMERMAN HJ: **Air, Air, Everywhere: Pneumatosis Cystoides Coli**
• **after Colonoscopy [letter].** *Gastrointest Endosc* 1990, 36:75–76. [103].
MEDINA E, ORTI E, TOME A, QUILES F, CANELLES P, MERTINEZ A: **Segmental Tuberculosis**
• **of the Colon Diagnosed by Colonoscopy.** *Endoscopy* 1990, 22:188–190. [90].
MERCHANT AA, CHENG EH: **Delayed Splenic Rupture after Colonoscopy [letter].** *Am*
• *J'Gastroenterol* 1990, 85:906–907. [97].
MINOLI G: **Development and Validation of an Endoscopic Severity Index for Crohn's Disease [letter].** *Gastrointest Endosc* 1990, 36:168.
MODIGLIANI R, MARY JY, SIMON JF, *ET AL*: **Clinical, Biological, and Endoscopic Picture**
• **of Attacks of Crohn's Disease. Evolution on Prednisolone. Groupe D'Etude Therapeutique Des Affections Inflammatoires Digestives.** *Gastroenterology* 1990, 98:811–818. [64].
MOHAMED AR, AL KARAWI M, YASAWY MI: **Schistosomal Colonic Disease.** *Gut* 1990,
• 31:439–442. [93].
NAKAGAWA K, MOMONO S, SASAKI Y, FURUSAWA A, UJIIE K: **Endoscopic Examination for**
• **Fistula.** *Endoscopy* 1990, 22:208–211. [44].
NELSON AM: **Delayed Hemorrhage Following 'Hot Biopsy' of a Diminutive**
• **Colonic Polyp.** *Gastrointest Endosc* 1990, 36:418. [106].
NIV Y: **Enema Preparation for Proctosigmoidoscopy Does not Cause Mucosal**
• **Changes.** *Endoscopy* 1990, 22:199–200. [11].
OKADA M, IMAMURA K, YAO T, SAKURAI T, IWASHITA A, MURAYAMA H: **The Evolution of**
• **the Lesion in the Solitary Rectal Ulcer Syndrome.** *Gastrointest Endosc* 1990, 36:621–623. [78].
OLAISON G, SJODAHL R, TAGESSON C: **Glucocorticoid Treatment in Ileal Crohn's**
• **Disease: Relief of Symptoms But not of Endoscopically Viewed Information.** *Gut* 1990, 31:325–328. [67].
PANOS RG, POELKA FG, NOGUERAS JJ: **Peutz-Jeghers Syndrome — a Call for**
• **Intraoperative Enteroscopy.** *Am Surg* 1990, 56:331–333. [94].
PARITHIVEL VS, ROSARIO PG, SUBBARAO M: **Shifting Blue Hue Sign.** *Gastrointest Endosc*
• 1990, 36:422–422. [27].
PFEIL SA, WEAVER MG, ABDUL-KARIM FW, YANG P: **Colonic Lipomas: Outcome of**
• **Endoscopic Removal.** *Gastrointest Endosc* 1990, 36:435–438. [104].
PIETROPAOLO V, MASONI L, FERRARA M, MONTORI A: **Endoscopic Dilation of Colonic**
• **Postoperative Strictures.** *Surg Endosc* 1990, 4:26–30. [41].
PUYMONTBRUN T, GANANSIA R, LEMARCHAND N, DELECHENAULT P, DENIS J: **Anal Ulcerations**
• **Due to Cytomegalovirus in Patients with AIDS — Report of 6 Cases.** *Dis Col Rectum* 1990, 33:1041–1043. [89].
RABINOVITZ M, SCHADE RR, DINDZANS VJ, BELLE SH, VAN THIEL DH, GAVALER JS: **Colonic**
• **Disease in Cirrhosis. an Endoscopic Evaluation in 412 Patients.** *Gastroenterology* 1990, 99:195–199. [32].
RAWLINSON J, TATE JJ, SHEPHERD DF, ROYLE GT, BRUNTON FJ: **Through the Colonoscope**
• **— a Radiologist's View.** *Clin Radiol* 1990, 41:253–257. [56].
REX DK, LEHMAN GA, HAWES RH, O'CONNOR KW, SMITH JJ: **Performing Screening**
• **Flexible Sigmoidoscopy Using Colonoscopies: Experience in 500 Subjects.** *Gastrointest Endosc* 1990, 36:486–488. [46].
REX DK, WEDDLE RA, LEHMAN GA, *ET AL*: **Flexible Sigmoidoscopy Plus Air Contrast**
•• **Barium Enema Versus Colonoscopy for Suspected Lower Gastrointestinal Bleeding.** *Gastroenterology* 1990, 98:855–861. [59].
ROBERTS PL, MARTIN FM, SCHOETZ DJ, MURRAY JJ, COLLER JA, VEIDENHEIMER MC: **Bleeding Stomal Varices - the Role of Local Treatment.** *Dis Colon Rectum* 1990, 33:547–549.
ROBERTS SR, CHANG C, CHAPMAN T, KOONTZ PG JR, EARLY GL: **Colonoscopic Removal of**
• **a Gallstone Obstructing the Sigmoid Colon.** *J Tenn Med Assoc* 1990, 83:18–19. [29].
ROCKEY DC, WEBER JR, WRIGHT TL, WALL SD: **Splenic Injury Following Colonoscopy.**
• *Gastrointest Endosc* 1990, 36:306–309. [98].
ROGERS BH: **Colonoscopy with Fluoroscopy [editorial].** *Gastrointest Endosc* 1990,
• 36:71–72. [37].
RUTGEERTS P, GEBOES K, VANTRAPPEN G, BEYLS J, KERREMANS R, HIELE M: **Predictability**
• **of the Postoperative Course of Crohn's Disease.** *Gastroenterology* 1990, 99:956–963. [66].

SAITO H, OSHIMI K, NAGASAKO K, *ET AL*: **Endoscopic Appearance of the Colon and**
- **Small Intestine of a Patient with Hemorrhagic Enteric Graft-vs-host Disease.** *Dis Col Rectum* 1990, **33**:695. **[81].**

SAKURAI Y, ITOH M, TSUCHIYA H, *ET AL*: **Acute Cholecystocolic Fistula Detected by**
- **Colonoscopy [letter].** *Gastrointest Endosc* 1990, **36**:163–164. **[28].**

SAUNDERS DR, HAGGITT RC, KIMMEY MB, SILVERSTEIN FE: **Morphological Consequences**
- **of Bisacodyl on Normal Human Rectal Mucosa: Effect of a Prostaglandin E1 Analog on Mucosal Injury.** *Gastrointest Endosc* 1990, **36**:101–104. **[12].**

SCHWARTZ AE, VANAGUNAS A, KAMEL PL: **Endoscopy to Evaluate Gastrointestinal**
- **Bleeding in Marathon Runners.** *Ann Intern Med* 1990, **113**:632–633. **[60].**

SCUDERA PL, KOIZUMI J, JACOBSON IM: **Brush Cytology Evaluation of Lesions Encountered During ERCP.** *Gastrointest Endosc* 1990, **36**:281–284.

SHEMESH O, BORNSTEIN IB, WEISSBERG N, BRAVERMAN DZ, RUDENSKY B: ***Listeria* Septicemia after Colonoscopy in an Ulcerative Colitis Patient Receiving ACTH [letter].** *Am J Gastroenterol* 1990, **85**:216.

SHIMAMOTO C, HIRATA I, OHSHIBA S, FUJIWARA S, NISHIO M: **Churg-Strauss Syndrome**
- **(Allergic Granulomatous Angiitis) with Peculiar Multiple Colonic Ulcers.** *Am J Gastroenterol* 1990, **85**:316–319. **[82].**

SLIMAK G, FLEISCHER D: **Blood-red Residual after Cherry-flavored Magnesium**
- **Citrate [letter].** *Gastrointest Endosc* 1990, **36**:79–80. **[10].**

SMEKTALA R, BÖDDEKER W, HAARMANN W: **Therapeutic and Diagnostic Colonoscopy as Emergency Treatment for Acute Pseudo-obstruction of the Large Bowel.** *Coloproctology* 1990, **12**:14–19.

SOON JC, SHANG NS, GOH PM, RAUFF A: **Perforation of the Large Bowel During**
- **Colonoscopy in Singapore.** *Am Surg* 1990, **56**:285–288. **[101].**

SPIGELMAN AD, WILLIAMS CB, ANSELL JK, RUTTER KR, PHILLIPS RK: ***Pneumatosis Coli*: a**
- **Source of Diagnostic Confusion.** *Br J Surg* 1990, **77**:155–155. **[50].**

STERMER E, LEVY N: **Ileus as a Complication of Colonoscopy [letter].** *Am J*
- *Gastroenterol* 1990, **85**:333–334. **[102].**

STOLTE M, RITTER M, BORCHARD F, KOCHSCHERRER G: **Collagenous Gastroduodenitis on**
- **Collagenous Colitis.** *Endoscopy* 1990, **22**:186–187. **[74].**

STROCCHI A, BOND JH, ELLIS C, LEVITT MD: **Colonic Concentrations of Hydrogen**
- **and Methane Following Colonoscopic Preparation with an Oral Lavage Solution.** *Gastrointest Endosc* 1990, **36**:580–582. **[96].**

SULLIVAN MJ: **Variable Stiffening Device for Colonoscopy.** *Gastrointest Endosc* 1990,
- **36**:642–643. **[36].**

TANDON RK, ATMAKURI SP, MEHRA NK, MALAVIYA AN, TANDON HD, CHOPRA P: **Is Solitary**
- **Rectal Ulcer a Manifestation of a Systemic Disease.** *J Clin Gastroenterol* 1990, **12**:286–290. **[79].**

THOMAS WM, JACKSON J, LAMONT GL, HARDCASTLE JD: **Early Incontinence Following Flexible Sigmoidoscopy.** *Br J Surg* 1990, **77**:887.

TRIADAFILOPOULOS G, SARKISIAN M: **Dilatation of Radiation-induced Sigmoid Stricture**
- **Using Sequential Savary-guilliard Dilators — a Combined Radiologic-endoscopic Approach.** *Dis Col Rectum* 1990, **33**:1065–1067. **[40].**

UNGER SW, SARANTO JR, FURLONG RJ, SCOTT JS: **Single Session Panendoscopy.**
- **Indications and Expectations for Yield.** *Am Surg* 1990, **56**:144–147. **[33].**

VAN TILBURG AJ, LAM HG, SELDENRIJK CA, *ET AL*: **Familial Occurrence of Collagenous**
- **Colitis. A Report of Two Families.** *J Clin Gastroenterol* 1990, **12**:279–285. **[76].**

VANNER SJ, MACDONALD PH, PATERSON WG, PRENTICE RS, DA COSTA LR, BECK IT: **A**
- **Randomized Prospective Trial Comparing Oral Sodium Phosphate with Standard Polyethylene Glycol-based Lavage Solution (Golytely) in the Preparation of Patients for Colonoscopy.** *Am J Gastroenterol* 1990, **85**:422–427. **[3].**

VILIEN M, RYTKONEN M: **Golytely Preparation for Folonoscopy-1.5 Liters is Enough**
- **for Outpatients.** *Endoscopy* 1990, **22**:168–170. **[1].**

WAYE JD: **Colonoscopy Without Fluoroscopy [editorial].** *Gastrointest Endosc* 1990,
- **36**:72–73. **[38].**

WAYE JD: **Endoscopy in Inflammatory Bowel Disease: Indications and**
- **Differential Diagnosis.** *Med Clin North Am* 1990, **74**:51-65. **[63].**

WAYE JD: **Colonoscopy Without Fluoroscopy [editorial].** *Gastrointest Endosc* 1990, **36**:72.

WILCOX CM, FORSMARK CE, CELLO JP: **Utility of Droperidol for Conscious Sedation in**
- **Gastrointestinal Endoscopic Procedures.** *Gastrointest Endosc* 1990, **36**:112–115. **[14].**

WILCOX CM, OSTROFF JW: **Colonoscopic Diagnosis of Paraprosthetic-enteric Fistula**
- **[letter].** *Gastrointest Endosc* 1990, **36**:166–167. **[61].**

WILLIAMS CB, BAILLIE J, GILLIES DF, BORISLOW D, COTTON PB: **Teaching Gastrointestinal**
- **Endoscopy by Computer Simulation: a Prototype for Colonoscopy and ERCP.** *Gastrointest Endosc* 1990, **36**:49–54. **[55].**

ZINBERG J, MOLINAS S, DAS KM: **Double-blind Placebo-controlled Study of Olsalazine**
- **in the Treatment of Ulcerative Colitis.** *Am J Gastroenterol* 1990, **85**:562. **[70].**

Diagnostic and Therapeutic Technology Assessment. Rigid and Flexible
- **Sigmoidoscopies.** *JAMA* 1990, **264**:89–92. **[45].**

Endoscopy: general issues

ALLESCHER HD, NEUHAUS H, HAGENMULLER F, CLASSEN M: **Effect of N-Butylscopolamine on Sphincter of Oddi Motility in Patients During Routine Ercp - a Manometric Study.** *Endoscopy* 1990, **22**:160–163.

BIGARD MA: **Disinfection of Endoscopic Equipment: Desirability and Possibilities [editorial] (in French).** *Gastroenterol Clin Biol* 1990, **14**:131–133.

COTTON PB, BAILLIE J: **British Endoscopy - Recent Highlights [Editorial].** *Gastrointest Endosc* 1990, **36**:413–415.

CREMER M, DEVIERE J, BAIZE M, MATOS C: **New Device for Endoscopic Cystoenterostomy.** *Endoscopy* 1990, **22**:76–77.

DEVIERE J, MOTTE S, DUMONCEAU JM, SERRUYS E, THYS JP, CREMER M: **Septicemia after Endoscopic Retrograde Cholangiopancreatography.** *Endoscopy* 1990, **22**:72–75.

FRANCESCHI D, STELLATO TA: **Microcomputer Image Processing in Gastrointestinal Endoscopy.** *Am Surg* 1990, **56**:128–130.

GIRARDI A, PIAZZA I, GIUNTA G, PAPPAGALLO G: **Retroperitoneal, Mediastinal and Subcutaneous Emphysema as a complication of Routine Upper Gastrointestinal Endoscopy.** *Endoscopy* 1990, **22**:83–84.

GRAHAM DY, MICHALETZ PA: **Does the Endoscope Control Head Need to be Disinfected Between Examinations?** *Gastrointest Endosc* 1990, **36**:88.

GRIFFIN SM, CHUNG SCS, LEUNG JWC, LI AKC: **Effect of Intranasal Oxygen on Hypoxia and Tachycardia During Endoscopic Cholangiopancreatography.** *Br Med J [Clin Res]* 1990, **300**:83.

HANSON PJB, GOR D, JEFFRIES DJ, COLLINS JV: **Elimination of High Titre HIV from Fibreoptic Endoscopes.** *Gut* 1990, **31**:657–659.

HIMAL HS: **Investigation of Obstructive Jaundice: Endoscopic Retrograde Cholangiopancreatography (ERCP) or CT Scan of the Abdomen.** *Am Surg* 1990, **56**:192–193.

JUETTNER FM, RATZENHOFER B, FRIEHS G, HACKL A: **Short-term Anesthesia with Midazolam and Flumazenil During Intraluminal Afterloading of Esophageal and Bronchial- Neoplasms in Ill, Inoperable Patients [letter].** *Endoscopy* 1990, **22**:97–98.

KANTROWITZ PA, VENNES JA, OVERHOLT BF: **Assuring Quality of Endoscopic Procedures Done Outside a Hospital [editorial].** *Gastrointest Endosc* 1990, **36**:313–314.

KÖHLER L, VESTWEBER KH, MENNIGEN R, SOMMER H, TROIDL H: **Whole Gut Irrigation and Prepacol® Laxative Preparation for Colonoscopy: a Comparison.** *Br J Surg* 1990, **77**:527–529.

LACHTER J, JACOBS R, LAVY A, WEISLER A, SUISSA A, ENAT R, EIDELMAN S: **Topical Pharyngal Anesthesia for Easing Endoscopy: a Double-blind, Randomized, Placebo-controlled Study.** *Gastrointest Endosc* 1990, **36**:19–21.

LADAS SD, GIORGIOTIS C, PIPIS P, PAPAIOANNOU C, TASSIOS P, KARRA E, RAPTIS SA: **Sedation for Upper Gastrointestinal Endoscopy - Time for Reappraisal [letter].** *Gastrointest Endosc* 1990, **36**:417–418.

LANCASTER JF, GOTLEY D, BARTOLO DC, LEAPER DJ: **Hypoxia and Hypotension During Endoscopy and Colonoscopy.** *Aust N Z J Surg* 1990, **60**:271–274.

LORENZ R: **Allergic Reaction to Contrast Medium after Endoscopic Retrograde Pancreatography [letter].** *Endoscopy* 1990, **22**:196.

MARATKA Z, SCHAPIRO M: **Terminology and Its Application to Computer-aided Data Processing in Digestive Endoscopy [editorial].** *J Clin Gastroenterol* 1990, **12**:130–131.

MARK JS, SPIRO H: **Informed Consent for Colonoscopy — a Prospective Study.** *Arch Intern Med* 1990, **150**:777–784.

MOMSEN OH: **Hiatal Hernia Causing an Unusual Complication of Gastroscopy [letter].** *Endoscopy* 1990, **22**:60–61.

MURRAY AW, MORRAN CG, KENNY GNC, ANDERSON JR: **Arterial Oxygen Saturation During Upper Gastrointestinal Endoscopy: the Effects of a Midazolam/pethidine Combination.** *Gut* 1990, **31**:270–273.

MYERS JO, RAGLAND JJ, CANDELARIA LA: **Fiberoptic Endoscopy of the Gastrointestinal Tract in Surgical Training.** *Surg Gynecol Obstet* 1990, **170**:283–286.

NIV Y: **Enema Preparation for Proctosigmoidoscopy Does not Cause Mucosal Changes [letter].** *Endoscopy* 1990, **22**:199–200.

PECORA AA: **Hypoventilation During Endoscopy: a Questionable Cause for Arterial Desaturation [letter].** *J Clin Gastroenterol* 1990, **12**:242.

PÖLLATH M, RÖSENER M, SELBACH K-D, FEUSTEL H: **Changes in Water and Electrolyte Balance of Patients During the First Hour after Irrigation.** *Coloproctology* 1990, **12**:38–44.

RANA S, PAL LS: **Upper Gastrointestinal Endoscopy — is Premedication or Topical Anesthesia Necessary? [letter].** *Gastrointest Endosc* 1990, **36**:317–318.

RAYMOND JM, LABADIE JC, FAYON E, BUI F, BALDIT C, DUMAS F, COUZIGOU P, BÉRAUD C, AMOURETTI M: **Evaluation of Decontamination Procedures used in Digestive Endoscopy Units in the Gironde Department (in French).** *Gastroenterol Clin Biol* 1990, **14**:134–139.

RIKIMARU T *ET AL*: **New Method of Endoscopic Measurement [letter].** *Lancet* 1990, **335**:672.

ROSARIO MT, COSTA NF: **Combination of Midazolam and Flumazenil in Upper Gastrointestinal Endoscopy.** *Gastrointest Endosc* 1990, **36**:30–33.

SANDERSON JD, TAYLOR RFH, PUGH S, VICARY FR: **Specialized Gastrointestinal Units for the Management of Upper Gastrointestinal Haemorrhage.** *Postgrad Med J* 1990, **66**:654–656.

SAUTER G, GRABEIN B, HUBER G, MANNES GA, RUCKDESCHEL G, SAUERBRUCH T: **Antibiotic Prophylaxis of Infectious Complications with Endoscopic Retrograde Cholangiopancreatography - a Randomized Controlled Study.** *Endoscopy* 1990, **22**:164–167.

SCHEERES DE, SIMON I, PONSKY JL: **Endoscopic Retrograde Cholangiopancreatography in a General Surgery Practice.** *Am Surg* 1990, **56**:185–191.

SCHOLER SG, SCHAFER DF, POTTER JF: **The Effect of Age on the Relative Potency of Midazolam and Diazepam for Sedation in Upper Gastrointestinal Endoscopy.** *J Clin Gastroenterol* 1990, **12**:145–147.

SCHULZ H-J: **Future of Gastroenterological Endoscopy.** *Z Klin Med* 1990, **45**:892–893.

SCOTT B: **Endoscopic Demands in The 90's.** *Gut* 1990, **31**:125–126.

SIVAK MV JR: **Privileges to Perform Endoscopy.** *Gastrointest Endosc* 1990, **36**:73–74.

THORPE JH: **Medicare and Endoscopy Reimbursement [letter].** *Am J Gastroenterol* 1990, **85**:100.

UNGER SW, SARANTO JR, FURLONG RJ, SCOTT JS: **Single Session Panendoscopy: Indications and Expectations for Yield.** *Am Surg* 1990, **56**:144–147.

VELLACOTT KD, KENOGBON J, GRIFFITHS G, MASON J: **Endoscopic Retrograde Cholangiopancreatography Using a Mobile Image Intensifier.** *Ann R Coll Surg Engl* 1990, **72**:132–134.

VILIEN M, RYTKONEN M: **Golytely Preparation for Colonoscopy - 1.5 Liters is Enough for Outpatients.** *Endoscopy* 1990, **22**:168–170.

WELLS ST, BAILLIE J: **The Design and Production of Videotapes for Endoscopic Teaching.** *Gastrointest Endosc* 1990, **36**:83–84.

WILCOX CM, FORSMARK CE, CELLO JP: **Utility of Droperidol for Conscious Sedation in Gastrointestinal Procedures.** *Gastrointest Endosc* 1990, **36**:112–115.

List of journals scanned

The *Index Medicus* abbreviation is given in parentheses

Acta Chirurgica Scandinavica (Acta Chir Scand)
Acta Radiologica (Acta Radiol)
American Journal of Clinical Pathology (Am J Clin Pathol)
American Journal of Diseases of Children (Am J Dis Child)
American Journal of Gastroenterology (Am J Gastroenterol)
American Journal of Pathology (Am J Pathol)
American Journal of Roentgenology (AJR)
American Journal of Surgery (Am J Surg)
American Journal of Surgical Pathology (Am J Surg Pathol)
American Surgeon (Am Surg)
Annals of Internal Medicine (Ann Intern Med)
Annals of Surgery (Ann Surg)
Annals of the Royal College of Surgeons of England (Ann R Coll Surg Engl)
Archives of Disease in Childhood (Arch Dis Child)
Archives of Internal Medicine (Arch Intern Med)
Archives of Surgery (Arch Surg)
Australian and New Zealand Journal of Medicine (Aust N Z J Med)
Australian and New Zealand Journal of Surgery (Aust N Z J Surg)

British Journal of Radiology (Br J Radiol)
British Journal of Surgery (Br J Surg)
British Medical Bulletin (Br Med Bull)
British Medical Journal (Br Med J)

Canadian Journal of Surgery (Can J Surg)
Canadian Medical Association Journal (Can Med Assoc J)
Cancer (Cancer)
Cancer Research (Cancer Res)
Clinical Radiology (Clin Radiol)
Colo-Proctology (Coloproctology)

Deutsche Medizinische Wochenschrift (Dtsch Med Wochenschr)
Digestion (Digestion)
Digestive Diseases and Sciences (Dig Dis Sci)
Diseases of the Colon and Rectum (Dis Colon Rectum)

Endoscopy (Endoscopy)
European Journal of Radiology (Eur J Radiol)
European Journal of Surgical Oncology (Eur J Surg Oncol)
Experimental and Molecular Pathology (Exp Mol Pathol)

Gastroenterologie Clinique et Biologique (Gastroenterol Clin Biol)
Gastroenterology (Gastroenterology)
Gastroenterology Clinics of North America (Gastroenterol Clin North Am)
Gastrointestinal Endoscopy (Gastrointest Endosc)
Gastrointestinal Radiology (Gastrointest Radiol)
Gut (Gut)

Hepato-Gastroenterology (Hepatogastroenterology)
Hepatology (Hepatology)
Histopathology (Histopathology)

International Journal of Colorectal Disease (Int J Colorect Dis)
International Journal of Pancreatology (Int J Pancreatol)
Italian Journal of Gastroenterology (Ital J Gastroenterol)

JAMA — Journal of the American Medical Association (JAMA)
Journal of Clinical Gastroenterology (J Clin Gastroenterol)
Journal of Clinical Pathology (J Clin Pathol)
Journal of Gastroenterology and Hepatology (J Gastroenterol Hepatol)
Journal of Hepatology (J Hepatol)
Journal of Pathology (J Pathol)
Journal of Pediatric Gastroenterology and Nutrition (J Pediatr Gastroenterol Nutr)
Journal of Pediatric Surgery (J Pediatr Surg)
Journal of Surgical Research (J Surg Res)
Journal of the Royal College of Surgeons of Edinburgh (J R Coll Surg Edinb)

Lancet (Lancet)
Liver (Liver)

Mayo Clinic Proceedings (Mayo Clin Proc)
Medical Clinics of North America (Med Clin North Am)
Medicine (Medicine [Baltimore])

New England Journal of Medicine (N Engl J Med)

Pancreas (Pancreas)
Pediatrics (Pediatrics)
Postgraduate Medical Journal (Postgrad Med J)
Presse Medicale (Presse Med)

Radiology (Radiology)
Revista Española de las Enfermedades del Aparato Digestivo (Rev Esp Enferm Apar Dig)

Scandinavian Journal of Gastroenterology (Scand J Gastroenterol)
Surgery (Surgery)
Surgery, Gynecology and Obstetrics (Surg Gynecol Obstet)

World Journal of Surgery (World J Surg)

Zeitschrift für Klinische Medizin (Z Klin Med)

© Current Science Ltd ISBN 1-870485-32-7 ISSN 0952-6293

Index to subjects

AIRMAIL

Affix Stamp

CURRENT SCIENCE
SUBSCRIPTIONS
34 - 42 CLEVELAND STREET
LONDON W1P 5FB
UNITED KINGDOM

NO POSTAGE
NECESSARY
IF MAILED
IN THE
UNITED STATES

BUSINESS REPLY MAIL
FIRST CLASS PERMIT NO. 33925 PHILADELPHIA, PA

Postage Will Be Paid By Addressee

CURRENT SCIENCE
20 NORTH 3rd STREET
PHILADELPHIA
PA 19106-2113
USA

AIRMAIL

Affix Stamp

CURRENT SCIENCE
SUBSCRIPTIONS
34 - 42 CLEVELAND STREET
LONDON W1P 5FB
UNITED KINGDOM

NO POSTAGE
NECESSARY
IF MAILED
IN THE
UNITED STATES

BUSINESS REPLY MAIL
FIRST CLASS PERMIT NO. 33925 PHILADELPHIA, PA

Postage Will Be Paid By Addressee

CURRENT SCIENCE
20 NORTH 3rd STREET
PHILADELPHIA
PA 19106-2113
USA

European Journal of Gastroenterology & Hepatology
Volume 3, 1991 (12 issues)

Yes! I want to keep updated on the latest developments in gastroenterology & hepatology

☐ **Personal** - (from personal funds) US$130

☐ **Institutional** US$255

Subscription rates include airspeed delivery
Subscriptions run on a calendar year basis
☐ Am Ex ☐ VISA ☐ MasterCard

Card no

Exp Date Amount payable ....

Signature .... Date ....

☐ Check enclosed payable to Current Science

☐ Please bill me (Institutional subscriptions ONLY)

Name ....

Address ....

....

....

Zip .... Country ....

if new address ☐ tick here

Return this form together with payment to address overleaf
Guarantee: Your money will be refunded if you write canceling your subscription within 30 days of receiving the first issue

Current Opinion in GASTROENTEROLOGY
Volume 7, 1991 (6 issues)

Yes! I want to keep updated on the latest developments in gastroenterology

☐ **Personal** - (from personal funds) US$100

☐ **Institutional** US$170

Subscription rates include airspeed delivery
Subscriptions run on a calendar year basis
☐ Am Ex ☐ VISA ☐ MasterCard

Card no

Exp Date Amount payable ....

Signature .... Date ....

☐ Check enclosed payable to Current Science

☐ Please bill me (Institutional subscriptions ONLY)

Name ....

Address ....

....

....

Zip .... Country ....

if new address ☐ tick here

Return this form together with payment to address overleaf
Guarantee: Your money will be refunded if you write canceling your subscription within 30 days of receiving the first issue

SUBSCRIBERS FROM USA & CANADA ONLY
You can use this card for change of address

European Journal of Gastroenterology & Hepatology
Volume 3, 1991 (12 issues)

Yes! I want to keep updated on the latest developments in gastroenterology & hepatology

☐ **Personal** - (from personal funds) £75

☐ **Institutional** £150

Subscription rates include airspeed delivery
Subscriptions run on a calendar year basis
☐ Am Ex ☐ VISA ☐ MasterCard

Card no

Exp Date Amount payable ....

Signature .... Date ....

☐ Cheque/Eurocheque enclosed payable to Current Science Ltd

☐ Bank transfer (details available on request)
Payment may be made in US$ at the current exchange rate
£ sterling must be drawn on a UK bank, US$ on a US bank

☐ Please send an invoice (Institutional subscriptions ONLY)

Name ....

Address ....

....

....

Postcode .... Country ....

if new address ☐ tick here

Guarantee: Your money will be refunded if you write cancelling your subscription within 30 days of receiving the first issue

Current Opinion in GASTROENTEROLOGY
Volume 7, 1991 (6 issues)

Yes! I want to keep updated on the latest developments in gastroenterology

☐ **Personal** - (from personal funds) £60

☐ **Institutional** £100

Subscription rates include airspeed delivery
Subscriptions run on a calendar year basis
☐ Am Ex ☐ VISA ☐ MasterCard

Card no

Exp Date Amount payable ....

Signature .... Date ....

☐ Cheque/Eurocheque enclosed payable to Current Science Ltd

☐ Bank transfer (details available on request)
Payment may be made in US$ at the current exchange rate
£ sterling must be drawn on a UK bank, US$ on a US bank

☐ Please send an invoice (Institutional subscriptions ONLY)

Name ....

Address ....

....

....

Postcode .... Country ....

if new address ☐ tick here

Guarantee: Your money will be refunded if you write cancelling your subscription within 30 days of receiving the first issue

SUBSCRIBERS FROM OUTSIDE USA & CANADA
You can use this card for change of address